# HANDBOOK OF GASTROENTEROLOGY

A Clinical Textbook Covering Luminal, Hepatobiliary, and Pancreatic Disease for ABIM Board Candidates



**Ramon C. Henson, MD**

**Trademark Disclaimer**

All brand names, product names, drug names, certification names, and registered trademarks mentioned in this textbook are the property of their respective owners. Their use in this publication does not imply endorsement, affiliation, or sponsorship by the trademark owner, nor does it imply that the trademark owner has reviewed, approved, or is in any way associated with this work. All trademarked names and registered marks appearing in this textbook are used solely for purposes of identification and educational reference, without any intent of trademark infringement.

**Medical Disclaimer**

This textbook is intended solely for educational and informational purposes and is designed to support the continuing professional development of licensed healthcare providers. The clinical content presented herein reflects information believed to be accurate and current at the time of publication; however, medicine evolves rapidly, and readers are advised that new research findings, updated clinical practice guidelines, and revised regulatory approvals may alter or supersede information contained in this work after its publication date.

Nothing in this publication constitutes medical advice, clinical guidance specific to any individual patient, or a substitute for the independent professional judgment of a licensed and qualified healthcare provider. No clinician-patient relationship is established, implied, or intended by the use of this textbook or any portion thereof. All clinical decisions, including but not limited to diagnosis, therapeutic selection, drug dosing, and patient monitoring, must be individualized based on thorough and direct assessment of the patient, the totality of current published evidence, applicable clinical practice guidelines, institutional protocols, and the informed professional judgment of the responsible clinician.

Drug information, dosages, treatment protocols, and therapeutic recommendations presented in this publication are offered for educational reference only and must be independently verified against current prescribing information, pharmacopeial references, and applicable regulatory approvals prior to clinical application. The author and publisher have made every reasonable effort to ensure the accuracy and completeness of the information presented; nevertheless, they expressly disclaim all liability for any adverse outcomes, clinical errors, patient harm, loss, or injury alleged to arise, directly or indirectly, from the use, misuse, or application of any information, recommendation, protocol, or clinical guidance contained in this publication.

# TABLE OF CONTENT

# PREFACE

Gastroenterology is a specialty defined by volume and velocity. A fellow on the inpatient consult service moves between a variceal bleed, an abnormal liver panel, a flare of ulcerative colitis, and a vague complaint of chronic diarrhea, often within the same afternoon, and is expected to arrive at each bedside already knowing which of a dozen overlapping clinical scores applies, what its cutoff means, and what to do next. This textbook was written for that specific moment: the point at which diagnostic reasoning has to convert into a specific, defensible clinical decision.

Two forces make that conversion harder than it should be. The first is sheer density. Modern gastroenterology and hepatology carry dozens of named scoring systems and classification schemes, from the Rockall and Glasgow-Blatchford scores in upper gastrointestinal bleeding to the Child-Pugh and Model for End-Stage Liver Disease indices in cirrhosis, from the Ranson and Bedside Index for Severity in Acute Pancreatitis criteria to the Mayo and Prague classifications used in inflammatory bowel disease and Barrett esophagus. Each was developed for a specific purpose, in a specific population, with a specific cutoff. Learning that a score exists is not the same as knowing, at two in the morning, which one governs the patient in front of you and what its threshold obligates you to do. The second force is the well-documented tendency, noted by experienced consultants and their trainees alike, toward vague consultative language: recommending that a team "consider" an intervention rather than specifying the intervention, its dose, its timing, and its trigger. Precision is what separates a consult note that changes management from one that simply restates the problem.

This book addresses both problems directly through its named proprietary feature, the GI Threshold Decision System, built into every chapter and consolidated at the back of the book in the GI Threshold Master Index. Each major clinical topic carries a Threshold Decision block that names the governing score or cutoff, states the decision it triggers, flags the look-alike scores or presentations most likely to be confused with it, and closes with a single memorable anchor. The intent is not to add another layer of memorization on top of the clinical chapters, but to make the threshold logic that already governs gastroenterology practice explicit, indexed, and fast to retrieve.

The chapters that surround this system are organized the way gastroenterology is actually practiced and taught: by organ system, moving from the esophagus through the stomach, small bowel, colon, pancreas, and liver, and closing with a dedicated chapter on acute gastrointestinal hemorrhage and vascular emergencies, the single most common reason a gastroenterologist is called to the bedside. Each chapter builds from definition and epidemiology through pathophysiology, clinical presentation, diagnostic workup, and evidence-based management, illustrated with the anatomical, histopathologic, endoscopic, and radiologic imagery that a clinical reference in this specialty requires, and grounded throughout in current society guidance from the American College of Gastroenterology, the American Gastroenterological Association, the American Association for the Study of Liver Diseases, and allied international bodies.

This book is a clinical reference, not an examination-preparation workbook. It contains no practice questions, board-style items, or knowledge checks of any kind. Its purpose is to be read, consulted, and trusted at the bedside, in clinic, and during preparation for board certification, by fellows, internal medicine residents and hospitalists, advanced practice providers, and practicing clinicians who need gastroenterology's threshold logic made explicit rather than assumed.

# CHAPTER 1: APPROACH TO THE GI PATIENT: HISTORY, EXAMINATION, AND DIAGNOSTIC REASONING

**Learning Objectives**

1. Elicit a gastrointestinal history that characterizes a presenting symptom by onset, quality, timing, and associated features sufficient to generate a working differential diagnosis.
2. Perform and interpret an abdominal and extraintestinal physical examination relevant to luminal, hepatobiliary, and pancreatic disease.
3. Organize the major gastrointestinal presenting complaints into structured diagnostic reasoning pathways.
4. Select an appropriate initial laboratory and imaging evaluation for common presenting symptoms.
5. Recognize alarm features that require expedited evaluation and apply threshold-based reasoning to triage the urgency of a gastroenterology consultation.

**Chapter Outline**

This chapter establishes the diagnostic scaffolding used throughout the remainder of the book: how to take a gastrointestinal history, how to examine the abdomen and its extraintestinal manifestations, how to reason from a presenting symptom to a differential diagnosis, how to select an initial laboratory and imaging evaluation, and how to recognize the features that convert a routine evaluation into an urgent one. These elements are sequenced deliberately: history and examination generate a differential diagnosis, presenting-symptom reasoning and initial testing narrow it, and threshold-based urgency assessment determines how quickly that narrowing must occur, a sequence that recurs, disease by disease, throughout the remainder of this book.

## History Taking in Gastroenterology

A gastrointestinal history is built around the presenting symptom, but its diagnostic value depends on the clinician's ability to convert a vague complaint into a structured set of discriminating features. A patient who reports abdominal pain has not yet given the clinician enough information to generate a differential diagnosis; the differential only emerges once the pain has been located, timed, characterized, and connected to precipitating and relieving factors. This process is deliberate rather than incidental, because the same complaint word conceals mechanistically distinct diseases whose treatments diverge sharply.

### Characterizing the Presenting Complaint

Onset establishes tempo: pain that began abruptly and reached maximal intensity within minutes suggests a vascular or perforative process, because ischemic and perforative injury generate visceral and then peritoneal pain rapidly, whereas pain that builds gradually over hours is more consistent with an inflammatory process such as appendicitis or cholecystitis, in which luminal obstruction and secondary inflammation accumulate before pain becomes severe. Location and radiation narrow the anatomic source because visceral afferents from foregut, midgut, and hindgut structures converge on spinal segments that project pain to characteristic surface regions before somatic peritoneal irritation localizes it further; epigastric pain radiating to the back suggests a retroperitoneal process such as pancreatitis or a penetrating posterior ulcer, while right upper quadrant pain radiating to the right scapula suggests biliary colic, because the referred pain follows the phrenic and lower thoracic dermatomal distribution shared with the diaphragmatic and hepatobiliary peritoneum.

Quality and timing add further discrimination. Colicky pain that waxes and wanes over minutes reflects intermittent smooth muscle contraction against a mechanical obstruction, as occurs with biliary colic or small bowel obstruction, and this pattern differs mechanistically from the constant, unremitting pain of an inflammatory or ischemic process in which afferent nociceptor stimulation is sustained rather than intermittent. The relationship of pain to meals is diagnostically informative because it identifies whether a lesion is provoked by the physiologic demands that a meal imposes: pain that worsens with eating suggests either mesenchymal ischemia, in which increased postprandial mesenteric blood flow demand cannot be met by a stenotic vessel, or biliary and pancreatic disease, in which cholecystokinin-mediated gallbladder contraction or pancreatic secretion provokes pain against an obstructed duct, whereas pain that improves with eating and recurs several hours later is more typical of duodenal ulcer disease, in which food buffers acid delivered to a duodenal mucosal defect.

**CLINICAL PEARL:** Ask every patient with abdominal pain a single sequencing question: did the pain start suddenly, over minutes, or did it build gradually over hours? This single answer separates the differential diagnosis into two broad mechanistic categories, vascular or perforative versus inflammatory or obstructive, before a single laboratory test has resulted.

**Past Medical, Surgical, and Family History**

Prior abdominal surgery reshapes the differential diagnosis of abdominal pain because adhesive disease becomes the leading cause of small bowel obstruction in a patient with a surgical scar, and a history of cholecystectomy shifts biliary-type pain toward the differential of sphincter of Oddi dysfunction or retained choledocholithiasis rather than acute cholecystitis, which requires an intact gallbladder. A history of inflammatory bowel disease changes the interpretation of a new symptom entirely, because abdominal pain, diarrhea, or bleeding in a patient with known Crohn disease or ulcerative colitis must be evaluated for both disease flare and for the complications specific to chronic inflammation, including stricture, fistula, and colitis-associated neoplasia, rather than being attributed reflexively to disease activity.

Family history carries particular weight in gastroenterology because several of the specialty's most consequential diagnoses are inherited or familial. A first-degree relative with colorectal cancer or an advanced adenoma diagnosed before age 60 changes screening recommendations for the patient in front of the clinician, and a family history of early-onset colorectal or endometrial cancer across multiple generations should prompt consideration of a hereditary cancer syndrome. Family history of celiac disease, inflammatory bowel disease, or autoimmune liver disease similarly raises pretest probability for conditions that share genetic susceptibility loci, even when the patient's own presentation is atypical.

### Medication, Substance, and Social History

Medication history is inseparable from gastrointestinal diagnosis because so much of the specialty's disease burden is iatrogenic or substance-related. Nonsteroidal anti-inflammatory drug use is the leading identifiable cause of peptic ulcer disease after Helicobacter pylori infection, and it acts through a mechanism distinct from acid hypersecretion, namely systemic prostaglandin suppression that impairs mucosal bicarbonate secretion and mucus production regardless of the route of administration. Anticoagulant and antiplatelet use changes both the presentation and the management of gastrointestinal bleeding, and a structured medication reconciliation, including over-the-counter and herbal preparations, is required before any bleeding evaluation proceeds. Alcohol use history requires a quantified, nonjudgmental approach, using either a standardized screening instrument or a direct quantification of drinks per week, because alcohol is a direct hepatotoxin whose contribution to liver disease is dose-dependent and because unrecognized alcohol use disorder identified during an inpatient admission carries a withdrawal risk that must be anticipated before it occurs.

**CAUTION:** A history of nonsteroidal anti-inflammatory drug or aspirin use is frequently underreported by patients who do not consider over-the-counter analgesics to be medications. Ask specifically about aspirin, ibuprofen, and naproxen use by name rather than asking generically about medications.

## The Gastrointestinal Physical Examination

The abdominal examination is performed in a fixed sequence, inspection, auscultation, percussion, and palpation, and the sequence itself is diagnostically meaningful, because palpation performed before auscultation can provoke bowel sounds that would not otherwise be present and can therefore obscure a true ileus.

### General Inspection and Vital Signs

Vital sign interpretation in gastrointestinal disease begins with the recognition that early compensated shock produces subtle findings before hypotension develops. Tachycardia frequently precedes any measurable drop in blood pressure in a young or previously healthy patient because compensatory vasoconstriction and increased heart rate maintain perfusion pressure until a substantial volume has been lost, meaning that a normal blood pressure does not exclude significant hemorrhage. Orthostatic vital signs, obtained by comparing supine and standing heart rate and blood pressure, detect this compensated state before resting vital signs become abnormal and should be checked in any patient with a history concerning for gastrointestinal blood loss.

## Abdominal Examination Technique

Inspection precedes hands-on examination and should note distension, visible peristalsis, surgical scars, and cutaneous stigmata such as caput medusae or spider angiomata that suggest chronic liver disease and portal hypertension before the abdomen has been touched. Auscultation characterizes bowel sounds as normal, hyperactive, hypoactive, or absent, and high-pitched, rushing sounds coinciding with cramping pain suggest mechanical obstruction, whereas absent bowel sounds after several minutes of listening suggest ileus or peritonitis. Percussion identifies the transition from tympany to dullness that localizes an enlarged liver or spleen, and the technique of shifting dullness, in which dullness in the flank converts to tympany when the patient rolls to the opposite side, is a bedside method for detecting ascites when at least 1,500 milliliters of fluid is present.

Palpation begins with light palpation in the quadrant farthest from the area of reported pain and proceeds toward the painful region last, both to build patient trust and to avoid provoking guarding that would obscure deeper findings. Specific maneuvers localize disease with reasonable precision: Murphy sign, in which inspiratory effort is arrested by pain when the examiner's fingers are held beneath the right costal margin, indicates cholecystitis because gallbladder inflammation causes the inflamed organ to contact the examining fingers during diaphragmatic descent; rebound tenderness and involuntary guarding indicate peritoneal irritation regardless of its underlying cause; and a positive psoas sign, in which passive hip extension provokes pain, suggests a retrocecal appendix or a retroperitoneal inflammatory process irritating the psoas muscle.

## Extraintestinal and Systemic Findings

**KEY POINT:** Jaundice becomes clinically detectable once total bilirubin exceeds approximately 2 to 3 milligrams per deciliter, and it is most reliably assessed in natural light examining the sclera, because scleral elastin has a particular affinity for bilirubin that produces earlier and more visible staining than skin.

Chronic liver disease produces a constellation of extraintestinal findings that reflect two convergent mechanisms, portal hypertension and impaired hepatic clearance of circulating estrogens. Spider angiomata, palmar erythema, and gynecomastia arise from the hyperestrogenic state that develops when a cirrhotic liver can no longer clear circulating estrogens efficiently, while caput medusae, splenomegaly, and ascites arise directly from portal hypertension as portosystemic collateral vessels dilate and splanchnic venous pressure rises. Asterixis, a flapping tremor elicited by asking the patient to extend the wrists and spread the fingers, reflects hepatic encephalopathy and results from the loss of normal postural muscle tone maintenance when circulating neurotoxins, most notably ammonia, are not adequately cleared by the liver or bypass it through portosystemic shunting.

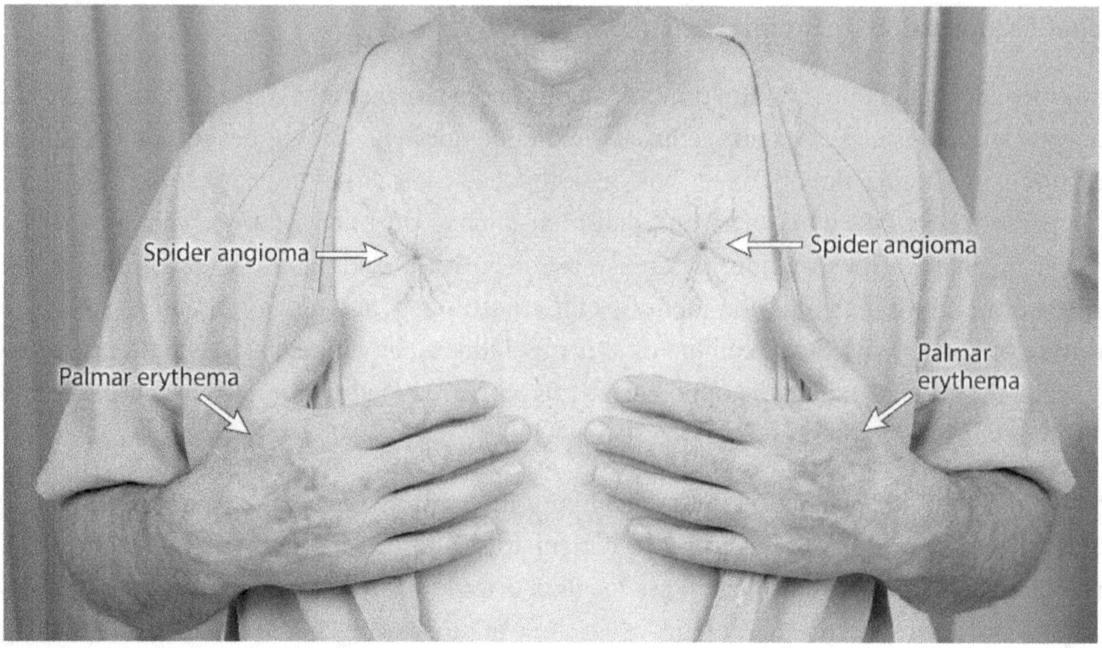


## Diagnostic Reasoning by Presenting Symptom

Four presenting complaints account for the large majority of gastroenterology consultation requests: abdominal pain, gastrointestinal bleeding or unexplained anemia, altered bowel habits, and abnormal liver chemistries. Organizing diagnostic reasoning around these four complaints, rather than around individual diseases, mirrors how patients actually present and how consultations are actually requested.

### Abdominal Pain

Abdominal pain is reasoned through location first and character second. Epigastric pain generates a differential spanning peptic ulcer disease, gastritis, pancreatitis, and, when radiating to the back, a penetrating posterior process; right upper quadrant pain generates a differential of biliary colic, acute cholecystitis, and choledocholithiasis, distinguished chiefly by duration, fever, and laboratory abnormality; right lower quadrant pain in an adult raises appendicitis foremost but must also account for terminal ileal Crohn disease, particularly in a younger patient without leukocytosis proportionate to the degree of pain; and diffuse pain with peritoneal signs of any origin represents a surgical emergency until proven otherwise, regardless of the specific diagnosis eventually reached.

Referred pain patterns add a further layer of reasoning beyond direct localization, because visceral pain is frequently perceived at a distance from its true origin as a consequence of shared spinal cord entry points between visceral and somatic afferent fibers. Left shoulder pain accompanying upper abdominal symptoms suggests diaphragmatic irritation, whether from splenic injury, a subphrenic abscess, or, less commonly, splenic flexure disease, because the diaphragm shares its sensory innervation with the C3 through C5 dermatomes that also supply the shoulder. Interscapular back pain accompanying epigastric discomfort should prompt consideration of a retroperitoneal or posterior process, including pancreatitis, a penetrating duodenal ulcer, or, in the appropriate vascular risk context, an aortic process that mimics gastrointestinal disease closely enough to be misattributed if the possibility is not actively considered.

Recognizing these referred patterns prevents two common reasoning errors: pursuing an exhaustive local workup of the site where pain is perceived when the true lesion lies elsewhere, and, conversely, dismissing a distant pain complaint as unrelated when it is in fact the only clue pointing toward the correct diagnosis.

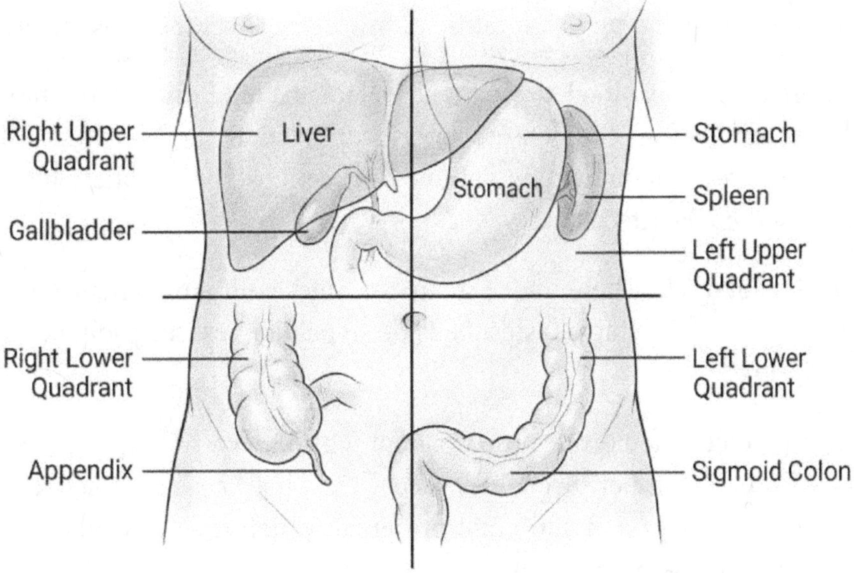


**Gastrointestinal Bleeding and Anemia**

Gastrointestinal bleeding is the single most common reason a gastroenterologist is asked to see a hospitalized patient, and the initial reasoning task is not to identify the bleeding source but to determine whether the patient is hemodynamically stable enough for the evaluation to proceed at a measured pace. Hematemesis and melena localize bleeding proximal to the ligament of Treitz with reasonable reliability, because blood exposed to gastric acid for a sufficient transit time is degraded to the black, tarry appearance of melena, whereas hematochezia usually indicates a colonic or distal source but can indicate a brisk upper source when transit time is fast enough that acid degradation has not occurred. Unexplained iron deficiency anemia, in the absence of overt bleeding, still requires a bidirectional endoscopic evaluation in most adults, because occult blood loss from an upper or lower source, most importantly colorectal neoplasia, must be excluded before iron deficiency is attributed to a nutritional or menstrual cause alone.

**THE GI THRESHOLD DECISION SYSTEM — Foundational Diagnostic Thresholds — Triaging Suspected Gastrointestinal Hemorrhage**

**Presentation Signature:** A patient reports melena, hematemesis, or hematochezia, or is found to have a hemoglobin substantially below their known baseline, and the receiving clinician must decide, before any imaging or endoscopy, how urgently the patient needs to be seen and stabilized.

**Threshold Point:** A shock index, defined as heart rate divided by systolic blood pressure, greater than 1.0 identifies a patient in compensated or overt hemorrhagic shock even when the systolic blood pressure remains within a numerically normal range, because the elevated ratio captures the tachycardic compensation that precedes measurable hypotension.

**The Call:** A shock index above 1.0, or any systolic blood pressure below 90 millimeters of mercury, mandates immediate large-bore intravenous access, crystalloid resuscitation, type and crossmatch, and involvement of the endoscopy and, where relevant, interventional radiology and surgical teams before further diagnostic workup proceeds; a shock index at or below 1.0 with a reassuring trajectory permits a more measured evaluation, including risk-stratification scoring, over the subsequent hours.

**Trap Logic:** A normal supine blood pressure does not exclude significant blood loss in a young, previously healthy patient whose compensatory vasoconstriction can maintain a normal resting blood pressure until 15 to 20 percent of circulating volume has been lost; orthostatic vital signs, not resting vital signs alone, detect this compensated state.

**Decision Anchor:** Calculate the shock index at first contact with any patient reporting gastrointestinal bleeding; a value above 1.0 is the single fastest bedside signal that resuscitation, not further history-taking, is the immediate priority.

In cases of suspected variceal hemorrhage in a patient with known or suspected cirrhosis, the threshold reasoning above is modified further, because variceal bleeding carries a distinct pretreatment pathway involving vasoactive medication and antibiotic prophylaxis before endoscopy, a distinction developed fully in the hepatology chapters of this book.

### Altered Bowel Habits and Diarrhea

Diarrhea is reasoned first by duration, because acute diarrhea lasting under two weeks is overwhelmingly infectious or medication-related and rarely requires extensive workup beyond stool studies in appropriately selected patients, whereas chronic diarrhea persisting beyond four weeks requires a structured evaluation for inflammatory, malabsorptive, motility-related, and secretory causes. Bloody diarrhea shifts the differential toward inflammatory bowel disease, infectious colitis from an invasive organism, or ischemic colitis, and the distinction among these three is guided by the tempo of onset, associated systemic symptoms, and the patient's vascular risk profile. Nocturnal diarrhea that awakens a patient from sleep is a discriminating feature favoring an organic rather than a functional cause, because functional bowel disorders characteristically spare sleep.

### Abnormal Liver Chemistries

Abnormal liver chemistries are reasoned by pattern before they are reasoned by magnitude. A hepatocellular pattern, in which aminotransferase elevation predominates over alkaline phosphatase elevation, points toward hepatocyte injury from viral, toxic, autoimmune, or metabolic causes, while a cholestatic pattern, in which alkaline phosphatase elevation predominates, points toward biliary obstruction or intrahepatic cholestasis and warrants imaging of the biliary tree before extensive serologic testing is pursued. The degree of aminotransferase elevation carries diagnostic weight of its own: elevations into the thousands are characteristic of acute viral hepatitis, ischemic hepatopathy, or drug-induced liver injury, while the modest elevations, typically two to five times the upper limit of normal, seen in metabolic dysfunction-associated steatotic liver disease reflect a fundamentally different and usually more indolent process.

**Dysphagia and Odynophagia**

Dysphagia is reasoned first by localizing the level at which the patient perceives difficulty and second by distinguishing solid-food from liquid-and-solid dysphagia, because these two axes point toward mechanistically distinct disease categories. Oropharyngeal dysphagia, in which the patient describes difficulty initiating a swallow, coughing, or nasal regurgitation within one to two seconds of swallowing, localizes to a neuromuscular or structural process above the upper esophageal sphincter and is evaluated primarily with a modified barium swallow study rather than upper endoscopy as the first test, because the process under investigation is one of coordinated muscular sequencing rather than luminal obstruction. Esophageal dysphagia, in which food sensation of sticking occurs several seconds after swallowing and is often localized retrosternally, is further divided by whether solids alone or both solids and liquids are affected from the outset: progressive dysphagia to solids that later includes liquids suggests a mechanical process, either a peptic stricture, a malignancy, or, in a younger patient with a history of atopy, eosinophilic esophagitis, whereas dysphagia to solids and liquids simultaneously from onset suggests a motility disorder such as achalasia, in which the lower esophageal sphincter fails to relax and peristalsis is disordered or absent. Odynophagia, pain with swallowing rather than difficulty swallowing, shifts the differential toward an infectious or pill-induced esophagitis, particularly in an immunocompromised patient, in whom candidal, viral, or medication-induced mucosal injury should be considered before a structural cause is pursued.

**KEY POINT:** New dysphagia to solid food in a patient over 50, particularly when accompanied by weight loss, warrants prompt upper endoscopy rather than an empiric trial of acid suppression, because the leading concern at this age is esophageal or gastric cardia malignancy rather than reflux alone.

Case Presentation: A 61-year-old man presents to clinic reporting three months of progressive difficulty swallowing solid food, initially with dense foods such as bread and steak and now extending to softer solids, without difficulty swallowing liquids. He reports an unintentional 12-pound weight loss over the same period and denies heartburn. He has a 30-pack-year smoking history and drinks alcohol regularly. Applying the reasoning developed in this section, progressive solid-food dysphagia that has not yet involved liquids, occurring in a patient over 50 with substantial smoking and alcohol exposure and accompanied by unintentional weight loss, localizes to a mechanical esophageal process and carries a pretest probability of malignancy high enough that empiric acid suppression would be an inappropriate first step. Upper endoscopy is scheduled urgently rather than electively, and at the time of the procedure a circumferential, friable mass is identified in the mid-esophagus, biopsies of which confirm squamous cell carcinoma. This case illustrates why the level, progression pattern, and associated features of dysphagia, rather than the symptom of dysphagia alone, determine both the urgency and the initial test selected, and why an empiric therapeutic trial is the wrong first move whenever alarm features accompany a new swallowing complaint.

## Initial Laboratory and Imaging Evaluation

### Core Laboratory Panel

A complete blood count with differential, a comprehensive metabolic panel, and a lipase measurement form the core initial panel for most gastrointestinal presentations, because together they screen for anemia and infection, assess renal and hepatic function, and evaluate for pancreatic injury without requiring the clinician to anticipate every possible diagnosis in advance. Liver chemistries should be interpreted as a panel rather than in isolation, because the ratio of aminotransferase elevation to alkaline phosphatase elevation, together with the bilirubin and albumin, characterizes both the pattern and the chronicity of liver injury more informatively than any single value.

### Selecting the Initial Imaging Study

Imaging selection follows the presenting complaint rather than a fixed protocol. Abdominal ultrasound is the preferred initial study for suspected biliary disease because it visualizes gallstones with high sensitivity and assesses bile duct caliber without ionizing radiation, while contrast-enhanced computed tomography is preferred for suspected pancreatitis complications, suspected bowel obstruction, or undifferentiated acute abdominal pain because it evaluates the bowel, mesentery, and solid organs simultaneously. Magnetic resonance cholangiopancreatography is reserved for cases in which ductal anatomy must be characterized noninvasively before deciding whether therapeutic endoscopic retrograde cholangiopancreatography is warranted, because unlike ultrasound and computed tomography, it visualizes the pancreaticobiliary ductal system directly without the procedural risk that endoscopic retrograde cholangiopancreatography itself carries.

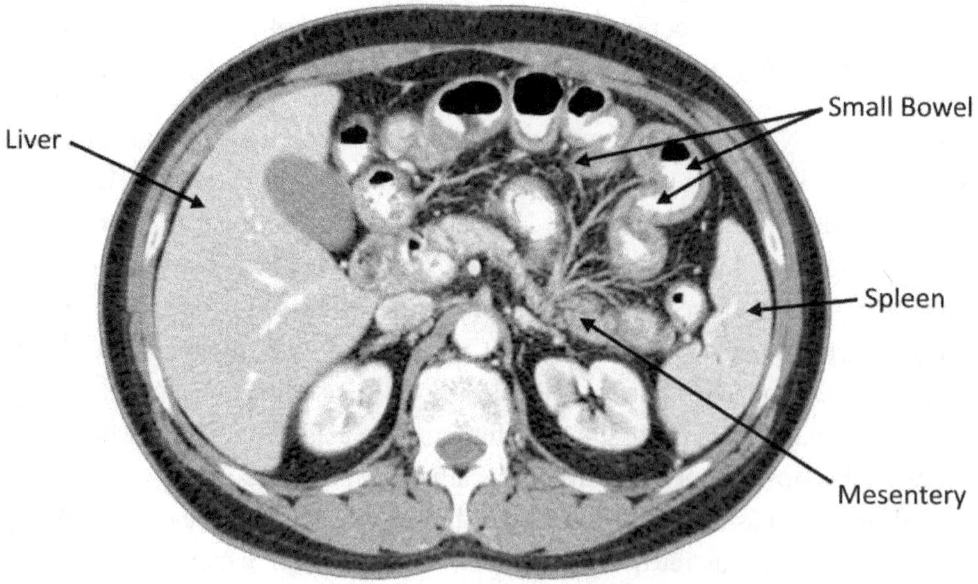


**CAUTION:** In a patient on anticoagulation who requires urgent endoscopy for suspected gastrointestinal hemorrhage, do not routinely delay the procedure to normalize coagulation parameters when hemorrhage is life-threatening; reversal strategy and procedural timing should be coordinated jointly with the requesting team rather than defaulting to a fixed waiting period, because delayed endoscopy in this setting carries its own measurable risk.

## Point-of-Care Ultrasound in the Initial Evaluation

Point-of-care ultrasound, performed by the evaluating clinician at the bedside rather than scheduled through radiology, has an expanding role in the initial gastroenterology assessment because it answers a focused binary question quickly rather than attempting a comprehensive survey. A bedside assessment for free intraperitoneal fluid, using the same views employed in trauma evaluation, can confirm ascites in a patient with clinical findings that are equivocal on examination and can guide safe site selection for a subsequent diagnostic or therapeutic paracentesis by identifying a fluid pocket away from bowel loops and the inferior epigastric vessels. Bedside evaluation of the inferior vena cava diameter and its respiratory variation provides a rapid, repeatable estimate of intravascular volume status in a patient with suspected gastrointestinal hemorrhage, complementing rather than replacing the shock index and orthostatic vital signs described earlier in this chapter, particularly when serial assessment is needed to track the response to resuscitation over the following hours. Point-of-care ultrasound does not replace a formal, radiology-performed study when the clinical question requires the fuller anatomic detail, Doppler characterization, or documentation that a formal study provides, and its appropriate role is to answer an immediate bedside question rapidly, not to substitute for definitive imaging when the diagnosis remains uncertain.

## Role of Endoscopy in the Initial Evaluation

Endoscopy is both diagnostic and therapeutic in gastroenterology in a way that distinguishes it from most other diagnostic tests, because upper endoscopy and colonoscopy permit direct mucosal visualization, tissue sampling, and, when indicated, immediate hemostatic or resection intervention within a single procedure. The timing of endoscopy is itself a clinical decision governed by the presenting complaint: suspected upper gastrointestinal hemorrhage in a hemodynamically stable patient is generally evaluated within 24 hours, whereas variceal hemorrhage or hemodynamic instability accelerates that timeline further, a distinction developed with its own threshold logic in the hepatology and hemorrhage chapters.

## Role of Tumor Markers and Specialized Serologic Testing

Tumor markers such as carcinoembryonic antigen and carbohydrate antigen 19-9 have limited value as screening or diagnostic tools in the initial evaluation because their sensitivity and specificity are insufficient to rule a malignancy in or out, and both are elevated by a range of benign inflammatory and hepatobiliary conditions; their appropriate use is as a baseline value for later surveillance once a malignant diagnosis has already been established by tissue or imaging, not as a first-line diagnostic test. Specialized serologic testing is more useful when it is deployed selectively against a specific pretest probability generated by the history: tissue transglutaminase immunoglobulin A, paired with a total immunoglobulin A level to exclude selective immunoglobulin A deficiency, is appropriate when malabsorptive symptoms, unexplained iron deficiency, or a family history of celiac disease is present; antineutrophil cytoplasmic and antinuclear antibodies are appropriate when autoimmune hepatitis or a hepatobiliary autoimmune process is suspected from a hepatocellular or cholestatic pattern of injury; and fecal calprotectin is appropriate when chronic diarrhea raises the question of inflammatory rather than functional bowel disease, because an elevated fecal calprotectin substantially raises the pretest probability that colonoscopy will identify mucosal inflammation, while a low value makes clinically significant inflammatory bowel disease unlikely enough to support a functional diagnosis without proceeding immediately to endoscopy.

## Nutritional and Functional Status Assessment at the Initial Encounter

Gastrointestinal disease frequently announces itself through nutritional and functional decline before a specific diagnosis is apparent, and a structured assessment of both at the initial encounter changes management independent of the eventual diagnosis, because a malnourished or frail patient tolerates both disease and procedural intervention differently than a well-nourished, functionally independent one.

### Screening for Malnutrition and Unintentional Weight Loss

Unintentional weight loss exceeding approximately 5 percent of body weight over six to twelve months is a threshold long used to distinguish clinically significant weight loss from ordinary fluctuation, and when present alongside a gastrointestinal symptom it should prompt a more expedited diagnostic pathway regardless of which specific symptom brought the patient to attention, because the mechanisms that produce involuntary weight loss, whether malabsorption, obstruction, chronic inflammation, or occult malignancy, are disproportionately serious relative to the same symptom occurring with a stable weight. A brief, validated nutritional screening tool, combined with serum albumin and prealbumin interpreted in the context of the patient's inflammatory state rather than as isolated nutritional markers, given that both are negative acute-phase reactants whose levels fall during any systemic inflammatory process independent of true nutritional status, identifies patients who require formal dietitian involvement before a procedural or surgical intervention is undertaken.

### Functional Status, Frailty, and Procedural Risk

Functional status, most efficiently assessed through a brief measure such as gait speed or the patient's ability to perform basic activities of daily living, predicts tolerance of both the underlying gastrointestinal disease process and any procedural intervention that its evaluation requires, and a frail patient identified at the initial encounter benefits from a modified diagnostic pathway, prioritizing the tests most likely to change management while deferring lower-yield testing that carries procedural risk disproportionate to its expected benefit in a patient with limited physiologic reserve. Frailty assessment is not a reason to withhold indicated diagnostic evaluation, including endoscopy, from an older or debilitated patient, but it is a reason to sequence that evaluation deliberately, optimizing volume status, correcting reversible metabolic derangements, and involving anesthesia colleagues proactively when moderate to deep sedation is anticipated in a patient whose baseline reserve is diminished.

**EVIDENCE:** Prospective cohort data in older endoscopy patients associate formal frailty assessment prior to sedated procedures with fewer cardiopulmonary complications and shorter recovery times, supporting frailty screening as a routine, low-cost component of the initial evaluation rather than a specialized add-on reserved for the visibly debilitated patient.

Documenting functional status and nutritional risk at the initial encounter also creates a reference point against which later decline can be measured objectively, which matters in chronic gastrointestinal disease, where a gradual downward trajectory over several encounters is easy to miss when each visit is compared only to the clinician's general impression rather than to a recorded baseline.

## Recognizing Red Flags and Determining Urgency

Certain features, regardless of the presenting complaint that carries them, identify a patient who requires expedited evaluation rather than routine outpatient referral.

### Alarm Features Requiring Expedited Evaluation

Unintentional weight loss, dysphagia, iron deficiency anemia, a palpable abdominal mass, persistent vomiting, and gastrointestinal bleeding at any age constitute alarm features that lower the threshold for endoscopic or cross-sectional evaluation regardless of the patient's age, because each reflects a mechanism, whether obstruction, malignancy, or occult blood loss, that is unlikely to resolve without intervention and is disproportionately associated with serious underlying pathology when present. Age itself modifies the interpretation of otherwise benign-appearing symptoms: new-onset dyspepsia or a change in bowel habits in a patient over 60 carries a materially higher pretest probability of malignancy than the identical symptom in a patient in their twenties, independent of any alarm feature.

### Triage of the GI Consult Request

A gastroenterology consultation request should be evaluated for urgency within minutes of receipt rather than queued by order of arrival, because a subset of requests, though not phrased urgently by the requesting team, describe a patient whose condition will deteriorate measurably within hours if evaluation is delayed. Requests describing active hematemesis, melena with hemodynamic change, suspected ascending cholangitis, or a new finding of severe acute pancreatitis warrant same-hour evaluation, while requests describing chronic, stable symptoms, an incidental imaging finding, or a request for outpatient follow-up planning can be triaged to routine same-day or next-day evaluation without compromising the patient.

### THE GI THRESHOLD DECISION SYSTEM — Foundational Diagnostic Thresholds — Ascending Cholangitis and the Urgency of Biliary Sepsis

**Presentation Signature:** A patient with known or suspected biliary obstruction develops fever, right upper quadrant pain, and jaundice, either together or in an incomplete combination, in the setting of a dilated or obstructed bile duct on imaging.

**Threshold Point:** The Tokyo Guidelines diagnostic criteria for acute cholangitis require evidence of systemic inflammation, evidence of cholestasis, and imaging evidence of biliary dilation or an identifiable obstructing cause; the presence of hypotension, altered mental status, or organ dysfunction in this setting defines the severe grade of the disease.

**The Call:** Suspected acute cholangitis of any severity requires prompt blood cultures and broad-spectrum antibiotics targeted at enteric organisms, and moderate to severe disease, or disease that fails to respond within 24 hours to antibiotics alone, requires urgent biliary drainage, most commonly by endoscopic retrograde cholangiopancreatography, performed emergently rather than electively.

**Trap Logic:** The classic Charcot triad of fever, jaundice, and right upper quadrant pain is present together in only a minority of confirmed cases; relying on the complete triad before initiating antibiotics or arranging urgent drainage delays treatment in patients who present with an incomplete but still diagnostic combination of findings.

**Decision Anchor:** In suspected cholangitis, antibiotics are started on clinical suspicion before culture results return, and severity grading, not diagnostic certainty alone, determines whether drainage is urgent or can be arranged semi-electively after a trial of antibiotics.

**EVIDENCE:** Multisociety guidance on acute cholangitis supports early, severity-stratified biliary drainage as the intervention most consistently associated with improved outcomes, reinforcing that antibiotics alone are inadequate definitive therapy once obstruction is confirmed.

Case Presentation: A 58-year-old man presents to the emergency department with two days of right upper quadrant pain, fever to 38.9 degrees Celsius, and darkening of his urine. He has a history of gallstones documented on ultrasound three years earlier that were never treated surgically. On examination he is tachycardic with a heart rate of 108 beats per minute, blood pressure 104/68 millimeters of mercury, and scleral icterus is visible in natural light. His abdomen is tender in the right upper quadrant without rebound or guarding. Initial laboratory evaluation reveals a white blood cell count of 16,200 per microliter, total bilirubin of 4.8 milligrams per deciliter, alkaline phosphatase of 410 units per liter, and aspartate and alanine aminotransferase values approximately three times the upper limit of normal, a cholestatic-predominant pattern. Applying the reasoning developed in this chapter, the combination of fever, jaundice, and right upper quadrant pain in a patient with known gallstone disease and a cholestatic laboratory pattern raises immediate concern for acute cholangitis, and the elevated heart rate relative to blood pressure, though not yet frankly hypotensive, signals early physiologic compromise that argues against a purely elective evaluation pathway. Blood cultures are drawn, broad-spectrum antibiotics covering enteric gram-negative organisms are administered within the hour, and right upper quadrant ultrasound confirms a dilated common bile duct with a visualized stone at the distal duct. Because the patient meets criteria for moderate-grade cholangitis with evidence of a defined obstructing stone, urgent endoscopic retrograde cholangiopancreatography with sphincterotomy and stone extraction is arranged rather than a trial of antibiotics alone, and the patient defervesces within 24 hours of drainage. This case illustrates the chapter's central principle: the initial history, examination, and laboratory pattern generated a specific, threshold-driven decision, urgent drainage rather than antibiotics alone, well before a definitive diagnosis had been confirmed by cholangiography.

## Special Populations and Diagnostic Pitfalls in the Initial Evaluation

The diagnostic reasoning developed above assumes a physiologically typical adult, and that assumption fails in several recurring populations whose altered anatomy, altered physiology, or altered symptom reporting changes both the differential diagnosis and the acceptable diagnostic tools.

### Pregnancy and the Gravid Abdomen

Pregnancy displaces the abdominal viscera progressively as the uterus enlarges, so that the point of maximal tenderness in appendicitis migrates cephalad and laterally as gestation advances, meaning that right lower quadrant tenderness, the classic finding in a nonpregnant adult, may instead localize to the right flank or right upper quadrant by the third trimester. Physiologic changes of pregnancy independently alter several of the reasoning tools developed earlier in this chapter: heart rate rises by 10 to 15 beats per minute at baseline, which shifts the shock index threshold and makes tachycardia a less specific marker of hemorrhage; alkaline phosphatase rises two- to fourfold from placental production alone, which removes it as a reliable marker of cholestasis unless interpreted alongside gamma-glutamyl transferase, an enzyme not produced by the placenta; and the differential diagnosis for right upper quadrant pain and abnormal liver chemistries must expand to include pregnancy-specific entities such as intrahepatic cholestasis of pregnancy and the hemolysis, elevated liver enzymes, and low platelet count syndrome, both of which carry management implications distinct from any diagnosis considered in a nonpregnant patient. Imaging selection is also constrained: ultrasound and, when necessary, magnetic resonance imaging without gadolinium are preferred, and computed tomography is reserved for situations in which the diagnostic benefit clearly outweighs the radiation exposure to the fetus.

### Older Adults and Atypical Presentations

Older adults, and particularly those who are frail or who have diabetic autonomic neuropathy, mount a blunted febrile and leukocytotic response to intra-abdominal infection, so that a normal temperature and a normal white blood cell count do not carry the same reassurance in a patient in their eighties that they carry in a patient in their thirties. Pain itself is frequently underreported or attributed by the patient to a chronic musculoskeletal condition, and a clinician who anchors on the patient's own minimization of symptom severity will systematically underestimate the acuity of processes such as mesenteric ischemia and perforation, both of which carry disproportionately high mortality in this population precisely because recognition and intervention are delayed. Polypharmacy compounds the diagnostic challenge, because anticoagulants alter the presentation and management of bleeding, opioids blunt the abdominal examination's sensitivity by masking peritoneal signs, and multiple concurrent medications increase the probability that a new gastrointestinal symptom is itself a drug effect rather than a new primary diagnosis.

### Immunocompromised and Critically Ill Patients

**CAUTION:** In a neutropenic or heavily immunosuppressed patient, abdominal pain and fever should never be attributed to a benign cause without imaging, because typhlitis and other necrotizing processes can progress rapidly and produce minimal localizing signs in a host whose inflammatory response is itself suppressed.

Immunocompromised patients, whether from chemotherapy-induced neutropenia, solid organ or hematopoietic stem cell transplantation, or advanced human immunodeficiency virus infection, present with a differential diagnosis that a nonimmunocompromised approach will not capture, including cytomegalovirus colitis, graft-versus-host disease of the gastrointestinal tract, and opportunistic infections that mimic inflammatory bowel disease both endoscopically and histologically. The physical examination in this population is also less reliable, because a suppressed inflammatory response can produce a soft, minimally tender abdomen even in the presence of a serious intra-abdominal process, which shifts diagnostic weight toward a lower threshold for cross-sectional imaging whenever the history is concerning, independent of examination findings that would otherwise permit observation in an immunocompetent patient. A low threshold for imaging in this population is not defensive medicine; it reflects a genuine shift in the pretest probability that physical examination alone can be trusted. That distinction matters clinically.

## Documenting the Initial Assessment and the Gastroenterology Consult Recommendation

The reasoning developed in this chapter is only as useful as the recommendation it produces, and a substantial body of experience among practicing consultants identifies imprecise, hedged recommendation language, rather than diagnostic error, as the most common reason a gastroenterology consult fails to change management in a timely way.

### Structuring a High-Value Consult Note

A consult note that changes management states, in order, the question being answered, the key findings that support the assessment, the specific diagnosis or working differential, and a numbered, dated, and dosed set of recommendations rather than a narrative paragraph that the primary team must parse for actionable content. Recommendations should specify the test or intervention, its timing, and the threshold that would trigger escalation, so that the primary team can act on the note without paging the consulting service again to clarify what was actually being recommended. Anticipating the next decision point, rather than only addressing the question as originally asked, is what distinguishes a consultation that shapes the remainder of the admission from one that answers a single narrow question and is filed away.

### From Vague Language to a Specific, Actionable Plan

Phrases such as "consider imaging" or "follow up as needed" transfer the burden of clinical decision-making back to a team that requested the consult specifically because it lacked the expertise to make that decision, and this pattern is identified repeatedly as a source of delayed care and repeat consultation. The corrective habit is straightforward to state and requires deliberate practice to apply consistently: replace every recommendation to "consider" a test with a recommendation to obtain a specific test, replace every recommendation to "monitor" a laboratory value with a specific value and a specific interval at which it should be rechecked, and replace every recommendation regarding medication with the specific agent, route, and confirm-against-formulary dosing range rather than a general instruction to treat.

## Patient Education and Shared Decision-Making at the Initial Visit

**PATIENT EDUCATION:** Patients retain diagnostic and procedural information more reliably when it is delivered in plain language, paired with the specific next step and its timing, and confirmed with teach-back rather than delivered as a list of medical terms without an accompanying plan.

The initial gastroenterology encounter is also the point at which the clinician establishes whether the patient understands why a given test is being recommended and what result would change the plan, and skipping this step produces the same downstream inefficiency as an imprecise consult note, because a patient who does not understand why colonoscopy has been recommended for anemia, rather than for a colon symptom, is less likely to complete the preparation adequately or keep the appointment. Explaining the reasoning in plain terms, for example that unexplained anemia requires looking directly at the lining of the stomach and colon because blood loss from those areas can occur without any pain or visible bleeding, closes the same gap between reasoning and action at the patient level that a precise, dosed recommendation closes at the level of the referring team. Shared decision-making becomes particularly relevant when a diagnostic pathway carries genuine alternatives, such as choosing between empiric acid suppression and prompt endoscopy for dyspepsia in a patient without alarm features, and documenting that the alternatives, their respective risks, and the patient's preference were discussed protects both the therapeutic relationship and the medical record.

Case Presentation: A 44-year-old woman is referred to gastroenterology clinic for iron deficiency anemia identified on routine laboratory testing performed for fatigue, with a hemoglobin of 9.8 grams per deciliter and a ferritin of 8 nanograms per milliliter. She reports no overt bleeding, has regular menstrual cycles that she does not consider unusually heavy, and has no abdominal pain, weight loss, or change in bowel habits. Her referring physician's note reads only "please evaluate anemia." Applying the structured reasoning developed in this chapter, unexplained iron deficiency anemia in an adult, even in the absence of overt bleeding or alarm features, warrants a bidirectional endoscopic evaluation because occult blood loss from an upper or lower gastrointestinal source, including colorectal neoplasia, must be excluded before the anemia is attributed to menstrual loss or dietary insufficiency alone; her age places her within standard average-risk colorectal cancer screening eligibility independent of the anemia, reinforcing rather than replacing the indication for colonoscopy. The consultation note documents this reasoning explicitly rather than restating the referral question, and closes with a specific, actionable plan: upper endoscopy and colonoscopy scheduled within the next two to four weeks, celiac serology sent prior to the procedures given the overlapping differential of malabsorptive iron deficiency, oral iron repletion initiated at a dose and formulation confirmed against current dosing guidance, and a follow-up hemoglobin and ferritin recheck at eight weeks with an explicit threshold, an inadequate rise, that would prompt reassessment of the repletion strategy or the diagnostic conclusion. This second case illustrates the chapter's closing principle: a consultation is complete not when a diagnosis has been reasoned through, but when that reasoning has been translated into a plan specific enough that the requesting team does not need to ask what happens next.

| Presenting Complaint | Leading Diagnostic Considerations | First-Line Test |
|---|---|---|
| Epigastric pain radiating to back | Pancreatitis, penetrating posterior ulcer | Lipase, contrast-enhanced CT |
| Right upper quadrant pain with fever | Acute cholecystitis, cholangitis | Right upper quadrant ultrasound |
| Melena or hematemesis | Peptic ulcer, variceal hemorrhage, gastritis | Hemoglobin, type and screen, upper endoscopy |
| Hematochezia | Diverticular bleeding, colitis, hemorrhoidal bleeding | Colonoscopy after hemodynamic assessment |
| Chronic diarrhea over four weeks | Inflammatory bowel disease, celiac disease, microscopic colitis | Stool studies, fecal calprotectin, celiac serology |
| Cholestatic liver chemistries | Choledocholithiasis, malignant biliary obstruction, PSC | Right upper quadrant ultrasound, MRCP |

**THE GI THRESHOLD DECISION SYSTEM — Foundational Diagnostic Thresholds**

**Presentation Signature:** This chapter's threshold instances addressed the two earliest decision points in gastroenterology practice: whether a bleeding patient requires immediate resuscitation, and whether a febrile, jaundiced patient requires emergent biliary drainage.

**Threshold Point:** A shock index above 1.0 and the Tokyo Guidelines severity grading for cholangitis both convert a qualitative clinical impression into a quantitative, reproducible decision point.

**The Call:** Both thresholds trigger action, resuscitation or drainage, before a definitive diagnosis is confirmed, because gastroenterology's highest-acuity presentations do not permit the clinician to wait for diagnostic certainty.

**Trap Logic:** Normal resting vital signs and an incomplete symptom triad are the two most common reasons these thresholds are missed or applied too late; orthostatic vital signs and severity grading, not the presence or absence of a classic triad, should drive the decision.

**Decision Anchor:** Every subsequent chapter in this book carries its own threshold instances built on this same structure: name the presentation, name the threshold, name the call, name the trap, and anchor the decision in a single memorable rule.

## Summary and Key Concepts

A gastrointestinal history is organized around onset, location, quality, timing, and relationship to meals, each of which narrows the differential diagnosis mechanistically rather than incidentally.

The abdominal examination follows a fixed sequence, inspection, auscultation, percussion, and palpation, and specific maneuvers such as Murphy sign and shifting dullness localize disease with reasonable bedside precision.

Extraintestinal stigmata of chronic liver disease reflect two convergent mechanisms: hyperestrogenism from impaired hepatic clearance, and portal hypertension from portosystemic collateral formation.

The four dominant gastroenterology presenting complaints, abdominal pain, bleeding or anemia, altered bowel habits, and abnormal liver chemistries, each have structured, pattern-based diagnostic reasoning pathways.

A shock index above 1.0 identifies compensated hemorrhagic shock before resting vital signs become abnormal, and severity-graded criteria for cholangitis determine whether drainage is urgent or can be sequenced after a trial of antibiotics.

Alarm features and consult urgency should be assessed within minutes of a patient's presentation or a consult request's receipt, not after routine evaluation has already been queued.

# CHAPTER 2: ENDOSCOPIC, RADIOLOGIC, AND FUNCTIONAL DIAGNOSTIC MODALITIES

**Learning Objectives**

1. Compare the diagnostic and therapeutic capabilities of upper endoscopy, colonoscopy, and endoscopic ultrasound.
2. Select the appropriate cross-sectional imaging modality for a given gastrointestinal or hepatobiliary indication.
3. Interpret the major endoscopic classification systems used to standardize findings across esophagitis, Barrett esophagus, and inflammatory bowel disease.
4. Describe the indications, technique, and complication profile of endoscopic retrograde cholangiopancreatography.
5. Apply functional and motility testing appropriately in the evaluation of esophageal and anorectal disorders.

**Chapter Outline**

This chapter surveys the diagnostic toolkit that the remainder of the book assumes: upper and lower endoscopy, endoscopic ultrasound and endoscopic retrograde cholangiopancreatography, cross-sectional and functional imaging, and the motility studies used when a structural evaluation has been unrevealing. Each modality is presented with its governing indication, its limitations, and the classification systems that make its findings reproducible across observers. The chapter closes with a practical, three-question framework for choosing among competing modalities, intended to be applied at the bedside rather than memorized as an abstract hierarchy.

## Upper Endoscopy and Colonoscopy

Upper endoscopy and colonoscopy remain the two highest-yield procedures in gastroenterology because both provide direct mucosal visualization, targeted biopsy, and immediate therapeutic intervention within a single encounter, a combination that distinguishes endoscopy from almost every other diagnostic modality used in internal medicine.

### Indications and Technique for Upper Endoscopy

Upper endoscopy visualizes the esophagus, stomach, and duodenum and is indicated for dysphagia, odynophagia, suspected upper gastrointestinal bleeding, iron deficiency anemia, refractory dyspepsia with alarm features, and surveillance of known Barrett esophagus or prior gastric or esophageal neoplasia. The procedure is performed under conscious sedation or, increasingly, propofol-based monitored anesthesia care, and a systematic examination proceeds from the esophagus through a retroflexed view of the gastric cardia and fundus before advancing to the antrum, pylorus, and duodenal bulb and second portion, a sequence designed to ensure that no mucosal surface, including the areas most prone to being overlooked such as the gastric cardia on forward view alone, is missed. A pre-procedure checklist confirming indication, consent, allergy status, and anticoagulation management reduces the likelihood that a preventable process error, rather than a true procedural complication, is the reason a case does not proceed as planned.

Magnetic resonance defecography avoids ionizing radiation and additionally visualizes the pelvic floor musculature and adjacent pelvic organs, which is valuable when multicompartment pelvic floor dysfunction, involving the bladder or vaginal vault in addition to the rectum, is suspected, whereas fluoroscopic defecography remains more widely available and provides a dynamic, real-time assessment that some centers find more physiologically representative of an actual evacuation effort.

The choice between catheter-based and wireless capsule pH monitoring, and between pH-only and combined pH-impedance monitoring, is guided by the specific clinical question. A wireless capsule affixed to the esophageal mucosa allows monitoring extended to 96 hours without the discomfort of a transnasal catheter, which improves the likelihood that the recorded days represent the patient's typical dietary and positional pattern rather than a day altered by the catheter's presence, while a transnasal catheter, though less comfortable, permits simultaneous impedance measurement, which detects nonacid and weakly acidic reflux events that pH monitoring alone would miss entirely. Impedance-pH monitoring is particularly valuable when reflux symptoms persist despite adequate acid suppression, because it distinguishes patients whose ongoing symptoms correlate with nonacid reflux, who require a different management strategy than escalating acid suppression further, from patients whose symptoms do not correlate with any detected reflux event at all, in whom a functional esophageal disorder rather than reflux disease itself becomes the leading explanation.

Case Presentation: A 39-year-old woman reports six months of recurrent, dull right upper quadrant pain occurring roughly one hour after meals, lasting thirty to sixty minutes, and occasionally waking her at night. She has no fever, jaundice, or weight loss. Transabdominal ultrasound shows no gallstones, a normal-caliber common bile duct, and a normal-appearing gallbladder wall. Basic laboratory studies, including liver chemistries and lipase, are unremarkable. Applying the modality-selection reasoning developed in this chapter, biliary-type pain with a structurally normal ultrasound and no gallstones does not exclude a gallbladder-origin process, because functional gallbladder disorders occur in the absence of stones or wall thickening; the appropriate next test is hepatobiliary scintigraphy with calculation of the gallbladder ejection fraction after cholecystokinin stimulation, not an empiric trial of acid suppression, which targets an entirely different organ and would not be expected to help a gallbladder-origin process. Scintigraphy demonstrates a gallbladder ejection fraction below the accepted threshold for normal contraction, and, critically, the injection of cholecystokinin during the study reproduces her typical pain, a finding that correlates with a favorable response to cholecystectomy. She is referred for laparoscopic cholecystectomy, and her symptoms resolve postoperatively. This case demonstrates the chapter's broader principle in a second clinical context: selecting the modality that is physiologically designed to answer the question at hand, functional gallbladder emptying rather than structural biliary anatomy, reaches the correct diagnosis when a structurally normal study has already, appropriately, excluded the more common explanations.

### Indications and Technique for Colonoscopy

Colonoscopy visualizes the colon and terminal ileum and serves simultaneously as a diagnostic tool for bleeding, altered bowel habits, and inflammatory bowel disease evaluation and as the primary modality for colorectal cancer screening and polypectomy, a dual role that no radiologic test can replace because polypectomy performed at the time of detection prevents the malignant transformation that screening is designed to interrupt. Adequate bowel preparation is the single largest determinant of colonoscopy quality, because a poorly prepared colon reduces adenoma detection rate measurably and is the most common reason a procedure must be repeated sooner than the interval that would otherwise be recommended; a validated preparation-quality scale should be documented for every procedure so that the recommended surveillance interval reflects the true completeness of the examination rather than an assumed adequacy. Terminal ileal intubation, performed routinely rather than selectively, adds diagnostic value beyond colorectal cancer screening alone, since it can identify terminal ileal Crohn disease or backwash ileitis that would otherwise go undetected until symptoms prompted a dedicated small bowel evaluation.

**KEY POINT:** Cecal intubation with photographic documentation of the cecal landmarks, appendiceal orifice and ileocecal valve, and adequate bowel preparation are the two quality benchmarks that most directly determine whether a colonoscopy can be trusted to have excluded significant pathology.

### Endoscopic Classification Systems

Standardized classification systems convert a subjective endoscopic impression into a reproducible score that guides management and communicates severity across observers. The Los Angeles classification grades erosive esophagitis by the extent and confluence of mucosal breaks, and the distinction between grades matters clinically because higher grades warrant a longer initial course of acid suppression and a lower threshold for repeat endoscopy to confirm healing. The Prague classification describes Barrett esophagus by its circumferential and maximal extent, expressed as C and M values, and this measurement directly determines the interval and technique of surveillance biopsy. The Forrest classification stratifies the endoscopic appearance of a bleeding peptic ulcer, from active spurting hemorrhage through a visible vessel, adherent clot, flat pigmented spot, and a clean ulcer base, and this grading determines both the need for endoscopic hemostatic therapy and the intensity of subsequent inpatient monitoring, because the rebleeding risk associated with each Forrest grade differs by an order of magnitude between the highest- and lowest-risk categories. The Mayo endoscopic subscore and the more granular Ulcerative Colitis Endoscopic Index of Severity quantify mucosal inflammation in ulcerative colitis and are used both to confirm remission objectively, rather than by symptom resolution alone, and to guide treatment escalation when mucosal healing lags behind symptomatic improvement.

Figure 2.1: Los Angeles Classification of Erosive Esophagitis

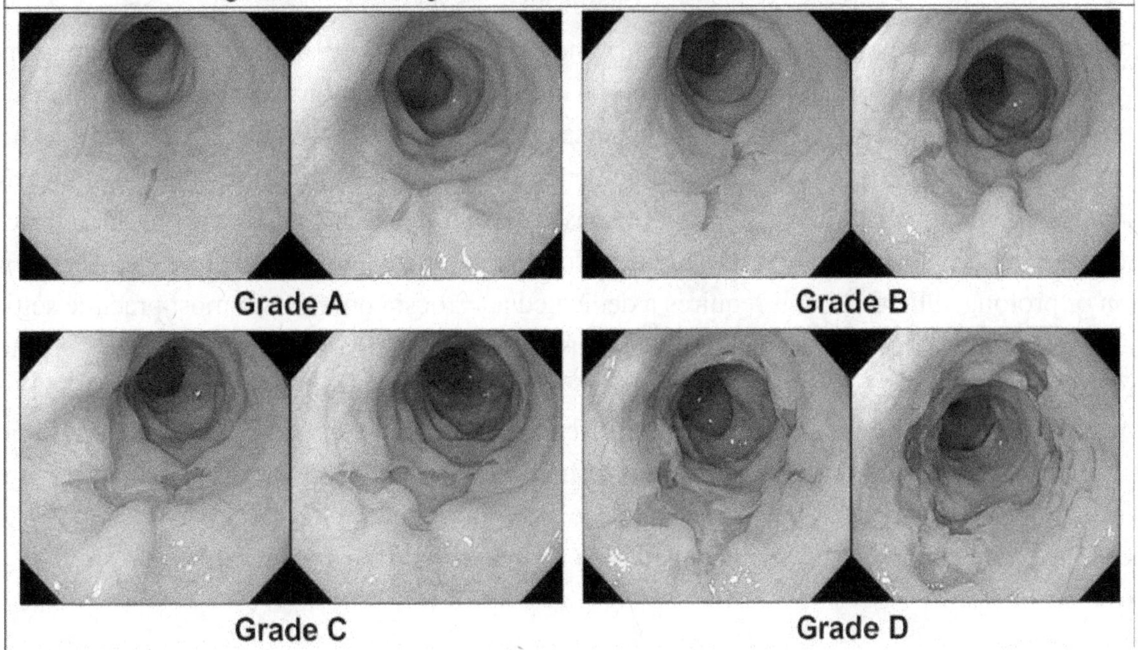


## Complications and Safety of Upper Endoscopy and Colonoscopy

Both procedures carry a low but nonzero complication rate that should be disclosed and understood in proportion to its actual frequency rather than either minimized or overstated. Perforation is the most serious complication of diagnostic endoscopy and occurs more frequently during therapeutic maneuvers, such as dilation, polypectomy, or stricture treatment, than during purely diagnostic examination, and its risk rises further in the setting of altered anatomy from prior surgery, active severe inflammation, or a stricture requiring forceful instrumentation. Post-polypectomy bleeding, either immediate or delayed by up to two weeks, results from incomplete thermal sealing of the resection site or from a coagulum that dislodges as healing progresses, and the risk is stratified by polyp size, location, and the resection technique used, information that should guide both the choice of technique and the post-procedure instructions given to the patient regarding activity and anticoagulation resumption. Cardiopulmonary events related to sedation, rather than to the endoscopic maneuver itself, account for a substantial proportion of overall procedural morbidity, which is why pre-procedure risk stratification, including a focused airway and cardiopulmonary assessment, is performed for every patient regardless of the indication for the procedure. These risks should be disclosed as part of informed consent using absolute rather than purely relative terms, since a relative risk figure alone can distort a patient's understanding of a complication that remains, in absolute terms, uncommon.

**CAUTION:** Post-polypectomy bleeding can present up to two weeks after the procedure and is easily mistaken for a new, unrelated source of bleeding if the recent colonoscopy is not specifically elicited in the history.

## Sedation Options and Anesthesia Considerations

Sedation strategy affects both patient experience and procedural safety, and the choice among moderate sedation with a benzodiazepine and opioid combination, deeper sedation with propofol administered by an anesthesia provider, and, occasionally, unsedated or minimally sedated examination should be individualized to the procedure's anticipated complexity, the patient's comorbidity burden, and airway risk factors rather than applied uniformly. Propofol-based monitored anesthesia care provides faster onset, faster recovery, and a more reliably immobile field for therapeutic maneuvers such as endoscopic mucosal resection or prolonged ERCP, but it requires a dedicated anesthesia provider in most practice settings and carries its own respiratory depression risk that must be weighed against these benefits, particularly in patients with obstructive sleep apnea, morbid obesity, or significant cardiopulmonary disease. A structured pre-procedure assessment, including an American Society of Anesthesiologists physical status classification and a focused airway examination, should be documented for every patient regardless of which sedation strategy is chosen, because the decision to proceed with moderate sedation rather than anesthesia-directed care is itself a clinical judgment that should be made deliberately rather than by default.

## Bowel Preparation Regimens and Quality Metrics Beyond Cecal Intubation

Split-dose bowel preparation, in which half of the prescribed preparation is taken the evening before the procedure and the remainder is completed within several hours of the scheduled start time, produces measurably better mucosal visualization than a single same-day or prior-evening dose because it minimizes the interval between preparation completion and colonic examination, during which small bowel and biliary secretions continue to accumulate and degrade an otherwise adequate preparation. Low-volume preparations combining a reduced volume of polyethylene glycol with an osmotic agent such as sodium sulfate or magnesium citrate improve patient tolerance and completion rates relative to older four-liter regimens without sacrificing preparation quality, which matters directly for diagnostic yield, since a patient who does not complete the preparation cannot receive its benefit regardless of the regimen prescribed.

Adenoma detection rate, the proportion of average-risk screening colonoscopies in which at least one adenoma is identified, is the single quality metric most strongly associated with interval colorectal cancer risk, meaning that an endoscopist whose adenoma detection rate falls below established benchmarks is associated with a measurably higher rate of cancers diagnosed between recommended screening intervals in their patients. Withdrawal time, the minimum duration spent examining the mucosa during withdrawal of the colonoscope, functions as a structural safeguard supporting adequate adenoma detection rather than as a meaningful outcome in isolation, because a longer withdrawal time in the absence of careful, systematic mucosal inspection does not by itself improve detection, and these metrics are tracked collectively, along with cecal intubation rate and bowel preparation adequacy, as the standard quality benchmarks against which endoscopists and endoscopy units are measured.

### Emerging Endoscopic Imaging Technologies

Optical enhancement technologies, including narrow band imaging, and its manufacturer-specific equivalents such as flexible spectral imaging color enhancement and i-scan, filter or process the reflected light captured during standard white-light endoscopy to accentuate mucosal and vascular surface patterns without requiring dye application, and these technologies improve the detection and characterization of subtle neoplastic and preneoplastic lesions, including diminutive colorectal polyps and early Barrett-associated dysplasia, that can be difficult to distinguish from surrounding mucosa under white light alone. Chromoendoscopy, the application of a dye such as indigo carmine or methylene blue directly onto the mucosal surface, achieves a related goal through a different mechanism, pooling in mucosal crevices to accentuate surface topology, and has a particular role in surveillance colonoscopy for longstanding inflammatory bowel disease, where dysplasia can arise in a flat, endoscopically subtle pattern that random biopsy sampling alone is more likely to miss than targeted biopsy of a chromoendoscopy-identified abnormality. Confocal laser endomicroscopy extends optical characterization to the cellular level, providing real-time histologic-resolution imaging during the endoscopic procedure itself, though its adoption remains limited by cost, the specialized training required for interpretation, and the fact that conventional targeted biopsy with standard histopathology remains an adequate, more widely available alternative for most indications. Dye-based and virtual chromoendoscopy techniques are complementary rather than competing, and many endoscopists move fluidly between them within a single examination depending on the region being inspected and the specific concern being evaluated.

### THE GI THRESHOLD DECISION SYSTEM — Endoscopic Diagnostic Thresholds — Forrest Classification and Rebleeding Risk

---

**Presentation Signature:** A patient undergoes upper endoscopy for suspected peptic ulcer bleeding, and a bleeding or recently bled ulcer is identified, requiring the endoscopist to translate its appearance into a management and monitoring decision.

**Threshold Point:** Forrest Ia and Ib, active spurting or oozing hemorrhage, and Forrest IIa, a visible vessel, carry rebleeding rates high enough to mandate endoscopic hemostatic therapy at the index procedure; Forrest IIb, an adherent clot, is managed with either hemostatic therapy or intensive medical therapy depending on institutional practice, while Forrest IIc and III, a flat pigmented spot or a clean base, carry low enough rebleeding risk that hemostatic intervention adds risk without meaningful benefit.

**The Call:** Forrest Ia through IIa lesions receive dual or combination endoscopic hemostatic therapy at the index procedure and are admitted for at least 48 to 72 hours of monitoring given the peak rebleeding window; Forrest IIc and III lesions can be managed with acid suppression alone and considered for earlier discharge once hemodynamically stable.

**Trap Logic:** An adherent clot, Forrest IIb, is frequently either over-treated with aggressive clot removal that provokes bleeding from an underlying visible vessel, or under-treated by being mistaken for a low-risk lesion; its intermediate risk requires a deliberate, protocol-guided decision rather than a default in either direction.

**Decision Anchor:** The Forrest grade assigned at the index endoscopy, not the initial hemoglobin or the volume of blood reported by the patient, is the single strongest predictor of rebleeding risk and should drive both the decision to treat endoscopically and the length of inpatient monitoring.

## Endoscopic Ultrasound and Endoscopic Retrograde Cholangiopancreatography

### Endoscopic Ultrasound

Endoscopic ultrasound combines endoscopy with a high-frequency ultrasound transducer mounted at the tip of the endoscope, allowing visualization of structures immediately adjacent to the gastrointestinal lumen with a resolution that transabdominal imaging cannot achieve, including the layers of the bowel wall itself, the pancreas, and regional lymph nodes. Its principal diagnostic role is in the local staging of esophageal, gastric, and pancreatic malignancy, where it determines depth of tumor invasion and nodal involvement with greater accuracy than cross-sectional imaging alone, and in the evaluation of suspected choledocholithiasis when noninvasive imaging is equivocal, because its sensitivity for small common bile duct stones exceeds that of transabdominal ultrasound and approaches that of magnetic resonance cholangiopancreatography. Fine-needle aspiration or biopsy performed under endoscopic ultrasound guidance provides tissue diagnosis of pancreatic masses, submucosal lesions, and mediastinal or celiac lymphadenopathy with a safety profile favorable enough that it has largely replaced percutaneous biopsy for lesions within its reach.

Contrast-enhanced and elastographic techniques extend endoscopic ultrasound's diagnostic reach further by characterizing the internal vascularity and stiffness of a lesion rather than its size and shape alone, which improves the distinction between a solid pancreatic mass suspicious for adenocarcinoma and a mass-forming pattern of chronic pancreatitis, two entities that can appear similar on standard grayscale imaging but behave very differently after intravenous contrast administration because chronic pancreatitis typically retains vascularity in a pattern distinct from the hypoenhancing appearance characteristic of pancreatic adenocarcinoma. These adjuncts do not replace tissue diagnosis when malignancy remains a serious consideration, but they refine the pretest probability that guides how aggressively a nondiagnostic initial biopsy should be pursued.

### Endoscopic Retrograde Cholangiopancreatography

Endoscopic retrograde cholangiopancreatography combines endoscopy with fluoroscopic cannulation of the bile duct, the pancreatic duct, or both, and its modern role is almost exclusively therapeutic rather than diagnostic, because magnetic resonance cholangiopancreatography now performs the diagnostic characterization of ductal anatomy without the procedural risk that endoscopic retrograde cholangiopancreatography carries. Indications include choledocholithiasis requiring extraction, malignant or benign biliary strictures requiring stenting, sphincter of Oddi dysfunction in selected patients, and pancreatic duct disruption or stricture in selected cases of chronic pancreatitis. The procedure carries a meaningfully higher complication rate than upper endoscopy or colonoscopy, most importantly post-endoscopic retrograde cholangiopancreatography pancreatitis, which results from mechanical, hydrostatic, and chemical injury to the pancreatic duct orifice during cannulation and is mitigated by rectal nonsteroidal anti-inflammatory drug administration and, in higher-risk cases, prophylactic pancreatic duct stent placement. Operator volume and institutional case mix both influence success and complication rates meaningfully enough that regionalization of complex ERCP to higher-volume centers is increasingly favored for the technically demanding subset of cases, such as altered surgical anatomy or intrahepatic stone disease.

**CAUTION:** Endoscopic retrograde cholangiopancreatography should not be used as a diagnostic-only procedure when noninvasive imaging can answer the same question; its risk profile is justified by its therapeutic capability, not by diagnostic uncertainty alone.

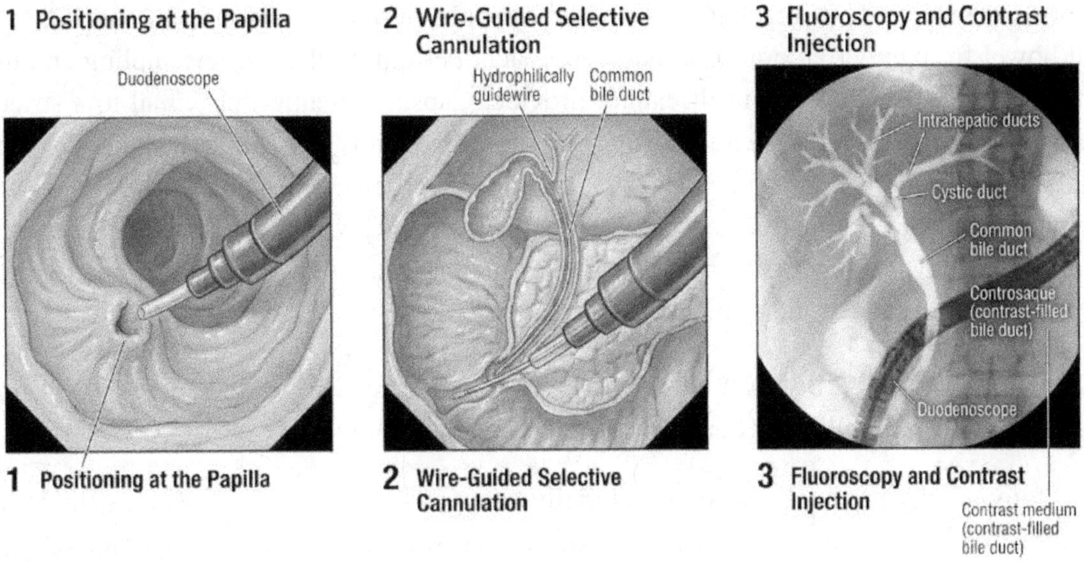


### Complications of ERCP and Risk Mitigation

Post-ERCP pancreatitis occurs in a meaningful minority of procedures and results from a combination of mechanical trauma to the papilla during cannulation, hydrostatic injury from contrast injection under pressure, and thermal or chemical injury when sphincterotomy or other papillary intervention is performed, with risk rising further in patients with a small, non-dilated bile duct, suspected sphincter of Oddi dysfunction, or a difficult, prolonged cannulation requiring multiple attempts. Rectal indomethacin or diclofenac administered immediately before or after the procedure reduces the incidence of post-ERCP pancreatitis and has become standard practice in patients without a contraindication, and prophylactic pancreatic duct stent placement provides additional risk reduction in the highest-risk subset of patients, such as those undergoing pancreatic sphincterotomy or difficult cannulation, though the stent itself requires either spontaneous passage confirmation or planned removal. Other recognized complications include bleeding after sphincterotomy, most often controlled endoscopically at the time it is recognized, cholangitis when biliary drainage is incomplete after an intervention, and, rarely, duodenal perforation related to the periampullary location of the procedure, each of which requires a distinct recognition and management pathway that the endoscopist and the admitting team should anticipate before the procedure rather than reason through only after a complication has already occurred.

### Capsule Endoscopy and Deep Enteroscopy

Capsule endoscopy visualizes the small bowel mucosa beyond the reach of standard upper endoscopy and colonoscopy by means of a swallowed, wireless recording device, and its principal indication is obscure gastrointestinal bleeding after a bidirectional endoscopic evaluation has been unrevealing, along with surveillance in selected small bowel Crohn disease and polyposis syndromes. Capsule endoscopy is purely diagnostic, and a positive finding requiring biopsy or therapeutic intervention is followed by device-assisted or deep enteroscopy, a technique using an overtube system to advance an endoscope deep into the small bowel from either an oral or a rectal approach, permitting the tissue sampling and therapeutic capability that capsule endoscopy itself cannot provide. Capsule retention proximal to a stricture is the procedure's most important complication, occurring more frequently in patients with known or suspected Crohn disease, which is why a patency capsule, a dissolvable device of matched dimensions, is used to confirm luminal patency before true capsule endoscopy in patients with risk factors for stricture, and why any patient with known severe stricturing disease is better served by cross-sectional enterography as the initial small bowel evaluation rather than capsule endoscopy.

## Cross-Sectional and Functional Imaging

### Computed Tomography and Its Gastrointestinal-Specific Protocols

Computed tomography protocol selection materially changes diagnostic yield, and a generic abdominal and pelvic study is frequently inadequate for a specific gastrointestinal question. Computed tomography enterography, which uses a large volume of neutral oral contrast to distend the small bowel and a dedicated enteric phase of contrast timing, is the preferred cross-sectional study for suspected small bowel Crohn disease because it distinguishes active inflammation, characterized by mural hyperenhancement and stratification, from chronic fibrostenotic change in a way that a standard protocol cannot. Triple-phase liver protocols, obtaining arterial, portal venous, and delayed phases, are required to characterize a hepatic lesion's enhancement pattern, because the timing of enhancement and washout, not the lesion's appearance on a single phase, is what distinguishes a benign hemangioma from hepatocellular carcinoma using standardized reporting criteria.

### Magnetic Resonance Imaging and Cholangiopancreatography

Magnetic resonance imaging offers superior soft tissue contrast without ionizing radiation and is preferred for hepatic lesion characterization when the diagnosis remains uncertain after computed tomography, for rectal cancer staging, and for pelvic fistula mapping in perianal Crohn disease, where its multiplanar capability delineates fistula tracts relative to the anal sphincter complex more precisely than any other noninvasive modality. Magnetic resonance cholangiopancreatography, a specific magnetic resonance sequence rather than a separate examination, produces a projectional image of the biliary and pancreatic ductal system analogous to a cholangiogram without instrumentation, and it has become the standard noninvasive test for characterizing choledocholithiasis, biliary strictures, and pancreatic duct anatomy before deciding whether therapeutic endoscopic retrograde cholangiopancreatography is warranted. Contraindications such as certain implanted devices and severe claustrophobia should be screened for before scheduling rather than discovered at the time of the scan, since a cancelled study delays the diagnostic pathway as much as an unavailable one.

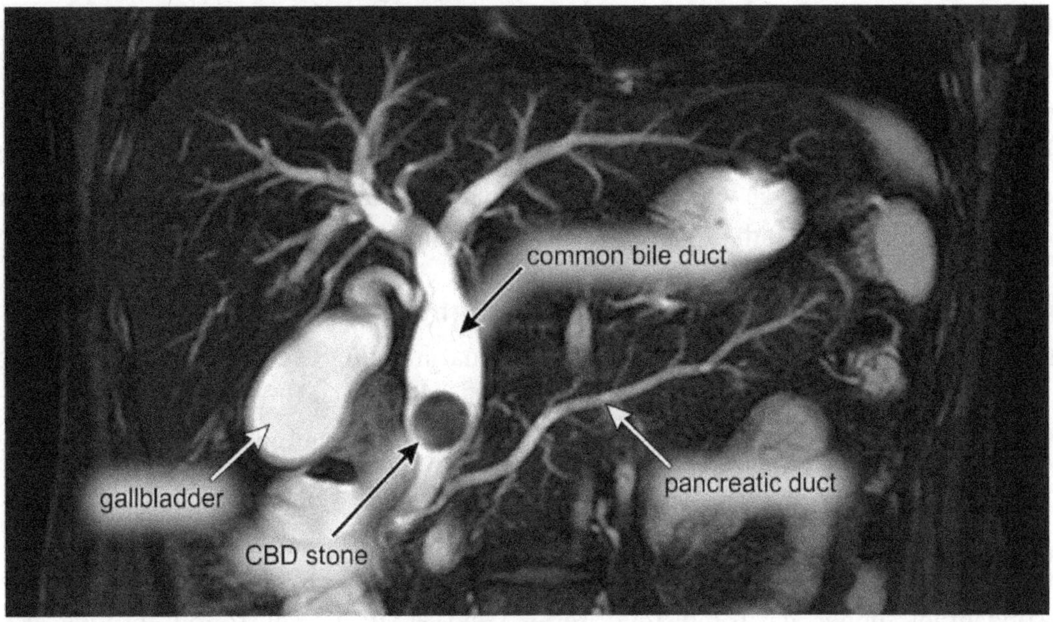


**Interpreting Discordant or Equivocal Findings Across Modalities**

Different modalities occasionally generate discordant impressions of the same lesion, and resolving that discordance requires understanding what each technique is and is not designed to detect rather than simply favoring whichever result was obtained most recently. A hepatic lesion that appears indeterminate on ultrasound but demonstrates a classic arterial-phase hyperenhancement with portal venous washout pattern on a dedicated triple-phase CT or MRI can be diagnosed as hepatocellular carcinoma using standardized imaging criteria without biopsy in a patient with cirrhosis, because the enhancement pattern itself, obtained on the appropriate modality, has been validated as diagnostic in this specific clinical context; the same lesion imaged only by ultrasound, a modality not designed to characterize enhancement kinetics, would appropriately remain indeterminate. Similarly, a common bile duct that appears mildly dilated on transabdominal ultrasound in an asymptomatic post-cholecystectomy patient, without a visualized stone, should prompt consideration of MRCP or endoscopic ultrasound to exclude a retained stone or stricture rather than either dismissal of the finding or immediate escalation to therapeutic ERCP, since a mildly dilated but otherwise unremarkable duct can also reflect a normal post-cholecystectomy anatomic change.

**KEY POINT:** When two imaging studies disagree, ask which modality was actually designed to answer the specific question at hand rather than treating both results as equally weighted evidence.

### Abdominal Ultrasound and Elastography

Abdominal ultrasound remains the first-line study for suspected biliary disease and for hepatic surveillance because it is inexpensive, avoids radiation, and detects gallstones with high sensitivity, though its accuracy for common bile duct stones and for detailed pancreatic evaluation is limited by bowel gas and body habitus in a way that magnetic resonance cholangiopancreatography and endoscopic ultrasound are not. Elastography, performed either by ultrasound-based shear wave technique or by magnetic resonance elastography, quantifies liver stiffness as a noninvasive surrogate for fibrosis stage, and its adoption has meaningfully reduced the number of liver biopsies performed for fibrosis staging alone, reserving biopsy for cases in which elastography and serologic fibrosis markers disagree or in which a specific histologic diagnosis, rather than fibrosis stage alone, is required.

## Radiologic and Nuclear Medicine Studies Unique to Gastroenterology

Several studies outside the endoscopic and cross-sectional imaging categories already discussed answer questions that neither endoscopy nor standard CT or MRI can address directly, and selecting among them requires understanding what physiologic process, rather than what anatomic structure, each is designed to visualize.

### Fluoroscopic Contrast Studies

Barium esophagram, upper gastrointestinal series, and small bowel follow-through use real-time fluoroscopic observation of contrast transit to characterize structural and motility abnormalities that a static cross-sectional image cannot capture, because swallowing and peristalsis are dynamic processes best evaluated in motion. A barium esophagram remains valuable in the initial evaluation of dysphagia when a motility disorder such as achalasia is suspected, as its characteristic bird's-beak narrowing at the gastroesophageal junction and dilated esophageal body provide a pattern-recognition diagnosis that directs the clinician toward confirmatory manometry, and it is also the preferred initial test for suspected postoperative leak or stricture after esophageal or gastric surgery, where its dynamic transit assessment and ability to use water-soluble contrast when perforation is a concern make it safer and more informative than endoscopy alone in the immediate postoperative period. A small bowel follow-through, while largely supplanted by CT and MR enterography for inflammatory bowel disease evaluation, retains a role in characterizing the length and degree of a small bowel stricture when enterography findings are equivocal or when a dedicated transit-time assessment is needed. These studies remain inexpensive, widely available, and free of the sedation risk that accompanies endoscopy, which sustains their role even in an era when endoscopic and cross-sectional alternatives exist for many of the same indications.

### Hepatobiliary Scintigraphy

Hepatobiliary scintigraphy, commonly referred to by the trade name of its radiotracer class as a HIDA scan, evaluates gallbladder function and biliary patency by tracking the hepatic uptake and biliary excretion of an intravenously administered radiotracer over a period of one to four hours, with delayed imaging or morphine augmentation used when standard timing is inconclusive. Its principal indication is confirming acute cholecystitis when ultrasound findings are equivocal, because nonvisualization of the gallbladder on scintigraphy, indicating cystic duct obstruction, has diagnostic performance for acute cholecystitis that exceeds ultrasound in ambiguous cases, and a secondary indication is quantifying gallbladder ejection fraction in the evaluation of suspected biliary dyskinesia, a functional gallbladder disorder considered when biliary-type pain occurs in the absence of gallstones and other structural pathology has been excluded. Because the test measures a physiologic process unfolding over time rather than a static anatomic snapshot, patient preparation, including an adequate fasting interval, materially affects result reliability, and a technically inadequate study should prompt repeat testing rather than an uncertain interpretation being carried forward into the clinical decision.

### PET-CT in Gastrointestinal Oncology

Positron emission tomography combined with computed tomography exploits the increased glucose metabolism of most malignant tissue to identify sites of disease with a sensitivity for detecting distant metastasis that anatomic imaging alone frequently lacks, and its principal gastroenterology-relevant role is in staging esophageal and gastric cancer prior to a planned curative resection, where identifying occult metastatic disease changes management from surgery to systemic therapy, and in evaluating an indeterminate hepatic or pancreatic lesion when other modalities have not resolved the diagnosis. Its limitations are equally important to recognize: PET-CT has limited sensitivity for peritoneal carcinomatosis and for tumors with low metabolic activity, including well-differentiated neuroendocrine tumors and mucinous adenocarcinoma, both of which are better evaluated by dedicated cross-sectional imaging or, in the case of neuroendocrine tumors, by somatostatin-receptor-based nuclear imaging rather than standard glucose-based PET. Physiologic FDG uptake in the stomach, small bowel, and colon can also obscure or mimic pathology, which is why PET-CT findings in the gastrointestinal tract are always interpreted alongside a correlative anatomic study rather than in isolation.

### Radiation Stewardship and Modality Selection

**KEY POINT:** When ultrasound or MRI can answer the clinical question as reliably as CT, they should be preferred, particularly in younger patients, in pregnancy, and in patients such as those with Crohn disease who are likely to require repeated imaging over a lifetime of disease monitoring.

Gastroenterology disproportionately involves patients who require serial imaging over years to decades, including those with chronic inflammatory bowel disease, cirrhosis under hepatocellular carcinoma surveillance, and pancreatic cystic lesions under interval follow-up, which makes cumulative radiation exposure a genuine clinical consideration rather than an abstract one. A deliberate strategy of substituting MRI or ultrasound for CT whenever their diagnostic performance is equivalent, reserving CT for indications in which its speed, availability, or superior evaluation of bowel and mesenteric detail is specifically required, measurably reduces lifetime radiation exposure in patients who will be imaged repeatedly, and this substitution strategy should be considered explicitly each time a follow-up study is ordered rather than defaulting to whichever modality was used previously.

## Communicating Diagnostic Findings to the Referring Team

A diagnostic study is only as valuable as the clarity with which its result is communicated to the team that ordered it, and the same precision principle developed in the previous chapter for consult recommendations applies equally to reporting a diagnostic finding: a report that states a finding without stating its clinical implication and the specific next step requires the referring team to independently interpret its significance, which reproduces the same delay that an imprecise consult recommendation produces. An endoscopy report describing a Forrest IIa visible vessel treated with combination hemostatic therapy is most useful to the admitting team when it also states explicitly that the patient remains at meaningfully elevated rebleeding risk for the next 48 to 72 hours and specifies the parameters, such as a defined drop in hemoglobin or new hemodynamic instability, that should prompt repeat endoscopy rather than simply documenting that hemostasis was achieved. The same principle applies to radiology results relayed verbally or through a preliminary report: stating that a finding is 'probably benign' without specifying the follow-up interval and the modality by which that follow-up should occur transfers an unresolved decision back to a team that sought imaging specifically to resolve it.

**EVIDENCE:** Structured, itemized reporting templates for both endoscopy and radiology have been associated in quality-improvement literature with more consistent adherence to recommended follow-up intervals than free-text narrative reports, reinforcing that format, not only content, affects whether a diagnostic finding translates into the intended next action.

## Cost, Access, and Practical Modality Selection

Diagnostic performance is not the only variable that determines which test is actually obtained, and a clinician who reasons only from a theoretical hierarchy of accuracy without accounting for local availability, scheduling delay, and cost risks recommending a pathway that cannot be executed in a clinically meaningful timeframe. Endoscopic ultrasound and specialized MRI sequences such as MRCP are concentrated at tertiary and academic centers in many regions, and a community-based clinician managing a patient with suspected choledocholithiasis may reasonably choose a diagnostic ERCP, accepting its higher procedural risk, when transfer or referral delay for MRCP would itself meaningfully postpone treatment of an actively symptomatic or septic patient. Conversely, when time pressure is not a factor, such as in the evaluation of a low-risk indeterminate hepatic lesion in an asymptomatic patient, deferring to the noninvasive, more widely reproducible study, even if it requires a modest scheduling delay, is the more appropriate choice. Cost considerations similarly shape real-world modality selection: an ultrasound-based elastography study is typically far less expensive than a liver biopsy, which reinforces its role as a first-line fibrosis assessment, while a PET-CT, considerably more expensive than conventional cross-sectional imaging, is reserved for the specific staging and problem-solving indications in which its unique information content justifies its cost, rather than being used as a routine surveillance tool.

## Wireless Motility Capsule and Breath Testing

The wireless motility capsule, a swallowed device that continuously records pH, pressure, and temperature as it transits the gastrointestinal tract, provides a single-test assessment of gastric, small bowel, and colonic transit time and is a useful alternative to nuclear medicine gastric emptying scintigraphy when a more comprehensive, whole-gut transit evaluation is needed, such as in a patient with diffuse dysmotility symptoms spanning multiple regions of the gut rather than isolated gastroparesis. Breath testing, using either lactulose or glucose substrate with measurement of exhaled hydrogen and methane, evaluates small intestinal bacterial overgrowth by detecting early, abnormal fermentation of the ingested substrate, and its interpretation requires attention to the timing and pattern of the rise in breath gases relative to substrate ingestion, because a rise that occurs too early to represent colonic fermentation, adjusted for individual mouth-to-cecum transit time, is what distinguishes a positive result from the normal physiologic fermentation that occurs once substrate reaches the colon in every individual.

## A Worked Framework for Modality Selection

Three questions, applied in sequence, resolve the large majority of modality-selection decisions encountered in practice. First, is the clinical question anatomic or functional: an anatomic question, such as whether a stone obstructs the bile duct, is answered by a structural test such as ultrasound, CT, or MRCP, while a functional question, such as whether the esophagus propels a swallowed bolus normally, requires a physiologic test such as manometry that a structural image cannot answer regardless of its resolution. Second, does the anticipated finding require immediate therapeutic capability or only diagnostic characterization: a patient with a high pretest probability of an obstructing common bile duct stone causing cholangitis is better served by proceeding to therapeutic ERCP directly, accepting its procedural risk, than by first obtaining a diagnostic MRCP that would only delay the drainage that is very likely to be required regardless of its result, whereas a patient with a low pretest probability benefits from the noninvasive diagnostic step first, since it may avoid an unnecessary procedure altogether. Third, what is the actual, local turnaround time for each candidate test, since the theoretically superior test obtained after a delay that allows a treatable condition to progress is not, in practice, the better choice for that specific patient at that specific institution. Applying these three questions in order, rather than defaulting to whichever test is most familiar or most readily ordered from habit, is the modality-selection discipline that this chapter's threshold-based reasoning is built to support.

**CLINICAL PEARL:** When uncertain which test to order, ask what the result would change. If neither a positive nor a negative result would alter the immediate management plan, the test is unlikely to be the right next step regardless of its accuracy.

## Functional and Motility Testing

### Esophageal Manometry and Ambulatory Reflux Monitoring

High-resolution esophageal manometry measures pressure along the entire length of the esophagus using closely spaced sensors and is the definitive test for esophageal motility disorders, generating a Chicago Classification diagnosis, such as achalasia, esophagogastric junction outflow obstruction, or a spastic or hypomotility disorder, based on integrated relaxation pressure and the pattern of peristalsis observed across a standardized set of swallows. Ambulatory pH or pH-impedance monitoring quantifies esophageal acid exposure over a 24- to 96-hour period, depending on the technology and catheter or wireless capsule used, and its principal role is confirming pathologic reflux in a patient being considered for antireflux surgery or in a patient with reflux symptoms that have not responded to empiric acid suppression, where a normal study substantially changes the diagnostic direction toward a functional or non-reflux esophageal disorder. The test requires a brief period of catheter or capsule placement that most patients tolerate without sedation, and its findings are reported using a standardized classification scheme specifically so that results remain comparable across different laboratories and equipment platforms.

### Anorectal Manometry and Defecography

Anorectal manometry measures resting and squeeze pressures of the anal sphincter complex along with rectal sensation and the coordination of rectal and sphincter pressures during a simulated defecation maneuver, and it is the key test distinguishing dyssynergic defecation, in which paradoxical sphincter contraction impairs evacuation despite normal colonic transit, from slow-transit constipation, in which the underlying problem is delayed colonic movement rather than an evacuation disorder, a distinction that changes treatment from pelvic floor biofunctional therapy in the former to prokinetic or secretagogue therapy in the latter. Defecography, performed by fluoroscopic or magnetic resonance imaging during an attempted evacuation, adds structural information, identifying rectocele, rectal prolapse, or intussusception that manometry alone cannot visualize, and is reserved for patients in whom a structural abnormality is suspected clinically or in whom manometry and biofeedback therapy have not resolved the symptom. Balloon expulsion testing is frequently performed alongside manometry as a rapid, complementary bedside screen, since an inability to expel a rectal balloon within a defined time supports a diagnosis of dyssynergic defecation even before the full manometric tracing has been formally analyzed.

**KEY POINT:** Functional and motility testing is appropriately sequenced after, not instead of, structural evaluation; endoscopy and cross-sectional imaging should exclude a mechanical or mucosal explanation for symptoms before a functional diagnosis is pursued.

### Diagnostic Modality Selection in Pregnancy and Special Populations

Endoscopy is generally considered safe during pregnancy when a strong indication exists, and upper endoscopy and colonoscopy performed with the lowest effective dose of sedation, avoiding agents with unfavorable fetal safety profiles and positioning the patient to avoid aortocaval compression in later pregnancy, should not be withheld from a pregnant patient with a clear indication such as significant gastrointestinal bleeding, because the risk of a missed or delayed diagnosis typically exceeds the procedural risk itself. Elective procedures, including screening colonoscopy and Barrett surveillance without alarm features, are appropriately deferred until after delivery, and ERCP, when required emergently for choledocholithiasis or cholangitis during pregnancy, is performed with fluoroscopy time minimized and abdominal shielding used, since the therapeutic benefit of urgent biliary drainage in this setting outweighs the radiation exposure when the alternative is ongoing biliary sepsis. Imaging selection in pregnancy follows the radiation stewardship principle discussed earlier in this chapter with particular force: ultrasound and non-gadolinium MRI are preferred whenever they can answer the clinical question, and CT is reserved for situations in which the diagnostic information it provides is not otherwise obtainable and is judged to meaningfully change management.

Case Presentation: A 34-year-old woman is referred for evaluation of progressive dysphagia to both solids and liquids over eighteen months, accompanied by regurgitation of undigested food and an 8-pound weight loss. Upper endoscopy performed at an outside facility was reported as normal, and a barium esophagram, obtained subsequently, demonstrates a dilated esophageal body with a smoothly tapered, bird's-beak narrowing at the gastroesophageal junction. Applying the reasoning developed in this chapter, dysphagia to solids and liquids from onset, in a patient with a structurally normal endoscopy, localizes to a motility disorder rather than a mechanical lesion, and the esophagram finding is characteristic enough to warrant high-resolution manometry as the next, confirmatory step rather than repeat endoscopy or empiric acid suppression. Manometry demonstrates absent peristalsis throughout the esophageal body and an integrated relaxation pressure above the upper limit of normal, confirming a Chicago Classification diagnosis of achalasia. The patient is referred for pneumatic dilation versus peroral endoscopic myotomy, with the specific choice guided by the manometric subtype and the patient's preference after both options are discussed. This case illustrates why a normal endoscopy does not exclude a motility disorder, and why esophagram findings, when characteristic, should direct the clinician to manometry rather than to a repeat structural evaluation that has already been adequately performed.

| Modality | Primary Indication | Key Limitation |
|---|---|---|
| Upper endoscopy | Dysphagia, suspected UGI bleeding, Barrett surveillance | Cannot assess motility or structures beyond the duodenum |
| Colonoscopy | CRC screening, altered bowel habits, LGIB | Preparation-dependent; limited small bowel access |
| Endoscopic ultrasound | Tumor staging, choledocholithiasis, tissue sampling | Operator-dependent; limited availability |
| ERCP | Therapeutic biliary/pancreatic duct intervention | Post-procedure pancreatitis risk |
| CT enterography | Small bowel Crohn disease activity | Ionizing radiation; oral contrast tolerance |

| | | |
|---|---|---|
| MRCP | Noninvasive ductal anatomy characterization | Cannot provide therapeutic intervention |
| High-resolution manometry | Esophageal motility disorders | Requires structurally normal endoscopy first |
| Anorectal manometry | Dyssynergic defecation vs. slow transit | Does not visualize structural lesions |

**THE GI THRESHOLD DECISION SYSTEM — Endoscopic and Imaging Diagnostic Thresholds**

**Presentation Signature:** This chapter's threshold instance addressed the moment an endoscopist has just identified a bleeding ulcer and must translate its appearance into a hemostasis and monitoring decision.

**Threshold Point:** The Forrest classification converts subjective endoscopic appearance into a graded, reproducible rebleeding risk estimate spanning active hemorrhage through a clean ulcer base.

**The Call:** High-risk Forrest grades receive endoscopic hemostatic therapy and extended monitoring; low-risk grades are managed medically with earlier discharge, and the intermediate adherent-clot grade requires deliberate, protocol-guided judgment rather than a reflexive default.

**Trap Logic:** Treating every visualized clot or lesion identically, rather than by its specific Forrest grade, both over-treats low-risk lesions and under-treats or mishandles the intermediate-risk adherent clot.

**Decision Anchor:** Assign a Forrest grade to every bleeding or recently bled ulcer at the index endoscopy; that grade, more than any other single data point, should determine the hemostasis and monitoring plan.

## Summary and Key Concepts

Upper endoscopy and colonoscopy combine diagnostic and therapeutic capability within a single encounter, distinguishing them from nearly every other diagnostic modality in gastroenterology.

Standardized endoscopic classification systems, including the Los Angeles, Prague, Forrest, and Mayo/UCEIS scores, convert subjective endoscopic impressions into reproducible, management-relevant grades.

Endoscopic ultrasound provides high-resolution local staging and tissue sampling, while ERCP has become an almost exclusively therapeutic procedure now that MRCP performs diagnostic ductal characterization noninvasively.

Cross-sectional imaging protocol selection, not merely the choice of modality, determines diagnostic yield; CT enterography, triple-phase liver protocols, and MRCP each answer a specific question that a generic study cannot.

Functional and motility testing, including esophageal manometry and anorectal manometry, is appropriately sequenced after structural evaluation has excluded a mechanical or mucosal explanation for symptoms.

The Forrest classification exemplifies the chapter's broader theme: an endoscopic finding becomes clinically useful only once it is converted into a graded, threshold-driven management decision.

# CHAPTER 3: GASTROESOPHAGEAL REFLUX DISEASE AND BARRETT ESOPHAGUS

## Postoperative Complications and Follow-Up After Antireflux Surgery

Dysphagia is expected transiently after fundoplication as postoperative edema resolves, and it should be anticipated and discussed with the patient before surgery rather than presenting as an unexpected complication in the recovery period; a dietary progression from liquids to soft foods over the initial weeks accommodates this expected phase. Dysphagia that persists beyond the expected postoperative window, or that develops after an initial period of normal swallowing, raises concern for a wrap that is too tight, has slipped, or has herniated into the chest, and evaluation with a barium esophagram, which visualizes the wrap's position and the pattern of contrast transit through it, is generally the appropriate first test, reserving repeat endoscopy or reoperation for cases in which the esophagram identifies a structural problem requiring correction. Gas-bloat syndrome, a sensation of inability to belch or vent swallowed air normally, is a recognized consequence of the fundoplication's mechanical effect on the gastroesophageal junction and, while it improves over time in most patients, should also be discussed preoperatively as an anticipated trade-off rather than framed only in terms of symptom relief.

## Learning Objectives

1. Explain the anatomic and physiologic mechanisms that normally prevent gastroesophageal reflux and how each can fail.
2. Distinguish typical from atypical and extraesophageal presentations of gastroesophageal reflux disease.
3. Select an appropriate diagnostic pathway for a patient with reflux symptoms, including when empiric therapy versus endoscopy versus ambulatory reflux monitoring is indicated.
4. Apply a stepwise, evidence-based approach to medical, endoscopic, and surgical management of gastroesophageal reflux disease.
5. Identify patients who require Barrett esophagus screening and apply the Prague classification and surveillance intervals correctly.
6. Stratify Barrett esophagus dysplasia grade to the appropriate endoscopic eradication or surveillance strategy.

This chapter develops gastroesophageal reflux disease from its underlying antireflux barrier physiology through typical and atypical presentation, diagnostic pathway selection, stepwise medical and procedural management, and its most consequential long-term complication, Barrett esophagus, including the dysplasia-stratified surveillance and eradication strategies that govern its management. The reasoning throughout links each decision to a specific threshold, whether a symptom duration, a Prague classification measurement, or a dysplasia grade, that converts clinical uncertainty into a defined next step. It closes with a set of clinical situations, refractory reflux, eosinophilic esophagitis, pregnancy, and scleroderma-spectrum disease, in which the general reasoning developed earlier in the chapter must be adapted to a specific population or an alternative diagnosis.

## Pathophysiology of the Antireflux Barrier

Reflux of gastric contents into the esophagus is prevented under normal circumstances by a coordinated barrier with several independent components, and disease develops when one or more of these components fails, either transiently or structurally. The lower esophageal sphincter, a specialized ring of tonically contracted smooth muscle at the gastroesophageal junction, maintains a resting pressure gradient that opposes the pressure difference between the abdominal cavity and the thorax, and transient lower esophageal sphincter relaxations, brief periods of inappropriate sphincter relaxation not triggered by swallowing, account for the majority of reflux episodes even in patients with a structurally normal, adequately toned sphincter at rest, meaning that reflux disease is frequently a disorder of inappropriate timing rather than of baseline sphincter weakness alone.

### The Crural Diaphragm and Hiatal Anatomy

The crural diaphragm functions as an external sphincter mechanically reinforcing the lower esophageal sphincter, contracting synchronously with inspiration to augment the antireflux barrier precisely when intra-abdominal pressure rises, and a hiatal hernia disrupts this reinforcement by displacing the gastroesophageal junction proximal to the diaphragmatic hiatus, separating the two sphincter mechanisms anatomically so that they can no longer act in unison. The size of a hiatal hernia correlates with the severity of reflux and with the likelihood of erosive disease, because a larger hernia both widens the diaphragmatic hiatus itself and creates a reservoir of gastric contents positioned to reflux across the now-displaced and functionally weakened gastroesophageal junction with less provocation than would be required in a patient without a hernia.

### Esophageal Clearance and Mucosal Defense

Even when reflux occurs, its clinical consequence depends on how quickly the refluxed material is cleared and how well the esophageal mucosa resists the injury that acid and pepsin, and in some patients bile, can produce during the period of contact. Peristaltic clearance, augmented by gravity in the upright position and by swallowed saliva, which carries bicarbonate that neutralizes residual acid, ordinarily restores a normal intraluminal pH within minutes of a reflux episode, and impaired peristalsis, whether from a primary motility disorder or from the acquired hypomotility seen in scleroderma-spectrum disease, prolongs acid contact time and worsens mucosal injury independent of the volume or frequency of reflux itself. Recumbency and nocturnal reflux are particularly injurious because both gravitational clearance and swallowing frequency fall during sleep, extending esophageal acid exposure time well beyond what the same volume of reflux would produce during waking hours.

**CLINICAL PEARL:** A patient whose reflux symptoms are predominantly nocturnal is more likely to have significant esophageal acid exposure and a higher risk of erosive disease than a patient with isolated postprandial daytime symptoms, because nocturnal reflux is cleared far less efficiently.

## Clinical Presentation: Typical, Atypical, and Extraesophageal

### Typical Esophageal Symptoms

Heartburn, a retrosternal burning sensation typically related to meals and posture, and regurgitation, the effortless return of gastric contents into the pharynx or mouth, together constitute the typical symptom complex with the strongest positive predictive value for gastroesophageal reflux disease, and a patient presenting with this combination in the absence of alarm features can often be managed with an empiric therapeutic trial rather than upfront endoscopy. The relationship of these symptoms to specific triggers, including large meals, recumbency after eating, and particular foods such as fatty meals, chocolate, caffeine, and alcohol, each of which lowers lower esophageal sphincter pressure or delays gastric emptying, supports the diagnosis further and also identifies specific, modifiable behavioral targets for initial management.

### Atypical and Extraesophageal Manifestations

Chronic cough, laryngitis with hoarseness, chronic throat clearing, and asthma that is poorly responsive to standard pulmonary therapy are the principal extraesophageal presentations attributed to reflux, and the mechanistic basis for this association is twofold: microaspiration of refluxate directly irritates the laryngeal and tracheobronchial mucosa, while a separate, vagally mediated esophagobronchial reflex can provoke bronchospasm and cough even without any refluxate reaching above the upper esophageal sphincter. Establishing reflux as the cause of an extraesophageal symptom is considerably harder than establishing it as the cause of typical heartburn, because the positive predictive value of these atypical symptoms for reflux disease is low and because a specialist in otolaryngology or pulmonology has often already evaluated and excluded other causes before the patient reaches gastroenterology, meaning that ambulatory reflux monitoring, ideally performed off acid suppression to establish a baseline, is frequently required to confirm a temporal association before extraesophageal symptoms are attributed definitively to reflux.

**CAUTION:** Do not attribute chronic cough or laryngitis to reflux disease by symptom pattern alone; the positive predictive value of these presentations for reflux is low, and objective testing or a structured, time-limited empiric trial with a clear endpoint should precede a durable diagnostic label.

### Multidisciplinary Evaluation of Suspected Laryngopharyngeal Reflux

A patient referred for suspected reflux-related laryngeal symptoms has typically already been evaluated by an otolaryngologist, who may have identified findings such as vocal cord edema or posterior laryngeal erythema on laryngoscopy that are frequently attributed to reflux but that also occur in patients with other causes of laryngeal irritation, including postnasal drip, voice overuse, and primary laryngeal disease, which limits the specificity of these laryngoscopic findings for reflux as the underlying cause. A coordinated approach in which gastroenterology confirms or excludes pathologic reflux objectively through pH-impedance monitoring, rather than the two specialties independently treating the same patient toward different endpoints, produces more efficient and more accurate care, and a structured, time-limited empiric trial, typically eight to twelve weeks of twice-daily proton pump inhibitor therapy with a predefined reassessment point, is a reasonable initial approach when objective testing is not immediately available, provided that a lack of response at the predefined endpoint prompts the coordinated workup described above rather than open-ended continuation of empiric therapy.

## Diagnostic Evaluation and Pathway Selection

### The Empiric Therapeutic Trial

A patient younger than 60 with typical heartburn and regurgitation and no alarm features, including dysphagia, odynophagia, unintentional weight loss, gastrointestinal bleeding, or iron deficiency anemia, is an appropriate candidate for an empiric trial of once-daily proton pump inhibitor therapy for four to eight weeks without preceding endoscopy, because the diagnostic and therapeutic yield of this approach in a low-risk population is high enough to make upfront endoscopy an inefficient use of a limited diagnostic resource. A robust symptomatic response to this trial supports the diagnosis and permits either continuation at the lowest effective dose or a structured attempt at discontinuation, while an inadequate response should prompt reassessment rather than an automatic dose escalation, because a substantial proportion of patients who fail an adequate proton pump inhibitor trial do not, in fact, have acid-mediated reflux disease as the explanation for their symptoms.

### Indications for Upfront Endoscopy

Any alarm feature, age 60 or older at symptom onset, symptoms refractory to an adequate empiric trial, or a plan to pursue long-term therapy in a patient who has not yet been endoscopically evaluated, shifts the pathway toward upfront upper endoscopy rather than continued empiric management, because each of these features raises the pretest probability of erosive disease, Barrett esophagus, or a mechanical or malignant process that a therapeutic trial alone would not detect. Endoscopy in this setting serves three simultaneous purposes: confirming or excluding erosive esophagitis using the Los Angeles classification described in the previous chapter, evaluating for Barrett esophagus in patients who meet screening criteria, and excluding an alternative or coexisting structural diagnosis, such as a peptic stricture or malignancy, that would change management entirely.

### Differentiating Nonerosive Reflux Disease From Functional Heartburn

Nonerosive reflux disease and functional heartburn present with an identical symptom, heartburn without endoscopically visible mucosal injury, but they are mechanistically distinct conditions that ambulatory reflux monitoring is specifically designed to separate. Nonerosive reflux disease is defined by pathologic esophageal acid exposure on monitoring despite a normal-appearing endoscopy, meaning that true pathologic reflux is occurring but has not yet, or does not, produce visible erosive injury, and these patients generally respond to acid-suppressive therapy in a manner similar to patients with erosive disease. Functional heartburn, by contrast, is defined by a normal esophageal acid exposure time on monitoring with a symptom pattern that does not correlate temporally with the reflux events that are recorded, indicating that visceral hypersensitivity, an exaggerated perception of normal physiologic esophageal events, rather than pathologic reflux itself, generates the symptom, and these patients respond poorly to escalating acid suppression because the underlying mechanism is not acid-mediated; management instead centers on neuromodulator therapy and pain-modulating approaches analogous to those used in other functional gastrointestinal disorders discussed later in this book. Making this distinction correctly prevents the common and frustrating pattern of a functional heartburn patient being escalated through multiple acid-suppressive regimens and, eventually, considered for antireflux surgery, none of which addresses the actual underlying mechanism.

Low-dose tricyclic antidepressants and, in select patients, other neuromodulator classes reduce esophageal hypersensitivity through central and peripheral mechanisms distinct from any effect on acid secretion, and their use in functional heartburn parallels their use in other pain-predominant functional gastrointestinal disorders covered elsewhere in this book, including functional dyspepsia and irritable bowel syndrome, reflecting a shared underlying mechanism, visceral hypersensitivity, that spans multiple regions of the gastrointestinal tract rather than being unique to the esophagus. Setting expectations explicitly with the patient before starting a neuromodulator is important clinically, because the medication class is more familiar to patients as an antidepressant than as a visceral pain treatment, and a patient who is not told clearly that a low, pain-modulating dose is being used for a gastrointestinal indication, not for depression, may discontinue the medication prematurely out of a mistaken belief that a psychiatric diagnosis is being implied.

### Ambulatory Reflux Monitoring in Diagnostic Uncertainty

Ambulatory pH or pH-impedance monitoring, described in the preceding chapter, is reserved for patients in whom the diagnosis remains uncertain after endoscopy, most commonly a patient with persistent symptoms and a normal or near-normal endoscopic examination, because a normal endoscopy does not exclude nonerosive reflux disease, in which esophageal acid exposure is pathologic despite the absence of visible mucosal injury. Monitoring performed off acid-suppressive therapy establishes whether pathologic acid exposure is present at all, which is the appropriate question in a patient naive to proton pump inhibitor therapy or being considered for antireflux surgery, while monitoring performed on therapy, using impedance to capture nonacid events, answers a different question, whether ongoing symptoms on treatment correlate with any detectable reflux event, acid or nonacid, which is the appropriate question in a patient already committed to long-term medical therapy whose symptoms have not adequately resolved.

**THE GI THRESHOLD DECISION SYSTEM — Esophageal Thresholds — When Reflux Symptoms Require Endoscopy Rather Than an Empiric Trial**

**Presentation Signature:** A patient presents with heartburn, regurgitation, or a combination of typical and atypical reflux symptoms, and the clinician must decide between an empiric therapeutic trial and upfront endoscopic evaluation.

**Threshold Point:** Age 60 or older at symptom onset, or the presence of any alarm feature, dysphagia, odynophagia, unintentional weight loss, gastrointestinal bleeding, or iron deficiency anemia, defines the threshold above which empiric therapy alone is an inadequate first step.

**The Call:** Patients meeting either threshold proceed to upper endoscopy before or instead of an extended empiric trial; patients meeting neither threshold may reasonably begin a four- to eight-week empiric proton pump inhibitor trial, with endoscopy reserved for an inadequate response or symptom recurrence after discontinuation.

**Trap Logic:** A partial or inconsistent symptomatic response to acid suppression is frequently misread as confirmation of the reflux diagnosis and grounds for dose escalation, when it should instead prompt reconsideration of whether acid-mediated reflux is the correct explanation for the symptom at all.

**Decision Anchor:** Age and alarm features, not symptom severity or duration alone, are what convert a reflux presentation from an empiric-trial candidate into an endoscopy-first candidate.

### The Relationship Between Helicobacter Pylori and Reflux Disease

Helicobacter pylori infection and gastroesophageal reflux disease interact in a way that is more nuanced than a simple causal relationship in either direction, and understanding this relationship prevents two opposite reasoning errors. Chronic Helicobacter pylori infection, particularly when it produces corpus-predominant gastritis, can reduce gastric acid output over time, and eradication of the infection in some patients unmasks or worsens preexisting reflux symptoms as acid secretion normalizes, an observation that has led some clinicians to worry, generally without sufficient evidence to withhold indicated treatment, that eradicating Helicobacter pylori will meaningfully worsen a patient's reflux disease. In practice, the indication to test for and treat Helicobacter pylori, discussed in detail in the next chapter, should be assessed on its own merits, most commonly a personal history of peptic ulcer disease or gastric malignancy risk factors, rather than being deferred or withheld because of a theoretical concern about worsening reflux symptoms, since the benefits of eradicating an infection with established malignancy and ulcer risk outweigh a modest and manageable risk of symptomatic reflux, which can itself be treated with standard acid-suppressive therapy if it emerges or worsens after eradication. Clinicians should present this relationship to patients in plain terms when it arises, since a patient who has read about the association online may otherwise decline indicated Helicobacter pylori testing or treatment out of an unfounded fear of worsening their reflux.

## Management of Gastroesophageal Reflux Disease

### Lifestyle and Behavioral Modification

Structured dietary counseling that identifies a patient's specific reflux triggers through a symptom diary, rather than issuing a generic list of foods to avoid, produces more durable behavior change, because a patient who has confirmed for themselves that a particular food reliably provokes symptoms is more likely to sustain avoidance than a patient handed a standardized list containing items that may not actually affect their own symptoms. Smoking cessation independently improves reflux symptoms by restoring lower esophageal sphincter tone, which nicotine transiently reduces, and by improving esophageal clearance, providing an additional, reflux-specific reason to support cessation efforts beyond the general health benefits already well established for this intervention.

Weight loss in patients who are overweight or obese produces a measurable reduction in reflux symptoms and esophageal acid exposure because excess intra-abdominal adiposity raises intragastric pressure and promotes both hiatal hernia formation and transient lower esophageal sphincter relaxations, making it one of the few reflux interventions with evidence for altering the underlying mechanical predisposition rather than only suppressing acid production. Elevating the head of the bed, avoiding recumbency within two to three hours of eating, and reducing or eliminating identified dietary triggers each address a specific mechanistic contributor described earlier in this chapter, delayed clearance during recumbency and lower esophageal sphincter relaxation provoked by particular foods, and should be recommended as a matter of course even when pharmacologic therapy is also initiated, rather than presented as an alternative to medication. This mechanical explanation is one reason weight loss produces more consistent symptomatic benefit in reflux disease than in many other chronic conditions where the connection to body weight is less direct.

### Pharmacologic Therapy

Proton pump inhibitors are the most effective acid-suppressive class available and are dosed once daily thirty to sixty minutes before the first meal of the day to align peak drug effect with the maximal density of actively secreting proton pumps, a timing detail that materially affects efficacy and is frequently misunderstood by patients who take the medication without regard to meal timing. Histamine-2 receptor antagonists provide a less potent but still clinically useful degree of acid suppression and retain a role as add-on nocturnal therapy for breakthrough symptoms in a patient already on a once-daily proton pump inhibitor, and as a lower-potency alternative in patients with mild, infrequent symptoms who do not require or desire more aggressive suppression. Potassium-competitive acid blockers, a newer class providing more rapid onset and more consistent acid suppression than traditional proton pump inhibitors by a mechanism that does not require conversion in an acidic intracellular compartment, are an emerging option particularly relevant in the initial healing phase of severe erosive esophagitis, confirmed against current dosing guidance and local availability.

**KEY POINT:** The most common reason for an apparent proton pump inhibitor failure is incorrect medication timing relative to meals, not true pharmacologic nonresponse; confirming and correcting dosing technique should precede any decision to escalate therapy or pursue further testing.

### Endoscopic and Surgical Antireflux Therapy

Surgical fundoplication, in which the gastric fundus is wrapped partially or completely around the distal esophagus to reinforce the antireflux barrier mechanically, is considered for patients with confirmed pathologic reflux who prefer to avoid long-term medication, who have a large hiatal hernia contributing to their symptoms, or whose reflux, particularly regurgitation, responds incompletely to medical therapy despite adequate acid suppression, since regurgitation is a mechanical rather than a purely acid-mediated phenomenon that pharmacologic acid suppression cannot fully address. Preoperative evaluation should confirm pathologic reflux objectively rather than relying on symptom report alone and should include esophageal manometry to exclude a significant motility disorder that would change the surgical approach or contraindicate a complete fundoplication, because a tight wrap performed in a patient with poor underlying esophageal peristalsis can produce severe postoperative dysphagia. Endoscopic and less invasive procedural alternatives, including transoral incisionless fundoplication and magnetic sphincter augmentation, offer intermediate options for appropriately selected patients who wish to avoid a full surgical fundoplication while still addressing the mechanical component of their disease.

**Figure 3.1: Normal Antireflux Barrier Anatomy and Hiatal Hernia**

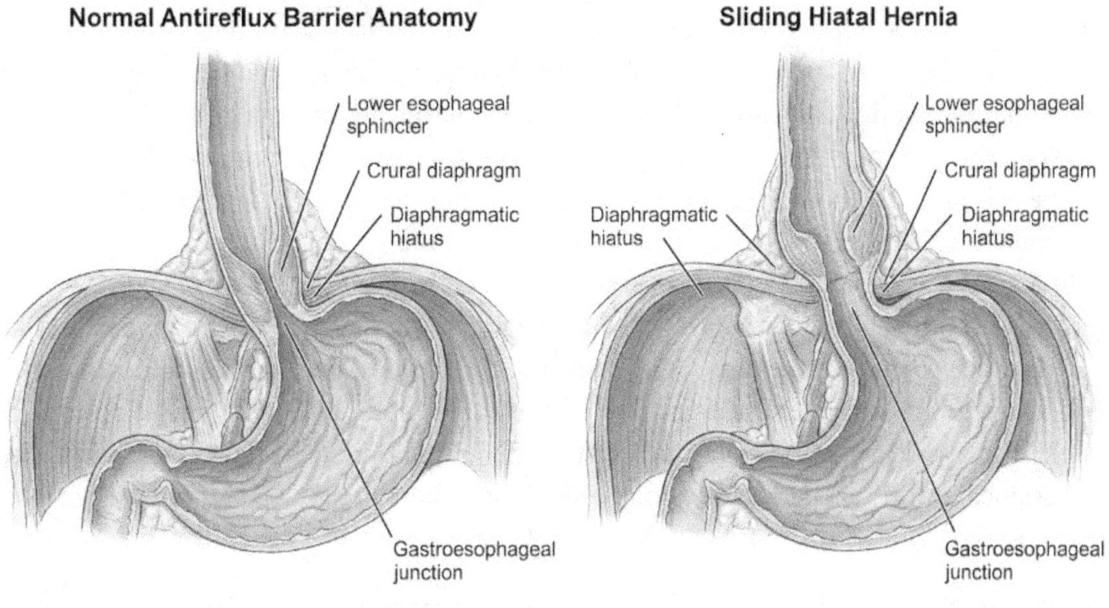

## Barrett Esophagus: Screening, Surveillance, and Dysplasia Management

### Screening Criteria and the Prague Classification

#### Epidemiology and Natural History

Barrett esophagus develops in a minority of patients with chronic reflux disease, and the annual rate of progression from nondysplastic Barrett esophagus to esophageal adenocarcinoma is low on a per-patient, per-year basis, information that is important to convey accurately during patient counseling because a diagnosis of Barrett esophagus, appropriately understood, warrants regular surveillance rather than the level of alarm that a cancer diagnosis itself would warrant. The overall incidence of esophageal adenocarcinoma has risen substantially in Western populations over recent decades, a trend attributed to rising rates of obesity and chronic reflux disease, and this population-level trend is part of why risk-stratified screening, rather than screening applied uniformly to every patient with reflux symptoms, is the current recommended approach, concentrating a limited endoscopic resource on the subset of patients most likely to benefit. Most patients who develop esophageal adenocarcinoma, notably, are not known to have Barrett esophagus at the time of their cancer diagnosis, either because they were never screened or because their cancer arose without a preceding diagnosis of Barrett esophagus having been made, a sobering reminder that current screening strategies, while risk-stratified and resource-efficient, do not capture the entire population ultimately affected by this malignancy.

#### Chemoprevention and Risk Factor Modification

Long-term proton pump inhibitor therapy in patients with confirmed Barrett esophagus is generally continued indefinitely, based on observational and mechanistic evidence that sustained acid suppression reduces ongoing chronic inflammatory injury to the metaplastic segment, a rationale distinct from and additional to its role in symptom control. Aspirin has been studied as a chemopreventive agent in Barrett esophagus based on epidemiologic associations between nonsteroidal anti-inflammatory drug use and reduced esophageal adenocarcinoma incidence, and while the evidence is not yet strong enough to recommend aspirin specifically for chemoprevention in a patient without an independent cardiovascular indication, it is a reasonable factor to weigh, alongside cardiovascular risk and bleeding risk, when a patient with Barrett esophagus is already being considered for aspirin therapy for another reason. Smoking cessation and weight management address two of the same modifiable risk factors relevant to reflux disease itself, discussed earlier in this chapter, and their benefit in Barrett esophagus specifically reinforces rather than duplicates the general lifestyle counseling that should already be part of every reflux patient's management.

Barrett esophagus, the replacement of normal squamous esophageal epithelium with metaplastic columnar epithelium as an adaptive response to chronic acid exposure, is screened for in patients with chronic gastroesophageal reflux disease symptoms of five or more years' duration who also carry at least one additional risk factor, including male sex, age over 50, White race, central obesity, a history of tobacco use, or a first-degree relative with Barrett esophagus or esophageal adenocarcinoma, because screening the entire population of reflux patients without risk stratification would identify far too few cases per procedure performed to be an efficient use of endoscopic resources. Once identified, the extent of Barrett esophagus is documented using the Prague classification, which records the circumferential extent, the C value, and the maximal extent, the M value, of columnar-appearing mucosa above the gastroesophageal junction, and this measurement, rather than a qualitative description, is what should populate the endoscopy report and guide the surveillance biopsy protocol.

**Surveillance Biopsy Protocol and Intervals**

Wide-area transepithelial sampling with computer-assisted analysis has been developed as a complementary or adjunctive sampling technique to standard forceps biopsy, using an abrasive brush to sample a larger surface area of the Barrett segment than discrete forceps biopsies can capture, and while it is not intended to replace the Seattle protocol outright, some practices use it as an adjunct to increase the likelihood of detecting dysplasia that random forceps sampling might miss, particularly in longer Barrett segments where the proportion of mucosa actually sampled by standard biopsy protocol is relatively small.

Surveillance biopsies follow the Seattle protocol, four-quadrant biopsies obtained at 1 or 2 centimeter intervals throughout the length of the Barrett segment along with targeted biopsy of any visible mucosal irregularity, because dysplasia in Barrett esophagus frequently arises in a patchy, endoscopically inconspicuous distribution that random, systematic sampling is more likely to detect than a limited number of biopsies obtained only from grossly abnormal-appearing areas. Surveillance intervals are determined by the presence and grade of dysplasia identified on biopsy rather than by the length of the Barrett segment alone: nondysplastic Barrett esophagus is surveilled at an interval determined by segment length, with longer segments surveilled more frequently than short segments, while any degree of confirmed dysplasia shortens the interval substantially or, in the case of high-grade dysplasia, prompts endoscopic eradication therapy rather than continued surveillance alone.

**THE GI THRESHOLD DECISION SYSTEM — Esophageal Thresholds — Barrett Dysplasia Grade and the Threshold for Eradication Therapy**

---

**Presentation Signature:** Surveillance biopsies from a segment of known Barrett esophagus return a pathology result describing the presence and grade of dysplasia, and this result must be translated into a specific surveillance or treatment decision.

**Threshold Point:** Indefinite for dysplasia and low-grade dysplasia occupy an intermediate risk zone requiring confirmation by an expert gastrointestinal pathologist and a repeat endoscopy, while confirmed high-grade dysplasia or intramucosal carcinoma crosses the threshold at which endoscopic eradication therapy, rather than continued surveillance, becomes the standard of care.

**The Call:** Confirmed low-grade dysplasia is managed with either endoscopic eradication therapy or intensified surveillance at a substantially shortened interval, a decision individualized to the patient; confirmed high-grade dysplasia is managed with endoscopic eradication therapy, typically radiofrequency ablation with or without endoscopic mucosal resection of any visible lesion, in essentially all appropriate surgical and endoscopic candidates.

**Trap Logic:** A single pathologist's read of indefinite for dysplasia or low-grade dysplasia carries substantial interobserver variability and should not, by itself, be treated as equivalent to a confirmed diagnosis; expert gastrointestinal pathology confirmation is required before the corresponding management threshold is applied.

**Decision Anchor:** Dysplasia grade, confirmed by an expert pathologist, not Barrett segment length or patient symptom severity, is the variable that determines whether the pathway is continued surveillance or endoscopic eradication therapy.

**Endoscopic Eradication Therapy**

Radiofrequency ablation delivers controlled thermal energy to the Barrett mucosa to a depth calibrated to destroy the metaplastic epithelium while sparing the deeper esophageal wall layers, and it is the primary eradication modality for flat, nonnodular dysplastic Barrett esophagus, typically requiring more than one treatment session spaced several months apart to achieve complete eradication of both dysplasia and the underlying intestinal metaplasia. Endoscopic mucosal resection is performed first, rather than ablation alone, whenever a visible nodule or irregularity is present within the Barrett segment, because resection provides a full-thickness histologic specimen that can confirm the depth of invasion and completeness of excision in a way that ablation, which destroys tissue rather than retrieving it, cannot, and understaging a nodular lesion by ablating it without first resecting and analyzing it risks leaving submucosally invasive carcinoma inadequately treated. Cryotherapy, delivering rapid freeze-thaw cycles to the mucosa through a spray or balloon catheter system, is an alternative ablative modality used in patients who have had an incomplete response to radiofrequency ablation or in whom radiofrequency equipment is unavailable, though it is used less commonly as first-line therapy given the more extensive outcome data supporting radiofrequency ablation. Endoscopic submucosal dissection, permitting en bloc resection of larger or more complex lesions than conventional mucosal resection can reliably remove in a single piece, is used selectively when a lesion's size or morphology raises particular concern for a deeper invasion that piecemeal resection would risk understaging.

Post-ablation care includes acid suppression at maximal tolerated dose to promote healing of squamous re-epithelialization over the ablated segment, and surveillance following successful eradication continues indefinitely, though at intervals longer than those used during active dysplasia management, because recurrence of intestinal metaplasia, including buried metaplasia beneath a neosquamous surface, has been described even after apparently complete eradication and macroscopically normal-appearing post-treatment mucosa.

**Patient Counseling at the Time of Barrett Esophagus Diagnosis**

**PATIENT EDUCATION:** Explain a new Barrett esophagus diagnosis in terms of a monitored condition with a low annual cancer risk, rather than as a cancer diagnosis itself, and pair the explanation with the specific surveillance interval and its rationale so the patient understands why routine, unhurried surveillance, rather than urgent action, is the correct response.

A new diagnosis of Barrett esophagus is frequently accompanied by disproportionate patient anxiety, because the word is often encountered by patients in the context of cancer risk before it is explained in the context of its actual, low annual progression rate, and a clinician who does not proactively frame the diagnosis accurately leaves that anxiety to be shaped by an internet search rather than by an informed conversation. Explaining the surveillance protocol concretely, including what the endoscopist looks for, how frequently surveillance will occur, and what a future finding of dysplasia would mean and require, gives the patient a specific mental model of their ongoing management rather than an open-ended sense of risk, and this framing also supports long-term adherence to surveillance, since a patient who understands why the interval matters is more likely to keep the appointment than a patient who received only the diagnosis without its accompanying plan. A brief written summary given to the patient at the visit reinforces the verbal explanation.

Case Presentation: A 57-year-old man with a 15-year history of heartburn, well controlled on a standard-dose proton pump inhibitor, undergoes surveillance upper endoscopy for previously documented nondysplastic Barrett esophagus with a Prague classification of C2M4. Biopsies obtained per the Seattle protocol return a report of low-grade dysplasia in two of twelve biopsy fragments, read by the local pathologist. Applying the reasoning developed in this chapter, a first finding of low-grade dysplasia falls within the intermediate-risk zone that requires confirmation by a second, expert gastrointestinal pathologist before a management threshold is applied, because interobserver variability at this grade is substantial enough that a single read should not, by itself, trigger eradication therapy. The specimens are sent for expert pathology review, which confirms the diagnosis of low-grade dysplasia. Given the confirmed diagnosis, the patient is counseled on both options, endoscopic eradication therapy with radiofrequency ablation or continued surveillance at a shortened interval, and after discussion of the modestly reduced but still present progression risk associated with each pathway, elects to proceed with radiofrequency ablation. This case illustrates the chapter's central management principle for Barrett esophagus: confirmation of the dysplasia grade by an expert pathologist is not an optional procedural formality but a threshold gate that must be passed before eradication therapy, rather than continued surveillance, becomes the appropriate next step.

## Long-Term Safety of Acid Suppression

Proton pump inhibitors are among the most widely prescribed medications in practice, and their long-term use has generated a substantial body of observational literature raising potential associations that require calibrated, evidence-proportionate counseling rather than either dismissal or alarm. Understanding which associations are mechanistically plausible and reasonably well supported, and which remain confounded or weakly supported, is part of the precise, actionable communication this book emphasizes throughout, because a patient who is either falsely reassured or unnecessarily frightened about long-term therapy is equally poorly served.

### Fracture Risk and Micronutrient Absorption

Profound acid suppression reduces the solubility and absorption of certain micronutrients, most notably calcium carbonate, which depends on an acidic gastric environment for optimal dissolution, and vitamin B12, whose release from dietary protein also depends on acid-peptic digestion, and observational data associate long-term proton pump inhibitor use with a modestly increased risk of hip and vertebral fracture, an association thought to involve both impaired calcium absorption and a possible direct effect on osteoclast function, although the absolute risk increase is modest and confounded in many studies by the underlying conditions that prompted long-term therapy in the first place. Patients on long-term therapy, particularly those with additional osteoporosis risk factors, benefit from routine calcium and vitamin D intake sufficiency assessment and age-appropriate bone density screening, applied as a standard component of long-term management rather than as a response to a specific new symptom. These effects are dose- and duration-dependent, reinforcing the general principle of using the lowest effective dose for the shortest duration consistent with the underlying indication.

### Enteric Infection and Microbiome Effects

Gastric acid serves a protective function against ingested pathogens by denaturing many organisms before they reach the small bowel, and profound acid suppression measurably increases the risk of enteric infection, most importantly Clostridioides difficile, both as a new infection and as a risk factor for recurrence after an initial episode has been treated, a mechanism distinct from and additive to antibiotic-associated risk. This risk is clinically relevant enough that ongoing proton pump inhibitor necessity should be specifically reassessed in any hospitalized patient being treated for Clostridioides difficile infection, and unnecessary acid suppression, meaning therapy continued without a clear ongoing indication, should be discontinued as part of that patient's overall management rather than continued reflexively because it was already on the medication list at admission. This risk should be part of the informed discussion whenever long-term therapy is initiated, not raised only after an infection has already occurred.

### Renal and Cardiovascular Associations

Observational studies have associated long-term proton pump inhibitor use with an increased risk of chronic kidney disease and, separately, with acute interstitial nephritis, an idiosyncratic hypersensitivity reaction that can occur at any point during therapy and should be considered in a patient on a proton pump inhibitor who develops unexplained renal function decline, particularly when accompanied by eosinophiluria or a temporal relationship to a change in dosing. Cardiovascular associations, including a proposed interaction with clopidogrel metabolism through shared hepatic cytochrome pathways, have been extensively studied without a conclusively demonstrated clinically significant interaction in most patients, and current guidance generally supports continuing indicated acid suppression in patients on dual antiplatelet therapy who have a clear gastroprotective indication, such as a history of upper gastrointestinal bleeding, rather than withholding a clearly indicated medication because of a theoretical interaction that has not been robustly confirmed. Shared decision-making, not automatic discontinuation, is the appropriate response to these associations.

**PATIENT EDUCATION:** When counseling a patient about long-term acid suppression, state plainly that the medication remains appropriate when a clear indication exists, that the absolute risks discussed in the literature are modest, and that the specific, actionable steps being taken, such as bone density monitoring or periodic reassessment of ongoing need, rather than vague reassurance alone.

Case Presentation: A 48-year-old woman undergoes laparoscopic Nissen fundoplication for reflux disease confirmed on preoperative pH-impedance monitoring, with normal preoperative manometry. Her reflux symptoms resolve completely, but at her six-week follow-up she reports new difficulty swallowing solid food that has progressively worsened rather than improved since surgery, well beyond the transient postoperative dysphagia she was counseled to expect. Applying the reasoning developed in this chapter, dysphagia that develops after an initial period of normal swallowing, rather than persisting continuously from the immediate postoperative period, is more consistent with a mechanical problem with the wrap, such as slippage, than with expected postoperative edema, which would be anticipated to improve rather than worsen over the same interval. A barium esophagram is obtained rather than proceeding directly to endoscopy, and it demonstrates a portion of the fundoplication wrap that has migrated above the diaphragm into the chest, a recognized complication known as wrap herniation. Given the progressive nature of her symptoms and the confirmed structural abnormality, she is referred back to her surgeon for evaluation for reoperation rather than being managed expectantly or with dilation, since a herniated wrap is a mechanical problem that dilation would not correct and might worsen. This case illustrates why postoperative dysphagia should be characterized by its trajectory, transient and improving versus new or progressive, before a management pathway, whether reassurance, esophagram, or referral back to the surgical team, is chosen.

## Refractory Reflux and Special Clinical Situations

### Evaluating the Patient Who Does Not Respond to Standard Therapy

#### Eosinophilic Esophagitis as a Reflux Mimic

Eosinophilic esophagitis is a chronic, immune-mediated esophageal disease driven predominantly by food antigen exposure, presenting most commonly in a younger adult with a personal or family history of atopy, and its symptom overlap with reflux disease, particularly dysphagia and a sensation of food sticking, means that it must be actively considered rather than assumed away in any patient with reflux-type symptoms that respond incompletely to acid suppression. Diagnosis requires esophageal biopsy demonstrating a peak eosinophil count above a defined threshold per high-power field on histology obtained from multiple esophageal levels, because eosinophilic infiltration can be patchy and biopsies confined to a single level or region can produce a false-negative result. Endoscopic features associated with eosinophilic esophagitis, including circumferential rings, longitudinal furrows, whitish exudates representing eosinophilic microabscesses, and, in longstanding disease, esophageal narrowing, should prompt biopsy even when the endoscopic appearance is subtle, since a meaningful proportion of confirmed cases have an endoscopically unremarkable-appearing esophagus. Its incidence has risen notably over recent decades, a trend that parallels rising rates of other atopic conditions and has increased clinical awareness enough that biopsy to exclude it is now considered a routine part of the evaluation of unexplained dysphagia, not a specialized or unusual step. Symptomatic overlap with reflux and the frequent coexistence of both conditions in the same patient mean that a therapeutic proton pump inhibitor trial and diagnostic biopsy are often pursued together rather than sequentially.

Management follows one of three general strategies, often used sequentially or in combination: proton pump inhibitor therapy, which produces histologic and symptomatic remission in a substantial subset of patients through a mechanism thought to involve acid-independent effects on esophageal epithelial barrier function rather than acid suppression alone; topical swallowed corticosteroid therapy, using either a compounded viscous formulation or an inhaler-derived corticosteroid swallowed rather than inhaled; and dietary elimination therapy, ranging from targeted elimination of the most commonly implicated food antigens to a more restrictive elimination and systematic reintroduction protocol performed with dietitian support. Esophageal dilation is reserved for patients with a fixed stricture or persistent narrowing despite adequate anti-inflammatory therapy, and it is performed cautiously, using smaller incremental dilations than would be used for a peptic stricture, because the inflamed, friable esophageal wall in active eosinophilic esophagitis carries an increased perforation risk during forceful dilation. Maintenance therapy, using whichever modality achieved remission at the lowest effective intensity, is generally continued indefinitely, since eosinophilic esophagitis is a chronic condition that recurs when treatment is withdrawn in most patients.

A patient whose reflux symptoms persist despite an adequate trial of once-daily proton pump inhibitor therapy, confirmed to be taken correctly relative to meals, requires a structured reassessment rather than an empiric increase to twice-daily dosing, because a substantial proportion of apparent treatment failures reflect either a nonacid mechanism that acid suppression cannot address or a diagnosis other than reflux disease altogether. Upper endoscopy, if not already performed, excludes erosive disease, eosinophilic esophagitis, which can mimic reflux symptoms and requires esophageal biopsy for diagnosis rather than endoscopic appearance alone, and other structural explanations, while ambulatory pH-impedance monitoring performed on therapy determines whether ongoing symptoms correlate with a detectable reflux event of any type. A patient with a symptom-reflux correlation on impedance testing despite adequate acid suppression is a candidate for antireflux surgery targeting the mechanical rather than the acid-secretory component of disease, while a patient without symptom-reflux correlation warrants evaluation for a functional esophageal disorder, in which visceral hypersensitivity rather than reflux itself generates the perceived symptom. This reassessment should be documented explicitly rather than implied. This sequencing prevents wasted procedural and testing resources on the wrong diagnostic branch.

**Reflux in Pregnancy and Other Special Populations**

Older adults with reflux disease warrant particular attention to polypharmacy interactions and to the possibility that new or worsening reflux symptoms reflect a medication effect rather than primary disease progression, since several classes of medications commonly prescribed in this population, including calcium channel blockers, anticholinergics, and certain osteoporosis medications, lower esophageal sphincter pressure or directly irritate the esophageal mucosa. A careful medication reconciliation, applying the same principle developed in the first chapter's discussion of medication history, frequently identifies a modifiable contributor before escalating acid-suppressive therapy is considered, and this review should specifically include bisphosphonates, which carry a well-recognized risk of pill esophagitis when taken without adequate water or without remaining upright for the required interval after ingestion, a mechanical rather than acid-mediated injury that acid suppression alone will not resolve.

Reflux symptoms are common in pregnancy as a consequence of progesterone-mediated lower esophageal sphincter relaxation combined with mechanically increased intra-abdominal pressure from the gravid uterus, and management is stepped, beginning with lifestyle modification and, when needed, agents with the most favorable pregnancy safety profile, typically starting with an antacid or sucralfate before proceeding to a histamine-2 receptor antagonist or proton pump inhibitor if symptoms remain inadequately controlled, a sequence that mirrors the general stepwise approach to reflux management while incorporating fetal safety as an explicit additional consideration at each step. In patients with scleroderma-spectrum disease, severe esophageal hypomotility from smooth muscle atrophy and fibrosis produces reflux disease that is often more severe and more resistant to standard therapy than reflux occurring with normal esophageal motility, because impaired clearance prolongs acid contact time regardless of how effectively acid secretion itself is suppressed, and antireflux surgery is generally avoided in this population because a fundoplication performed against a severely hypomotile esophagus risks converting reflux symptoms into severe, difficult-to-treat dysphagia. Endoscopy during pregnancy, when indicated for alarm features rather than for typical uncomplicated symptoms, follows the same safety considerations for sedation and positioning discussed in the previous chapter.

| Dysplasia Grade | Confirmation Required | Recommended Pathway |
|---|---|---|
| No dysplasia | Standard community pathology read | Surveillance interval by Prague segment length |
| Indefinite for dysplasia | Optimize acid suppression, repeat biopsy | Repeat endoscopy in 3-6 months |
| Low-grade dysplasia | Expert GI pathology confirmation | Eradication therapy or shortened-interval surveillance |
| High-grade dysplasia | Expert GI pathology confirmation | Endoscopic eradication therapy |

| | | |
|---|---|---|
| Intramucosal carcinoma | Expert GI pathology confirmation, EMR staging | Endoscopic eradication therapy after resection staging |

**THE GI THRESHOLD DECISION SYSTEM — Reflux and Barrett Esophagus Thresholds**

**Presentation Signature:** This chapter's threshold instances addressed the two central decision points in reflux and its most consequential complication: when to move from empiric therapy to endoscopy, and when to move from surveillance to eradication therapy.

**Threshold Point:** Age 60 and alarm features govern the first decision; confirmed dysplasia grade, established by expert pathology review, governs the second.

**The Call:** Both thresholds convert a continuous, uncertain clinical picture into a binary management pathway, endoscopy versus empiric trial, eradication versus continued surveillance, once the defining criterion is met.

**Trap Logic:** Partial treatment response and single-pathologist dysplasia reads are the two most common sources of misapplied thresholds in this chapter; both require a second, more definitive data point, confirmed nonresponse or expert pathology confirmation, before the threshold decision is finalized.

**Decision Anchor:** In reflux disease, age and alarm features decide the diagnostic pathway; in Barrett esophagus, confirmed dysplasia grade decides the management pathway. Neither decision should be made on an unconfirmed or preliminary data point.

## Summary and Key Concepts

The antireflux barrier depends on the lower esophageal sphincter, the crural diaphragm, esophageal clearance, and mucosal defense; failure of any one component, not acid production alone, produces disease.

Typical heartburn and regurgitation carry strong predictive value for reflux disease, while extraesophageal symptoms such as cough and laryngitis carry low predictive value and require objective confirmation.

Age 60 or older and alarm features define the threshold at which upfront endoscopy, rather than an empiric therapeutic trial, becomes the appropriate first diagnostic step.

Proton pump inhibitor timing relative to meals is the most common source of apparent treatment failure and should be corrected before therapy is escalated or further testing pursued.

Barrett esophagus screening targets patients with long-standing reflux symptoms plus additional risk factors, and the Prague classification standardizes documentation of segment extent.

Confirmed dysplasia grade, established by expert gastrointestinal pathology review rather than a single community read, is the threshold that determines whether a patient proceeds to endoscopic eradication therapy or continued surveillance.

Refractory reflux requires structured reassessment, including exclusion of eosinophilic esophagitis and on-therapy impedance testing, before therapy is escalated further or surgery is considered.

# CHAPTER 4: ESOPHAGEAL MOTILITY AND STRUCTURAL DISEASE

**Learning Objectives**

1. Classify esophageal motility disorders using the Chicago Classification and relate each pattern to its underlying pathophysiology.
2. Select the appropriate treatment for achalasia based on manometric subtype and patient factors.
3. Evaluate and manage peptic, malignant, eosinophilic, and caustic esophageal strictures, including safe dilation technique.
4. Recognize Zenker diverticulum, Schatzki ring, and esophageal webs and select the appropriate diagnostic and therapeutic approach for each.
5. Recognize esophageal perforation and Boerhaave syndrome promptly and apply threshold-based reasoning to the conservative-versus-surgical management decision.

**Chapter Outline**

This chapter addresses the structural and motility disorders of the esophagus that were introduced diagnostically in the first two chapters: the physiology and classification of esophageal motility disorders, the evaluation and stepwise management of achalasia, the evaluation and dilation of esophageal strictures from peptic, malignant, eosinophilic, and caustic causes, the recognition of Zenker diverticulum and Schatzki ring, and the emergency recognition and management of esophageal perforation. Each section links a specific diagnostic threshold, a manometric subtype, a stricture etiology, or a time-from-perforation interval, to a defined management pathway.

## Esophageal Motility Disorders: Pathophysiology and Classification

### Normal Peristalsis and the Chicago Classification Framework

Normal esophageal peristalsis depends on the coordinated, sequential contraction of striated muscle in the proximal esophagus and smooth muscle in the distal esophagus, transitioning through a physiologic zone of lower amplitude contraction where the two muscle types overlap, and on appropriate relaxation of the lower esophageal sphincter timed precisely to the arrival of the peristaltic wave so that the swallowed bolus passes into the stomach without resistance. High-resolution manometry captures this sequence as a continuous pressure topography plot, and the Chicago Classification interprets that plot using a hierarchical algorithm beginning with the integrated relaxation pressure, a measure of how completely the lower esophageal sphincter relaxes during swallowing, before proceeding to assess the pattern of peristalsis itself, because an elevated integrated relaxation pressure identifies a disorder of esophagogastric junction outflow before the classification scheme even considers whether peristalsis in the esophageal body is normal, weak, absent, or spastic. This hierarchical structure reflects the underlying physiology: outflow obstruction at the gastroesophageal junction is mechanistically the more fundamental abnormality, and disordered peristalsis in the body of the esophagus is frequently a secondary or independent finding that must be interpreted in that context rather than in isolation.

**Achalasia: Subtypes and Pathogenesis**

Achalasia results from the progressive, immune-mediated destruction of inhibitory neurons in the myenteric plexus of the distal esophagus and lower esophageal sphincter, and because these are specifically the neurons responsible for sphincter relaxation and for the normal, coordinated peristaltic wave, their loss produces the disease's defining combination of a lower esophageal sphincter that fails to relax appropriately and a body of the esophagus that cannot generate normal, propagating peristalsis. The Chicago Classification divides achalasia into three subtypes based on the pattern of pressurization observed in the esophageal body: Type I, with no significant pressurization and essentially absent contractility; Type II, with panesophageal pressurization reflecting simultaneous, disorganized compression of trapped contents throughout the esophageal body; and Type III, spastic achalasia, with premature, spastic contractions superimposed on the outflow obstruction. This subtyping carries direct treatment implications, because Type II achalasia responds most favorably to any of the standard treatment modalities, while Type III achalasia, given its spastic component, responds preferentially to a myotomy long enough to address the spastic segment, a distinction developed further in the management section of this chapter. This subtyping is determined at the time of initial diagnostic manometry, before any treatment decision is made.

**Figure 4.1: Chicago Classification Manometric Patterns**

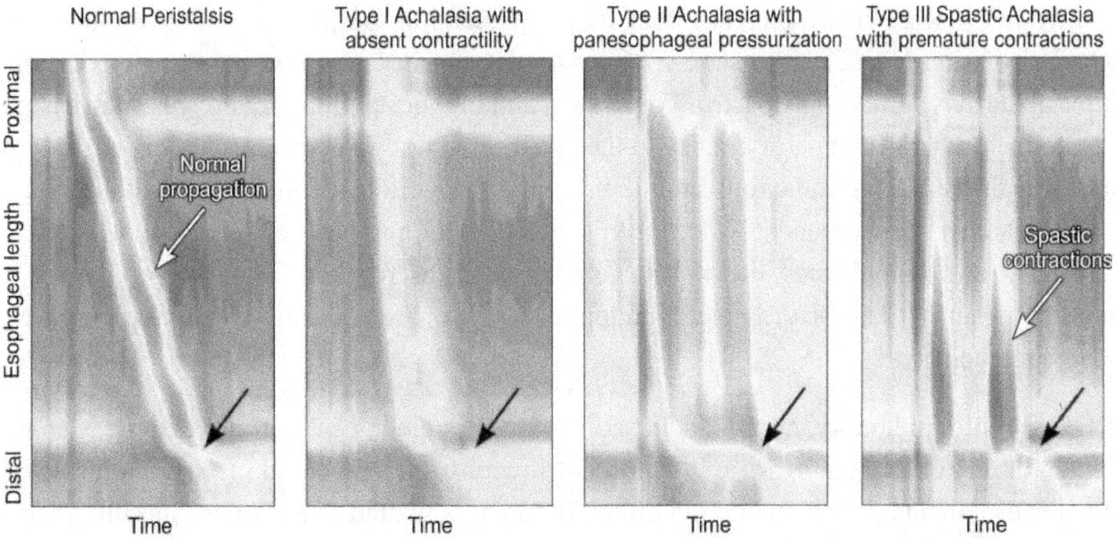


Normal Peristalsis | Type I Achalasia with absent contractility | Type II Achalasia with panesophageal pressurization | Type III Spastic Achalasia with premature contractions

## Esophagogastric Junction Outflow Obstruction and Spastic Disorders

Esophagogastric junction outflow obstruction describes a pattern of elevated integrated relaxation pressure without the fully absent or panesophageal-pressurized peristalsis that defines achalasia, and it represents a heterogeneous category that can reflect early or incompletely expressed achalasia, a mechanical process such as a subtle stricture or hiatal hernia effect not fully appreciated on endoscopy, or, in some cases, an artifact of the manometric catheter's position or the patient's technique during the study, which is why a diagnosis of esophagogastric junction outflow obstruction generally prompts confirmatory follow-up, either repeat manometry, a functional lumen imaging probe assessment of esophagogastric junction distensibility, or a period of clinical observation, rather than immediate committal to achalasia-specific therapy. Distal esophageal spasm and hypercontractile, or jackhammer, esophagus are distinguished from achalasia by normal or only mildly elevated integrated relaxation pressure combined with premature or excessively vigorous contractions in the esophageal body, and both are managed primarily with pharmacologic smooth muscle relaxants and, in refractory cases, peroral endoscopic myotomy targeting the spastic segment, reflecting a shared underlying mechanism of esophageal body hypercontractility distinct from the outflow-predominant pathophysiology of achalasia itself.

## Ineffective Esophageal Motility and Absent Contractility

Ineffective esophageal motility and absent contractility describe patterns of weak or entirely absent peristalsis in the esophageal body with a normal integrated relaxation pressure, distinguishing them from the outflow-predominant disorders discussed above, and they are frequently found incidentally during the workup of reflux disease or dysphagia rather than representing the primary explanation for a patient's symptoms in isolation. These patterns are commonly seen in association with systemic connective tissue disease, particularly scleroderma-spectrum disorders, and in longstanding, severe gastroesophageal reflux disease, where chronic inflammatory injury to the esophageal body's neuromuscular apparatus over years can itself impair peristaltic function, and their clinical significance lies primarily in the impaired esophageal clearance they produce, which, as discussed in the previous chapter, worsens reflux-related mucosal injury and complicates the risk-benefit calculation for antireflux surgery, since a poorly peristalsing esophagus tolerates a complete fundoplication poorly and often warrants a partial wrap instead if surgery is pursued at all.

**KEY POINT:** A structurally normal endoscopy never excludes a motility disorder; conversely, a manometric finding of esophagogastric junction outflow obstruction should prompt exclusion of a subtle mechanical cause, including a hiatal hernia effect, before it is treated as a primary motility diagnosis.

## Achalasia Epidemiology and the Problem of Diagnostic Delay

Achalasia is an uncommon disease, and its rarity, combined with the fact that its early symptoms, mild intermittent dysphagia and occasional regurgitation, overlap substantially with far more common conditions such as reflux disease, means that the average interval between symptom onset and confirmed diagnosis is measured in years rather than weeks in a meaningful proportion of patients, during which time many are treated empirically for reflux disease without symptomatic improvement, a pattern that itself should prompt reconsideration of the working diagnosis rather than continued escalation of acid-suppressive therapy. This diagnostic delay carries clinical consequence beyond prolonged symptoms alone, because progressive esophageal body dilation and the loss of any residual peristaltic function that occurs with longstanding, untreated disease can complicate later treatment and is associated with poorer outcomes after eventual intervention, reinforcing why the reasoning developed in the first chapter, treating dysphagia to both solids and liquids as a signal to pursue manometry rather than an extended empiric reflux trial, has consequences that extend well beyond diagnostic efficiency alone.

## Clinical Evaluation of Suspected Motility Disorders

### Symptom Pattern and Initial Testing Sequence

Dysphagia to both solids and liquids from onset, as developed in the first chapter's diagnostic reasoning framework, is the symptom pattern that should raise suspicion for a motility disorder and prompt the specific evaluation sequence developed in this chapter, beginning with upper endoscopy to exclude a mechanical or mucosal cause, since motility testing is only interpretable, and only indicated, once a structural explanation has been reasonably excluded. A barium esophagram, obtained either before or after endoscopy depending on institutional workflow, frequently provides pattern-recognition clues that anticipate the manometric diagnosis, including the classic bird's-beak narrowing and progressive esophageal body dilation of achalasia, or the corkscrew appearance sometimes seen in distal esophageal spasm, and these findings, while not diagnostic on their own, appropriately direct the clinician toward confirmatory high-resolution manometry as the definitive next step rather than toward repeat endoscopy or an empiric trial of acid suppression.

A timed barium esophagram, in which the height and width of a retained barium column are measured at fixed intervals, most commonly one and five minutes, after the patient swallows a standardized volume, provides an objective, reproducible measure of esophageal emptying that complements manometry's assessment of contractile pattern, and it is particularly useful in achalasia both for establishing a pretreatment baseline against which treatment response can be objectively compared and for identifying incomplete treatment response even when a patient's subjective symptom burden has improved, since symptom report and objective emptying do not always move in parallel.

### High-Resolution Manometry Interpretation in Practice

Interpreting a manometry study requires attention to more than the final Chicago Classification diagnosis alone, because the raw pressure topography plot and the pattern of the patient's response across the standardized set of test swallows carry information relevant to treatment planning, particularly the length and location of any spastic segment in Type III achalasia or distal esophageal spasm, which directly determines how long a subsequent myotomy needs to extend to adequately address the abnormal segment. A functional lumen imaging probe, a catheter-mounted balloon that measures the cross-sectional area and distensibility of the esophagogastric junction during controlled volumetric distension, provides complementary information to manometry, particularly in equivocal cases or when manometry cannot be tolerated or completed, and its assessment of esophagogastric junction opening during a procedure itself has an emerging role in confirming the adequacy of a myotomy at the time it is performed.

**THE GI THRESHOLD DECISION SYSTEM — Esophageal Motility Thresholds — Achalasia Subtype and Treatment Selection**

**Presentation Signature:** A patient with confirmed achalasia on high-resolution manometry, having already been staged into a Chicago Classification subtype, requires selection among pneumatic dilation, Heller myotomy, and peroral endoscopic myotomy.

**Threshold Point:** Type II achalasia responds favorably to any of the three standard treatment modalities with comparable success rates, while Type III achalasia, given its spastic esophageal body component, responds preferentially to a myotomy of sufficient length to cover the spastic segment, a length that pneumatic dilation, which addresses only the lower esophageal sphincter itself, cannot provide.

**The Call:** Type II achalasia treatment selection is guided primarily by patient preference, local expertise, and anticipated need for a future antireflux procedure, since Heller myotomy is typically paired with a partial fundoplication while peroral endoscopic myotomy is not; Type III achalasia treatment is directed toward peroral endoscopic myotomy or a similarly extended surgical myotomy, tailored in length to the spastic segment identified on manometry.

**Trap Logic:** Offering pneumatic dilation as a default first-line option without first confirming the Chicago Classification subtype risks under-treating Type III achalasia, whose spastic component a dilation targeting only the sphincter does not address.

**Decision Anchor:** Confirm the Chicago Classification subtype before selecting a treatment modality for achalasia; Type III achalasia specifically requires a myotomy of adequate length, not sphincter-directed dilation alone.

## Management of Achalasia and Related Motility Disorders

### Pneumatic Dilation, Peroral Endoscopic Myotomy, and Heller Myotomy

Pneumatic dilation uses a noncompliant balloon positioned fluoroscopically across the lower esophageal sphincter and inflated to a pressure sufficient to tear the circular muscle fibers of the sphincter, performed typically in a graduated series of increasing balloon diameters across separate sessions, and it achieves durable symptom relief in a substantial majority of appropriately selected patients, though repeat dilation is required in a meaningful minority over time. Laparoscopic Heller myotomy divides the circular muscle fibers of the lower esophageal sphincter and distal esophagus under direct surgical visualization, typically combined with a partial fundoplication to mitigate the reflux that an unopposed myotomy would otherwise produce, and it offers a more durable initial response than pneumatic dilation in most comparative studies, at the cost of a surgical procedure and its associated recovery. Peroral endoscopic myotomy achieves a comparable myotomy endoscopically, through a submucosal tunnel created endoscopically that allows the endoscopist to divide the circular muscle fibers from within the esophageal lumen without any external incision, and its principal advantage over Heller myotomy, beyond its incisionless approach, is the ability to extend the myotomy length flexibly to address a long spastic segment in Type III achalasia or distal esophageal spasm, a flexibility that has made it the preferred approach at many centers for spastic motility disorders specifically. Perforation is the most feared complication of pneumatic dilation, occurring in a small minority of procedures, and immediate post-procedure clinical assessment along with a low threshold for contrast imaging when a patient reports disproportionate pain helps ensure this complication, when it occurs, is recognized promptly rather than after a delay that would worsen its management, as described later in this chapter. Intraoperative endoscopy or a functional lumen imaging probe assessment at the time of myotomy helps confirm that the myotomy has adequately opened the esophagogastric junction before the operation concludes, reducing the likelihood of a technically incomplete procedure going unrecognized until symptoms fail to improve postoperatively.

### Pharmacologic and Endoscopic Botulinum Toxin Options

Botulinum toxin injected endoscopically into the lower esophageal sphincter inhibits acetylcholine release at the neuromuscular junction, producing temporary sphincter relaxation that provides symptomatic relief lasting weeks to several months before repeat injection is required, and its role is generally reserved for patients who are poor candidates for pneumatic dilation or myotomy because of significant comorbidity or limited life expectancy, or as a bridging measure while a patient is being optimized for a more durable procedure, rather than as first-line therapy in an otherwise appropriate surgical or endoscopic candidate, because its effect is temporary and repeated injection is associated with increased submucosal fibrosis that can complicate a subsequent myotomy if one is later pursued. Calcium channel blockers and nitrates, administered sublingually before meals, provide modest and often poorly tolerated symptomatic relief through direct smooth muscle relaxation and are generally reserved for patients unable to undergo any of the more definitive interventions. Its onset of effect is rapid, typically within days, making it a reasonable bridging option in a patient who needs symptomatic improvement before a definitive procedure can be arranged.

### Management of Distal Esophageal Spasm and Hypercontractile Esophagus

First-line management of distal esophageal spasm and hypercontractile esophagus centers on smooth muscle relaxants, most commonly a calcium channel blocker or, in refractory cases, a low-dose tricyclic antidepressant or other neuromodulator targeting the visceral hypersensitivity that frequently accompanies these disorders and contributes to symptom perception independent of the manometric abnormality itself, an overlap with the functional heartburn mechanism discussed in the previous chapter. Botulinum toxin injection into the distal esophageal body, distinct from the sphincter-directed injection used in achalasia, provides temporary relief in patients who do not respond adequately to pharmacologic therapy, and peroral endoscopic myotomy, extended in length to cover the spastic segment identified on manometry, is reserved for patients with severe, pharmacologically refractory symptoms given its greater invasiveness relative to the medical options, mirroring the length-tailored myotomy approach already described for Type III achalasia.

### Post-Treatment Surveillance and Long-Term Considerations

Gastroesophageal reflux disease is a recognized long-term consequence of both pneumatic dilation and myotomy, since each intervention deliberately weakens the same antireflux barrier discussed in the previous chapter, and patients treated for achalasia should be counseled about this trade-off explicitly and monitored for reflux symptoms after treatment, with a lower threshold for surveillance endoscopy than in the general population given emerging data suggesting an increased risk of Barrett esophagus in this population. Long-standing, poorly treated achalasia also carries a modestly increased lifetime risk of esophageal squamous cell carcinoma, related to chronic stasis and mucosal irritation from retained food and secretions in the dilated, poorly emptying esophageal body, which reinforces the value of achieving durable symptom and emptying improvement with definitive therapy rather than accepting a suboptimal treatment response indefinitely. This surveillance discussion should be initiated at the time treatment is planned, not deferred until reflux symptoms are already bothering the patient postoperatively.

### Anastomotic Strictures After Esophageal and Gastric Surgery

Strictures at a surgical anastomosis, most commonly following esophagectomy, gastrectomy with esophagojejunal reconstruction, or bariatric surgery, arise from a combination of localized ischemia at the anastomotic line and the normal fibrotic healing response, and they present with dysphagia in the postoperative period, an interval that ranges from weeks to several months after the index operation depending on the specific procedure and healing course. Dilation of an anastomotic stricture generally follows a more conservative increment than a routine peptic stricture given the surgically altered anatomy and the theoretical, though generally low in practice, risk of disrupting the anastomosis itself, and endoscopists performing these dilations benefit from reviewing the operative report beforehand to understand the specific anastomotic configuration and any surgical clips or staple lines in the region before instrumenting it. Anastomotic strictures frequently require more dilation sessions than peptic strictures to achieve a durable result, and persistent narrowing despite repeated dilation should prompt evaluation for anastomotic ischemia or, particularly following oncologic resection, local tumor recurrence at the anastomosis, both of which change management substantially from simple mechanical dilation alone.

## Esophageal Strictures: Peptic, Malignant, Eosinophilic, and Caustic

### Peptic Stricture Evaluation and Dilation Technique

Peptic strictures develop from chronic acid-mediated injury and fibrosis at the gastroesophageal junction or distal esophagus, typically in a patient with a long history of poorly controlled reflux disease, and endoscopic dilation, using either graduated bougie dilators passed over a guidewire or a through-the-scope balloon dilator, is the primary treatment, performed in incremental sessions rather than attempting to achieve full luminal caliber in a single session, following the widely applied rule of thumb that no more than three dilators of progressively increasing diameter, or an equivalent balloon diameter increase, should be used in a single session once resistance is encountered, because exceeding this increment materially raises perforation risk without proportionate benefit. Concurrent maximal acid suppression is essential both to promote healing of the stricture itself and to reduce the likelihood of recurrence, and a peptic stricture that fails to respond to an adequate course of dilation and acid suppression should prompt biopsy to exclude an underlying malignant or eosinophilic process that a purely peptic diagnosis would not explain. Sedation and topical pharyngeal anesthesia should be adequate to allow a controlled, unhurried dilation technique, since a struggling or inadequately sedated patient increases the risk of an uncontrolled dilator advancement.

**Malignant Stricture and Palliative Stenting**

A malignant esophageal stricture, most commonly from esophageal or gastric cardia adenocarcinoma or squamous cell carcinoma, presents with the progressive solid-food dysphagia pattern described in the first chapter and requires biopsy confirmation and staging before a management pathway is finalized, since the treatment of a potentially resectable malignancy diverges sharply from the treatment of unresectable or metastatic disease. Self-expanding metal stents provide effective palliation of dysphagia in patients with unresectable disease, restoring luminal patency without the incremental dilation approach used for benign strictures, since the goal in this setting is durable palliation rather than long-term luminal remodeling, while dilation alone, without stenting, is generally avoided as definitive management of a malignant stricture given its low durability and the availability of a more effective palliative option. Stent migration and tumor ingrowth or overgrowth are recognized causes of recurrent dysphagia after initially successful stenting and should be evaluated with repeat imaging or endoscopy rather than assumed to represent disease progression alone.

**Eosinophilic and Caustic Strictures**

Strictures related to eosinophilic esophagitis, discussed in the previous chapter, require the more cautious, smaller-increment dilation approach described earlier in this section given the increased perforation risk associated with the inflamed, friable esophageal wall characteristic of active disease, and effective anti-inflammatory therapy should be optimized alongside, rather than instead of, mechanical dilation, since dilation alone without addressing the underlying inflammation is likely to be followed by stricture recurrence. Caustic ingestion, whether accidental or intentional, produces a distinct injury pattern and management pathway: acute endoscopic evaluation, generally performed within the first 24 to 48 hours by an experienced endoscopist using minimal air insufflation, grades the depth and circumferential extent of the burn, and this grading determines both the risk of subsequent stricture formation and the timing of any dilation, which is deliberately delayed for several weeks after a severe caustic injury to allow the acute inflammatory phase to resolve, since dilation attempted during the acute phase, when the esophageal wall is maximally friable, carries substantially elevated perforation risk. Psychiatric evaluation is also indicated for any intentional caustic ingestion before the patient is discharged.

**CAUTION:** Early dilation attempted during the acute inflammatory phase of a caustic esophageal injury carries a materially elevated perforation risk; dilation of a caustic stricture is deliberately deferred until the acute phase has resolved, typically several weeks after the initial injury.

**Radiation-Induced Esophageal Stricture**

Esophageal strictures following radiation therapy for thoracic malignancy, most commonly lung or esophageal cancer itself, or following radiation to the mediastinum for lymphoma, develop from progressive fibrosis of the irradiated segment over months to years after treatment completion, typically presenting as gradually progressive solid-food dysphagia in a patient with a known radiation history, and this history is essential to elicit specifically, since a patient may not volunteer prior cancer treatment unprompted when presenting with a seemingly unrelated swallowing complaint. Management follows the same incremental dilation principle applied to peptic and caustic strictures, though radiation-associated tissue is often more fibrotic and less compliant than peptic tissue, generally requiring a more conservative, more gradual dilation approach with an even lower threshold to stop a session if resistance is encountered, and recurrence after dilation is common enough in this population that patients should be counseled from the outset that repeated dilation sessions over time are the expected course of management rather than a sign that the initial treatment failed.

**THE GI THRESHOLD DECISION SYSTEM — Esophageal Structural Thresholds — Safe Dilation Increments and Perforation Risk**

**Presentation Signature:** An endoscopist performing dilation of an esophageal stricture, benign or malignant, must decide how aggressively to dilate within a single session before stopping.

**Threshold Point:** The rule of three: no more than three sequentially larger dilators, or an equivalent balloon diameter increase, should be passed within a single session once resistance is first encountered, because perforation risk rises disproportionately beyond this increment.

**The Call:** Once resistance is encountered and three dilators of progressively increasing size have been passed, the session is concluded regardless of whether the target luminal diameter has been reached, with the plan to complete further dilation in a subsequent, staged session rather than in a single aggressive encounter.

**Trap Logic:** A tight, long-standing, or radiation-associated stricture can tempt an endoscopist toward a single, more aggressive dilation to minimize the number of procedures a patient undergoes; this trade-off favors the patient's convenience over their safety and should be resisted in favor of staged dilation.

**Decision Anchor:** The rule of three governs every stricture dilation regardless of etiology; eosinophilic and caustic strictures warrant an even more conservative increment given their additionally elevated baseline perforation risk.

**Older Adults and Polypharmacy-Related Esophageal Injury**

Pill esophagitis, direct mucosal injury from a medication tablet or capsule that lodges against the esophageal wall rather than passing promptly into the stomach, occurs disproportionately in older adults because of a combination of reduced saliva production, impaired esophageal motility from age-related or comorbid causes, and polypharmacy involving medications, including certain antibiotics, bisphosphonates, and potassium chloride, that are directly caustic to esophageal mucosa when contact time is prolonged. This injury frequently occurs at sites of physiologic esophageal narrowing or extrinsic compression, most commonly where the aortic arch crosses the esophagus, and typically presents with acute odynophagia rather than dysphagia, a distinction from the structural causes discussed elsewhere in this chapter that should prompt a focused medication history rather than an assumption of a primary structural or malignant process, particularly when the onset is acute and temporally associated with a new medication. Prevention, through patient counseling on taking pills with an adequate volume of water and remaining upright for a defined period afterward, is more effective than treatment after the fact and should be part of routine counseling whenever a medication with recognized esophageal toxicity is prescribed to a patient with any of the risk factors described above. Reviewing the medication list at every visit is a low-cost habit that prevents this diagnosis from being overlooked.

### Mid-Esophageal and Epiphrenic Diverticula

Diverticula arising in the mid-esophagus or just proximal to the diaphragm, epiphrenic diverticula, differ mechanistically from Zenker diverticulum in that they are more often true or traction-type diverticula associated with an underlying esophageal motility disorder, most commonly a spastic disorder or achalasia, rather than isolated cricopharyngeal dysfunction, meaning that identification of a mid-esophageal or epiphrenic diverticulum should prompt manometric evaluation for an underlying motility disorder rather than being treated as an isolated structural finding. Asymptomatic diverticula in this location, an increasingly common incidental finding given the frequency of cross-sectional imaging performed for unrelated indications, do not require intervention, while symptomatic diverticula, presenting with dysphagia, regurgitation, or aspiration, are managed surgically with diverticulectomy combined with myotomy addressing the underlying motility disorder, since treating the diverticulum alone without addressing the motility abnormality that produced it is associated with a higher rate of symptom recurrence. Surgical planning should always confirm the underlying motility diagnosis first.

## Esophageal Diverticula and Mucosal Rings

### Zenker Diverticulum

Zenker diverticulum is a false diverticulum arising through a specific area of anatomic weakness in the posterior pharyngoesophageal wall, Killian triangle, as a consequence of impaired relaxation and coordination of the cricopharyngeus muscle, the upper esophageal sphincter, and its clinical presentation, oropharyngeal dysphagia, regurgitation of undigested food hours after eating, halitosis, and, in advanced cases, aspiration pneumonia, reflects the diverticulum's location proximal to the true esophagus and its tendency to trap food and secretions. Diagnosis is established by barium esophagram, which is generally preferred over upper endoscopy as the initial test given the risk of inadvertent perforation of the diverticular sac if an endoscope is passed without prior knowledge of its location and orientation, and treatment, reserved for symptomatic patients, involves either open surgical or endoscopic cricopharyngeal myotomy with diverticulectomy or diverticulopexy, addressing the underlying cricopharyngeal dysfunction that permits the diverticulum to form and persist rather than treating the diverticular sac in isolation. If endoscopy is performed in a patient with a known or suspected Zenker diverticulum, the endoscopist proceeds under direct visualization with particular caution advancing past the pharyngoesophageal junction, since the diverticular opening can be mistaken for the true esophageal lumen if the anatomy is not anticipated in advance.

Figure 4.2: Zenker Diverticulum on Barium Esophagram

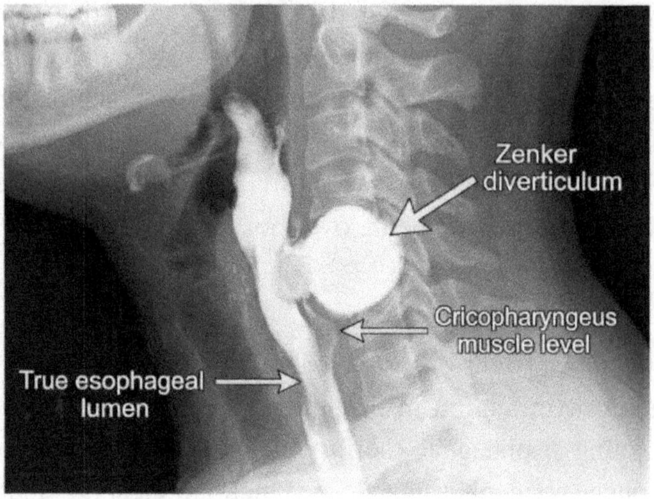


## Schatzki Ring and Esophageal Webs

A Schatzki ring is a thin, mucosal ring located at the squamocolumnar junction of the distal esophagus, strongly associated with a hiatal hernia and thought to arise from chronic reflux-related injury at this specific anatomic transition point, and its characteristic presentation, intermittent solid-food dysphagia, often precipitated classically by poorly chewed bread or meat and sometimes termed steakhouse syndrome when it causes acute food bolus impaction, distinguishes it from the progressive dysphagia pattern of a peptic or malignant stricture. Endoscopic dilation, frequently accomplished by simply passing a large-diameter endoscope or a single dilation session rather than the incremental staged approach required for a true stricture, provides durable relief in most patients, and acid suppression is generally recommended concurrently given the ring's association with reflux disease. Esophageal webs, thin mucosal folds typically located in the proximal esophagus, are associated in their classic though now uncommon presentation with iron deficiency anemia as part of Plummer-Vinson syndrome, and, like Schatzki rings, respond to simple endoscopic dilation once identified. Recurrence after dilation is common enough that a patient with a Schatzki ring should be counseled that repeat dilation over time is a normal part of managing this condition.

## Communicating Structural Esophageal Diagnoses to Patients

A structural esophageal diagnosis, whether a stricture, a diverticulum, or a motility disorder, benefits from the same concrete, plan-anchored explanation developed in earlier chapters, because a patient told only that they have 'a narrowing' or 'a spasm disorder' without an accompanying explanation of mechanism and next steps is left with an incomplete understanding that can generate either unwarranted anxiety or a false sense that the problem is trivial. Framing achalasia specifically as a disorder in which the muscle coordination that normally moves food into the stomach has been lost, rather than as a blockage in the usual sense, helps a patient understand why treatment targets the sphincter and esophageal muscle rather than removing an obstruction, and setting expectations about the durability and potential need for repeat intervention with pneumatic dilation, in particular, prevents a patient from interpreting a symptom recurrence years later as a treatment failure rather than an expected feature of the disease's natural history.

## Foreign Bodies and Esophageal Food Bolus Impaction

### Recognition and Urgency Stratification

Esophageal food bolus impaction, in which a poorly chewed piece of food, classically meat, becomes lodged and cannot pass into the stomach, is among the more common gastroenterology emergencies and, as noted earlier in this chapter, frequently reveals an underlying Schatzki ring, peptic stricture, or, particularly in a younger patient, eosinophilic esophagitis that had not previously been diagnosed, making the impaction itself both an acute problem to be managed urgently and a diagnostic opportunity to identify its underlying structural cause. A patient who is unable to handle their own secretions, evidenced by drooling or an inability to swallow saliva, has a complete obstruction and requires urgent, generally same-hour, endoscopic evaluation, while a patient who can tolerate liquids and manage secretions, suggesting a partial obstruction, can be observed for a brief period, since spontaneous passage occurs in some cases, though endoscopy is still generally pursued within 24 hours if spontaneous resolution does not occur, in order to both remove the impaction and evaluate the underlying cause. Glucagon and other pharmacologic agents intended to relax the lower esophageal sphincter and facilitate spontaneous passage have limited and inconsistent efficacy and should not substantially delay definitive endoscopic evaluation in a patient with a complete obstruction.

Recurrent food bolus impaction in the same patient is itself a diagnostic clue that should prompt active investigation for eosinophilic esophagitis if it has not already been diagnosed, since a substantial proportion of adults presenting with recurrent impaction, as opposed to a single isolated event, are ultimately found to have this condition on biopsy, and treating each episode as an isolated mechanical event without pursuing this underlying diagnosis leaves the patient at ongoing risk for further impactions that adequate anti-inflammatory therapy could prevent.

### Endoscopic Management and Sharp or Caustic Foreign Bodies

Endoscopic removal of a food bolus impaction can be accomplished either by gently advancing the bolus into the stomach, generally the preferred technique when no obstructing lesion prevents passage, or by retrieving it piecemeal using a snare or retrieval net when advancement is not safely possible, and biopsy of the surrounding esophageal mucosa to evaluate for eosinophilic esophagitis should be obtained at the same procedure whenever the underlying cause is not already established, since a second procedure dedicated solely to biopsy is an avoidable inconvenience for the patient. Sharp, pointed, or button-battery foreign bodies, more common in pediatric patients but occasionally encountered in adults, require more urgent endoscopic removal than a food bolus alone, given their risk of perforation or, in the specific case of button batteries, rapid caustic mucosal injury from generated electrical current, and any esophageal foreign body of this type is treated as a time-sensitive emergency regardless of whether the patient is symptomatic at the time of presentation. Meat tenderizer enzymes, historically used to dissolve an impacted meat bolus, are no longer recommended given the risk of esophageal wall injury from prolonged, uncontrolled enzymatic digestion of the tissue itself, and their use has been supplanted entirely by prompt endoscopic intervention.

**Figure 4.3: Endoscopic Dilation Technique for Peptic Stricture**

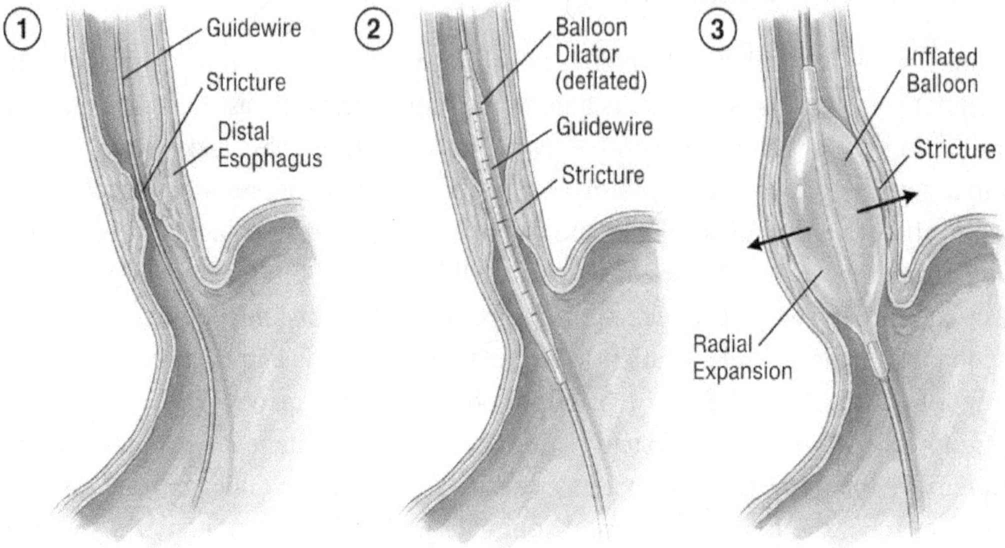


**CAUTION:** A suspected button battery lodged in the esophagus is a true emergency requiring removal as soon as it can be safely accomplished, since caustic injury from generated current can progress to full-thickness perforation within hours, a materially faster timeline than the urgency generally associated with a simple food bolus impaction.

### Coordinating Structural Esophageal Care Across Specialties

Severe structural esophageal disease frequently requires coordination across gastroenterology, thoracic or foregut surgery, speech-language pathology for swallowing assessment, and nutrition services, and applying the consult-precision principle developed in the first chapter to this coordination, specifying explicitly which service is responsible for which decision and by when, prevents the same diffusion of responsibility that an imprecise single consult note produces on a smaller scale. A patient recovering from esophageal perforation repair, for example, benefits from an explicit, jointly developed plan specifying the criteria and imaging study that will be used to confirm anastomotic or repair-site healing before oral intake resumes, rather than each specialty independently assuming the other has already established this plan, a gap that in practice is a recognized source of either unnecessarily prolonged nil-by-mouth status or premature, unsafe resumption of oral intake.

## Nutritional Support in Severe Esophageal Structural Disease

Patients with severe, unresolved dysphagia from any structural or motility cause discussed in this chapter, whether awaiting definitive treatment, recovering from esophageal perforation, or managing a stricture requiring multiple staged dilations, may develop clinically significant nutritional compromise if oral intake remains inadequate for an extended period, and proactive nutritional assessment, applying the screening principles introduced in the first chapter, should not be deferred until weight loss or laboratory evidence of malnutrition has already become apparent.

### Selecting a Nutritional Support Strategy

A modified, softer oral diet is sufficient for many patients with mild to moderate dysphagia and should be the first-line recommendation whenever oral intake remains safe and adequate, but a patient with severe dysphagia anticipated to persist for more than several days to a week, such as one recovering from esophageal perforation repair or undergoing staged dilation of a severe stricture, benefits from a more structured nutritional plan developed proactively with dietitian input rather than reactively once oral intake has already become inadequate. Enteral nutrition, when required, is generally preferred over parenteral nutrition whenever the gastrointestinal tract distal to the esophageal problem is functional, and a nasoenteric tube or, for anticipated longer-term need, a percutaneous gastrostomy or jejunostomy placed either endoscopically, radiologically, or surgically depending on the specific anatomic situation, provides this access; placement below an esophageal obstruction or stricture, when technically feasible, allows nutritional support to continue even while the esophageal problem itself is still being definitively treated.

## Esophageal Perforation and Boerhaave Syndrome

### Iatrogenic Perforation During Endoscopic Procedures

Iatrogenic perforation during upper endoscopy is uncommon during purely diagnostic examination but rises meaningfully during therapeutic maneuvers, particularly stricture dilation, and recognizing it at the time it occurs, rather than after the patient has left the procedure area, changes the management pathway substantially, since a perforation identified and treated immediately, before significant mediastinal or peritoneal contamination has occurred, is far more likely to be managed successfully with endoscopic closure alone. Any unexpected resistance, unusual pain reported by a sedated patient, or a visible defect in the wall during a therapeutic maneuver should prompt immediate assessment for perforation, including fluoroscopic contrast injection through the endoscope if available, rather than proceeding with the remainder of the planned procedure, and an endoscopist who identifies a perforation at the time of the causative procedure should attempt endoscopic closure with clips at that same session whenever technically feasible, since this immediate intervention frequently avoids the need for surgery altogether. Documentation of this real-time recognition and closure is important for subsequent care coordination.

### Recognition and Initial Management

Esophageal perforation, whether iatrogenic from endoscopic instrumentation, spontaneous as in Boerhaave syndrome, in which forceful vomiting against a closed glottis generates sufficient intraluminal pressure to rupture the esophageal wall, most classically at the left posterolateral distal esophagus, or related to foreign body impaction or caustic injury, presents with severe chest or upper abdominal pain, often accompanied by subcutaneous emphysema palpable in the neck or chest wall and, on auscultation, a crunching sound synchronous with the heartbeat known as Hamman sign, though this classic finding is present in only a minority of confirmed cases and its absence should not delay evaluation when the clinical scenario is otherwise suggestive. Initial management follows a sequence common to any suspected gastrointestinal perforation: the patient is made nil by mouth, broad-spectrum antibiotics covering oral and gastrointestinal flora are initiated promptly given the high risk of mediastinal contamination and subsequent mediastinitis, and a water-soluble contrast esophagram or contrast-enhanced computed tomography is obtained to confirm the perforation and characterize its size, location, and the degree of extraluminal contamination, information that directly determines the subsequent management pathway.

Regardless of whether primary repair, diversion, or nonoperative management is chosen, adequate drainage of any associated pleural effusion or mediastinal fluid collection, most commonly by image-guided or surgical chest tube placement, is a component of management that applies across all three pathways, since undrained contaminated fluid collections propagate ongoing sepsis independent of how the perforation defect itself is addressed, and this drainage decision should be made explicitly and early rather than deferred until a patient fails to improve on antibiotics alone.

**Conservative Versus Surgical Management Thresholds**

A small, contained perforation identified promptly, with minimal extraluminal contamination and without evidence of sepsis, can in selected cases be managed nonoperatively, with nil by mouth status, broad-spectrum antibiotics, and either close observation or endoscopic closure using clips or a covered esophageal stent to seal the defect, an approach increasingly favored at experienced centers for appropriately selected, hemodynamically stable patients. A perforation identified late, associated with substantial mediastinal or pleural contamination, or accompanied by hemodynamic instability or sepsis, requires surgical intervention, typically primary repair with tissue reinforcement when feasible or, in more extensive or delayed presentations, esophageal diversion or resection, because the physiologic consequences of ongoing mediastinal contamination in this subset of patients exceed what nonoperative management or endoscopic closure alone can adequately control. The time elapsed between perforation and diagnosis is itself an important variable in this decision, since a delay of more than 24 hours is associated with more extensive contamination and inflammation that generally favors a surgical rather than a purely conservative approach, independent of the perforation's size. Close multidisciplinary monitoring remains essential even when a nonoperative pathway is chosen. A multidisciplinary discussion involving surgery, gastroenterology, and, where relevant, critical care should occur promptly once imaging results are available, regardless of which pathway is ultimately chosen.

Case Presentation: A 68-year-old man is brought to the emergency department after an episode of forceful vomiting following a large meal and heavy alcohol intake, followed immediately by severe, tearing substernal chest pain radiating to the back. On examination he is tachycardic and diaphoretic, and crepitus is palpable over the lower neck. A chest radiograph shows pneumomediastinum. Applying the reasoning developed in this chapter, forceful vomiting followed immediately by severe chest pain and subcutaneous emphysema is the classic presentation of Boerhaave syndrome, and the patient is made nil by mouth, broad-spectrum antibiotics are started immediately, and a water-soluble contrast esophagram is obtained rather than proceeding directly to endoscopy, which risks extending the perforation. The esophagram confirms a distal esophageal perforation with a moderate volume of extraluminal contrast extending into the mediastinum. Given the presentation, now approximately six hours from symptom onset, combined with early hemodynamic compromise and a nontrivial degree of contamination on imaging, the patient is taken emergently for surgical repair rather than managed with endoscopic closure alone, and thoracic surgery performs primary repair with tissue flap reinforcement. This case illustrates the chapter's closing principle: the decision between conservative, endoscopic, and surgical management of esophageal perforation depends on an integrated assessment of contamination extent, time from perforation, and hemodynamic status, not on perforation size or mechanism alone.

Case Presentation: A 74-year-old man presents with several months of progressive difficulty initiating swallowing, intermittent regurgitation of undigested food several hours after meals, halitosis noted by his spouse, and one episode of aspiration pneumonia treated three months earlier. He denies odynophagia or weight loss. Applying the reasoning developed in this chapter, oropharyngeal-type symptoms, regurgitation of undigested food well after eating, and a history of aspiration pneumonia together suggest a pharyngoesophageal process such as Zenker diverticulum rather than a distal esophageal or gastric etiology, and a barium esophagram, rather than upper endoscopy, is obtained as the initial test given the risk of inadvertent perforation of an undiagnosed diverticular sac during blind endoscopic passage. The esophagram confirms a 3-centimeter posterior outpouching at the pharyngoesophageal junction consistent with Zenker diverticulum. Given his symptom burden, including a prior aspiration event, and the diagnosis now confirmed radiographically, he is referred for endoscopic cricopharyngeal myotomy with diverticulotomy, after which his regurgitation and aspiration risk resolve. This second case reinforces the chapter's diagnostic sequencing principle from a different structural disease: the correct initial test is determined by the specific anatomic process suspected from the history, not by defaulting to endoscopy as the reflexive first step for every esophageal complaint.

| Stricture Etiology | Dilation Approach | Key Additional Step |
|---|---|---|
| Peptic | Standard incremental dilation, rule of three | Maximal acid suppression |
| Malignant | Self-expanding metal stent preferred | Tissue diagnosis and staging first |
| Eosinophilic | Smaller-increment, cautious dilation | Concurrent anti-inflammatory therapy |
| Caustic (acute) | Defer dilation several weeks | Endoscopic burn grading at 24-48 hours |
| Schatzki ring | Single-session large-diameter dilation | Acid suppression for reflux association |

**Presentation Signature:** This chapter's threshold instances addressed subtype-based treatment selection in achalasia and safe-increment dilation across every stricture etiology.

**Threshold Point:** Chicago Classification subtype determines whether a sphincter-directed intervention alone is adequate or whether an extended myotomy is required; the rule of three defines the safe dilation increment per session across stricture types.

**The Call:** Both thresholds convert a structural or manometric finding into a specific, sequenced procedural plan rather than a single one-time intervention chosen by default.

**Trap Logic:** Treating achalasia subtypes interchangeably, and treating dilation increment as a convenience variable to be maximized in a single session, are the two most common ways these thresholds are misapplied.

**Decision Anchor:** Confirm subtype before treating achalasia; respect the rule of three before treating any stricture. Neither threshold should be bypassed for procedural convenience.

## Summary and Key Concepts

The Chicago Classification interprets high-resolution manometry hierarchically, assessing esophagogastric junction relaxation before esophageal body peristalsis, reflecting outflow obstruction as the more fundamental abnormality.

Achalasia subtype, not symptom severity, determines optimal treatment selection: Type II responds to any standard modality, while Type III requires a myotomy of adequate length to cover its spastic segment.

Esophageal stricture management follows the rule of three, no more than three progressively larger dilators per session, regardless of etiology, with eosinophilic and caustic strictures requiring even greater caution.

Zenker diverticulum is diagnosed by barium esophagram rather than endoscopy given perforation risk, and its treatment addresses the underlying cricopharyngeal dysfunction rather than the diverticular sac alone.

Schatzki ring and esophageal webs respond to simple, single-session dilation and are distinguished from true strictures by their thin, mucosal, non-fibrotic structure.

Esophageal perforation management is determined by an integrated assessment of contamination extent, time from perforation, and hemodynamic status, not by perforation size or mechanism alone.

# CHAPTER 5: PEPTIC ULCER DISEASE, HELICOBACTER PYLORI, AND GASTRITIS

**Learning Objectives**

1. Explain the physiologic balance between gastric acid secretion and mucosal defense that determines susceptibility to peptic injury.
2. Select an appropriate Helicobacter pylori testing strategy based on clinical context and apply current eradication regimens correctly.
3. Differentiate Helicobacter pylori-associated, nonsteroidal anti-inflammatory drug-associated, and idiopathic peptic ulcer disease and manage each appropriately.
4. Stratify nonsteroidal anti-inflammatory drug-related gastrointestinal risk and apply appropriate gastroprotective strategies.
5. Classify gastritis by etiology, including autoimmune gastritis, and recognize its associated complications.
6. Recognize clinical features that should prompt evaluation for Zollinger-Ellison syndrome in a patient with refractory or atypical peptic ulcer disease.

**Chapter Outline**

This chapter develops the physiology of gastric acid secretion and mucosal defense, the epidemiology, pathogenesis, testing, and treatment of Helicobacter pylori infection, the clinical presentation and management of peptic ulcer disease from both infectious and nonsteroidal anti-inflammatory drug causes, the classification of gastritis including its autoimmune and stress-related forms, and the recognition of Zollinger-Ellison syndrome as a cause of refractory ulcer disease. Each section connects a specific diagnostic or risk threshold to a defined management pathway, continuing the reasoning framework established in earlier chapters.

## Gastric Acid Physiology and Mucosal Defense

### Regulation of Gastric Acid Secretion

Gastric acid secretion by parietal cells is governed by three convergent stimulatory pathways acting on the same final common enzyme, the hydrogen-potassium adenosine triphosphatase, or proton pump, embedded in the parietal cell's secretory canaliculus: histamine, released from enterochromaffin-like cells and acting on the parietal cell's H2 receptor; acetylcholine, released from vagal and enteric neurons in response to the cephalic phase of digestion and gastric distension; and gastrin, released from antral G cells in response to luminal peptides and gastric distension, which acts both directly on the parietal cell and indirectly by stimulating histamine release from enterochromaffin-like cells, meaning that gastrin's effect is substantially amplified through this indirect histaminergic pathway rather than occurring through direct parietal cell stimulation alone. This three-pathway convergence explains why proton pump inhibitors, which act at the final common step shared by all three stimulatory inputs, achieve more complete and more consistent acid suppression than histamine-2 receptor antagonists, which block only one of the three convergent pathways and leave the gastrin- and acetylcholine-mediated components of secretion relatively intact.

**Figure 5.1: Convergent Pathways of Gastric Acid Secretion**

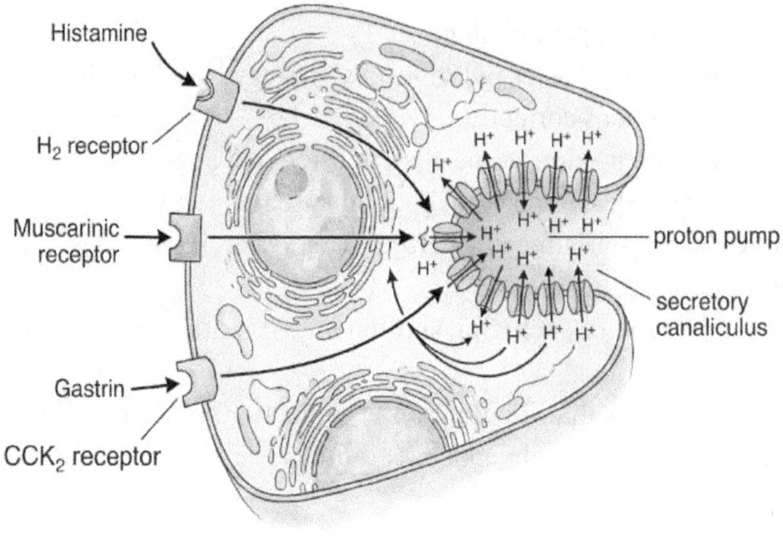


### Mucosal Protective Mechanisms

The gastroduodenal mucosa defends itself against the acidic, proteolytic luminal environment through a coordinated set of mechanisms operating at different levels: a surface mucus-bicarbonate layer that maintains a near-neutral pH gradient immediately adjacent to the epithelial surface despite a markedly acidic bulk luminal pH; rapid epithelial cell turnover and restitution that repairs superficial injury within hours; and robust mucosal blood flow that delivers bicarbonate and nutrients while clearing back-diffused hydrogen ions, a function that depends heavily on prostaglandin-mediated vasodilation. Prostaglandins, particularly those synthesized through the cyclooxygenase-1 pathway, are central to this entire protective system, stimulating mucus and bicarbonate secretion, maintaining mucosal blood flow, and promoting epithelial restitution simultaneously, which is precisely why nonsteroidal anti-inflammatory drugs, through their inhibition of cyclooxygenase-1-mediated prostaglandin synthesis, produce mucosal injury through a mechanism entirely independent of gastric acid output itself, a distinction that has direct treatment implications developed later in this chapter. This layered defense explains why injury to any single component can tip the balance toward ulceration even without a change in acid output itself.

### NSAID Effects Beyond the Stomach and Duodenum

While this chapter's discussion of nonsteroidal anti-inflammatory drug toxicity has focused on gastroduodenal injury, the same cyclooxygenase-1-mediated mechanism produces injury throughout the gastrointestinal tract, including small bowel enteropathy, which can cause occult blood loss, protein-losing enteropathy, or, in severe cases, diaphragm-like strictures from chronic small bowel ulceration and healing, and colonic injury, including exacerbation of underlying inflammatory bowel disease and an association with diverticular bleeding, both of which are frequently overlooked because clinical attention defaults to the stomach and duodenum when nonsteroidal anti-inflammatory drug-related gastrointestinal injury is suspected. This broader distribution of potential injury is part of why unexplained iron deficiency anemia or occult gastrointestinal blood loss in a patient on chronic nonsteroidal anti-inflammatory drug therapy, if a bidirectional endoscopic evaluation is unrevealing, should prompt consideration of small bowel evaluation using the capsule endoscopy or cross-sectional enterography techniques introduced in the second chapter, rather than concluding that the medication has been adequately investigated as a cause once upper and lower endoscopy alone have been completed. This whole-tract awareness reflects the same diagnostic discipline emphasized throughout this book: locate the mechanism, not just the most familiar anatomic site.

## Dyspepsia: Organic Versus Functional Presentation

Dyspepsia, encompassing epigastric pain, early satiety, postprandial fullness, and bloating, is one of the most common presenting complaints in general and gastroenterology practice, and the reasoning developed throughout this chapter, testing for Helicobacter pylori, evaluating for peptic ulcer disease, and, when refractory, considering rarer causes such as Zollinger-Ellison syndrome, applies specifically to the subset of dyspepsia patients with an organic explanation, which itself is a minority of all patients presenting with this symptom complex.

### Functional Dyspepsia as the More Common Outcome

The majority of patients ultimately diagnosed after a negative or unremarkable workup, including a Helicobacter pylori-negative status and a structurally normal upper endoscopy, are found to have functional dyspepsia, a disorder of gut-brain interaction characterized by visceral hypersensitivity and, in a subset of patients, impaired gastric accommodation to a meal, discussed in full detail in the following chapter alongside its specific management approach. Recognizing this expected outcome distribution in advance, rather than treating a negative organic workup as an unexpected or unsatisfying result, helps frame the diagnostic process for the patient from the outset: a negative workup for peptic ulcer disease and Helicobacter pylori infection is not a diagnostic failure but the anticipated result for most patients with this symptom complex, and it appropriately redirects management toward the functional disorder pathway developed in the next chapter rather than prompting an open-ended search for an organic cause that, in most patients, does not exist. Setting this expectation at the start of the workup, not only after a negative result arrives, improves the patient's experience of the diagnostic process.

### Extraintestinal Associations of Helicobacter Pylori

Beyond its well-established gastroduodenal disease associations, Helicobacter pylori has been linked to a number of extraintestinal conditions, most notably unexplained iron deficiency anemia and immune thrombocytopenic purpura, both of which can improve following successful eradication in appropriately selected patients, a relationship thought to involve chronic occult blood loss and altered iron absorption in the case of anemia, and molecular mimicry-driven immune dysregulation in the case of immune thrombocytopenic purpura, though the strength of evidence and the proportion of patients who respond to eradication varies across these associations. Current guidance supports testing for and treating Helicobacter pylori in a patient with unexplained iron deficiency anemia or immune thrombocytopenic purpura without an otherwise identified cause, as a low-risk, potentially high-yield intervention, even though the majority of patients with either condition will ultimately have a different or additional explanation identified through their broader workup. Discussing this rationale with the patient helps set realistic expectations about what eradication is and is not expected to accomplish for a coexisting hematologic finding.

## Helicobacter Pylori Infection

### Epidemiology and Transmission

Helicobacter pylori is among the most prevalent chronic bacterial infections worldwide, acquired predominantly in childhood through person-to-person transmission via oral-oral or fecal-oral routes, and its prevalence varies substantially by region, socioeconomic status, and birth cohort, with higher rates generally observed in populations with crowded childhood living conditions and lower access to clean water and sanitation, a pattern that has produced declining prevalence in many higher-income countries across successive birth cohorts even as the infection remains highly prevalent in other regions and populations. Once acquired, infection typically persists for the lifetime of the host in the absence of treatment, establishing chronic colonization of the gastric mucus layer and adjacent epithelium that, while often clinically silent for years or decades, drives a persistent inflammatory response with the disease consequences developed throughout this section.

### Pathogenesis and Disease Associations

Helicobacter pylori survives the acidic gastric environment through production of urease, which hydrolyzes urea into ammonia and buffers the immediate periplasmic environment, and it establishes chronic infection by adhering to gastric epithelial cells and triggering a sustained local and systemic immune response that, rather than clearing the organism, instead drives the chronic gastric inflammation responsible for the majority of the infection's disease associations. The pattern of gastritis produced by the infection determines much of its downstream clinical consequence: antral-predominant gastritis is associated with increased gastrin release and increased acid output, favoring duodenal ulcer formation, while corpus-predominant or pangastritis is associated with progressive parietal cell loss, reduced acid output, and an increased risk of gastric ulcer, atrophic gastritis, intestinal metaplasia, and, ultimately, gastric adenocarcinoma, a divergence that explains why the same infection produces markedly different clinical phenotypes across different patients depending on which gastric region bears the predominant burden of inflammation. Helicobacter pylori is also causally associated with gastric mucosa-associated lymphoid tissue lymphoma, a low-grade B-cell lymphoma that, in its early, localized stage, frequently regresses completely with eradication therapy alone, without chemotherapy or radiation, a treatment response unique among gastrointestinal malignancies and one that underscores the infection's role as a direct pathogenic driver rather than merely an epidemiologic association.

**Testing Strategies for Helicobacter Pylori**

Testing strategy is determined by whether the patient is already undergoing endoscopy for another indication and by whether the patient is currently on acid-suppressive or antibiotic therapy, both of which affect test performance substantially. In a patient already undergoing upper endoscopy, biopsy-based testing, including rapid urease testing, histology, or, when antibiotic resistance is a specific concern, culture with susceptibility testing, is efficient since it requires no additional procedure; in a patient not undergoing endoscopy, noninvasive testing with a urea breath test or a monoclonal stool antigen test is preferred over serology, because both directly detect active infection with high sensitivity and specificity, unlike serologic antibody testing, which cannot distinguish active from previously treated or resolved infection and therefore has a very limited role in the current diagnostic algorithm. Proton pump inhibitors suppress urease activity and bacterial density sufficiently to produce false-negative urea breath testing, biopsy-based testing, and stool antigen testing alike, which is why these medications should be held for at least one to two weeks, and bismuth or antibiotics for at least four weeks, before active testing is performed, a timing detail that, when overlooked, is a common and avoidable source of false-negative results and missed diagnoses. Serologic testing retains a narrow role only in specific circumstances, such as recent gastrointestinal bleeding, where active bleeding can reduce bacterial density enough to produce a false-negative result on the more direct tests, making a positive serology, interpreted with the important caveat that it cannot distinguish active from past infection, still occasionally useful in this specific bleeding context.

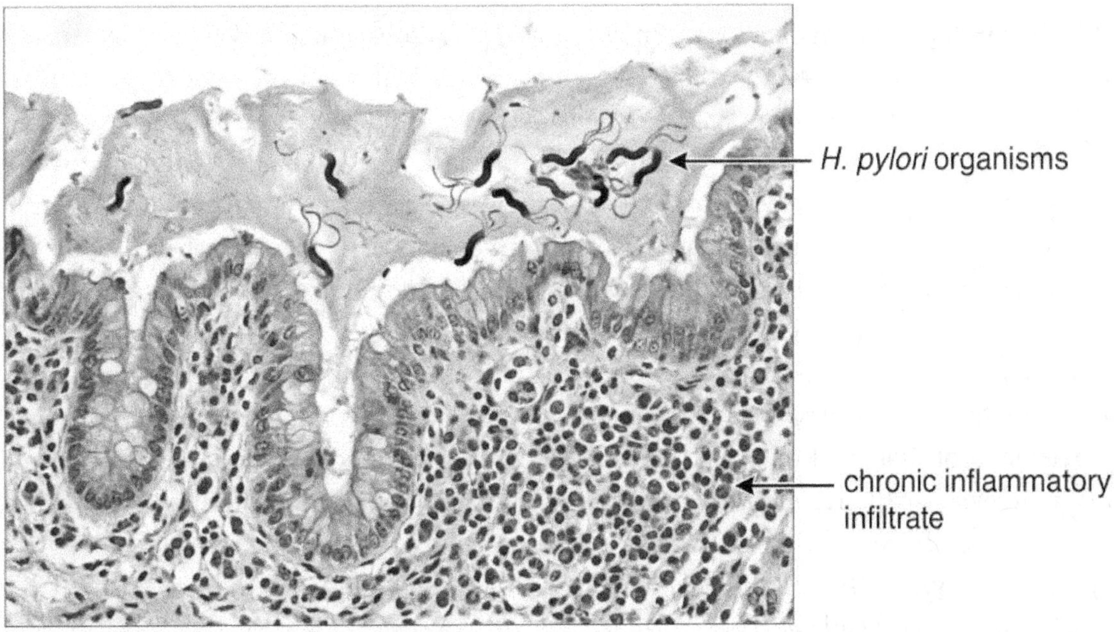


**Figure 5.2:** *Helicobacter pylori* on Histology

## THE GI THRESHOLD DECISION SYSTEM — Gastric Thresholds — Test-and-Treat Versus Endoscopy-First for Dyspepsia

**Presentation Signature:** A patient under age 60 presents with dyspepsia, and the clinician must decide between a noninvasive Helicobacter pylori test-and-treat strategy and upfront upper endoscopy.

**Threshold Point:** Age under 60 without alarm features defines the threshold below which a test-and-treat strategy, testing noninvasively for Helicobacter pylori and treating if positive, is an appropriate initial approach; age 60 or older, or any alarm feature, including bleeding, anemia, dysphagia, or unintentional weight loss, crosses the threshold requiring upfront endoscopy.

**The Call:** Patients below the age and alarm-feature threshold are tested noninvasively and treated if positive, with endoscopy reserved for those who test negative or whose symptoms persist despite eradication; patients meeting either threshold proceed directly to endoscopy, which then guides both biopsy-based Helicobacter pylori testing and evaluation for a structural or malignant cause.

**Trap Logic:** Applying a test-and-treat strategy in a patient with an alarm feature risks delaying the diagnosis of gastric malignancy, since a negative or successfully treated Helicobacter pylori result would otherwise be misread as reassurance that no further evaluation is needed.

**Decision Anchor:** Age and alarm features, applied identically to the reflux-versus-endoscopy threshold from the previous chapter, again determine whether a noninvasive strategy or upfront endoscopy is the correct first step in evaluating dyspepsia.

### Treatment Regimens and Antibiotic Resistance

First-line Helicobacter pylori eradication regimens have shifted substantially over recent years in response to rising clarithromycin resistance in many regions, and current guidance favors bismuth quadruple therapy, combining a proton pump inhibitor, bismuth subsalicylate, and two antibiotics, typically metronidazole and tetracycline, or non-bismuth concomitant or hybrid quadruple therapy over the older clarithromycin-based triple therapy in regions or patient populations with meaningful clarithromycin resistance prevalence or in patients with any prior macrolide exposure, since prior macrolide use for any indication is itself a risk factor for clarithromycin resistance and should be specifically elicited before regimen selection. Regimen duration of fourteen days, rather than the shorter seven- to ten-day courses used historically, improves eradication rates meaningfully and is now generally preferred, reflecting an evolution in practice driven directly by accumulating resistance and eradication-rate data rather than an arbitrary extension of treatment duration. Penicillin allergy status should also be confirmed and, where the history is unclear or the reaction described is inconsistent with a true immunoglobulin E-mediated allergy, clarified before amoxicillin-containing regimens are excluded unnecessarily, since amoxicillin-based regimens are generally preferred when tolerated and avoiding them without cause narrows the effective regimen options available.

### Confirming Eradication

Confirmation of eradication with a urea breath test or stool antigen test, performed at least four weeks after completing antibiotic therapy and after any proton pump inhibitor has been held for the interval described earlier in this section, should be obtained in essentially every treated patient rather than assumed based on symptomatic improvement alone, because a substantial minority of first-line regimens fail to achieve eradication given current resistance patterns, and a patient whose symptoms improve despite persistent infection, whether from placebo response or from unrelated symptom resolution, would otherwise remain infected and at ongoing risk for the disease associations described above. A patient who fails first-line therapy should not simply repeat the same regimen, since a repeated failed regimen both wastes a treatment opportunity and promotes further resistance; second-line therapy should use a different antibiotic combination, and susceptibility testing, obtained either through culture at the time of a repeat endoscopy or through molecular resistance testing where available, becomes increasingly valuable after a second treatment failure to guide a more targeted, evidence-based third-line regimen.

**KEY POINT:** Confirm Helicobacter pylori eradication in every treated patient using a urea breath test or stool antigen test at least four weeks after completing therapy; symptomatic improvement alone is not a reliable indicator of successful eradication.

### Patient Counseling on NSAID Risk and Alternatives

Many patients do not consider over-the-counter nonsteroidal anti-inflammatory drugs to carry the same risk profile as a prescription medication, a perception gap that directly parallels the underreporting pattern discussed in the first chapter's history-taking section, and effective counseling addresses this gap explicitly, explaining in plain terms that ibuprofen and naproxen purchased without a prescription carry the same mechanistic risk of gastrointestinal injury as any prescribed nonsteroidal anti-inflammatory drug at an equivalent dose and duration of use. Discussing specific alternatives, rather than only warning against continued use, gives the patient an actionable substitute: acetaminophen, when adequate for the level of pain being managed, carries no gastrointestinal toxicity; topical nonsteroidal anti-inflammatory drug formulations achieve therapeutic local tissue concentration for musculoskeletal indications with substantially lower systemic absorption and correspondingly lower gastrointestinal risk than oral formulations; and for patients who require ongoing oral nonsteroidal anti-inflammatory drug therapy despite these alternatives, the specific, dosed gastroprotective strategy determined by the risk-stratification framework in this chapter should be communicated as clearly as the medication itself, following the same precision-in-recommendation principle introduced in the first chapter. Written after-visit materials reinforcing this specific plan help sustain adherence beyond the visit itself.

### Idiopathic Peptic Ulcer Disease

A meaningful proportion of peptic ulcers are neither Helicobacter pylori-associated nor nonsteroidal anti-inflammatory drug-associated even after careful evaluation excludes both, a category termed idiopathic peptic ulcer disease, and this diagnosis appears to be increasing in relative frequency as Helicobacter pylori prevalence declines in many populations, meaning that a growing proportion of the ulcers a clinician encounters will not fit either of the two classic etiologic categories. Idiopathic ulcers tend to have a higher rate of recurrence and complication than Helicobacter pylori-associated ulcers treated with successful eradication, and management centers on long-term maintenance acid suppression, since there is no specific causative factor to eliminate, combined with the same systematic reassessment for occult nonsteroidal anti-inflammatory drug use, unrecognized Helicobacter pylori infection with a false-negative test, or a hypersecretory state described in the refractory ulcer disease discussion later in this chapter, since an ulcer labeled idiopathic after an incomplete workup is a different clinical situation than one genuinely idiopathic after all identifiable causes have been carefully excluded. Documenting the specific evaluation steps completed before assigning this label protects against the diagnosis being used as a default explanation when the workup was simply incomplete.

## Peptic Ulcer Disease

### Clinical Presentation and Differential Diagnosis

Epigastric pain is the dominant symptom of peptic ulcer disease, and its relationship to meals carries diagnostic weight, though imperfectly: duodenal ulcer pain classically improves with eating and recurs two to three hours later as acid is again delivered unbuffered to the ulcer base, while gastric ulcer pain is more variably related to meals and can be provoked or worsened by eating in some patients, a distinction useful as a general pattern but not reliable enough to substitute for endoscopic confirmation when the diagnosis carries management consequences. A substantial proportion of peptic ulcers, particularly among older adults and patients on chronic nonsteroidal anti-inflammatory drug therapy, are entirely asymptomatic until a complication, most commonly bleeding, brings the patient to medical attention, which is part of why nonsteroidal anti-inflammatory drug risk stratification, discussed below, matters even for patients without current dyspeptic symptoms. This distinction is useful but never definitive on its own.

### NSAID-Induced Ulcers and Risk Stratification

Nonsteroidal anti-inflammatory drug-induced ulcers arise through the cyclooxygenase-1 inhibition mechanism described earlier in this chapter, a mechanism entirely independent of Helicobacter pylori infection, and the two risk factors are additive rather than substitutive, meaning that a patient with both an active infection and ongoing nonsteroidal anti-inflammatory drug use carries a substantially higher ulcer risk than either factor alone would predict, which is why testing for and treating Helicobacter pylori is recommended before initiating chronic nonsteroidal anti-inflammatory drug therapy in appropriate candidates. Gastrointestinal risk from nonsteroidal anti-inflammatory drug use is stratified by the presence of prior ulcer history, particularly a prior complicated ulcer, age, concurrent use of anticoagulants, corticosteroids, or additional antiplatelet agents, and the specific agent and dose used, since cyclooxygenase-2 selective agents carry a meaningfully lower gastrointestinal risk than nonselective agents at equivalent anti-inflammatory efficacy, though this benefit must be weighed against the cardiovascular risk associated with cyclooxygenase-2 selective agents in appropriate patients.

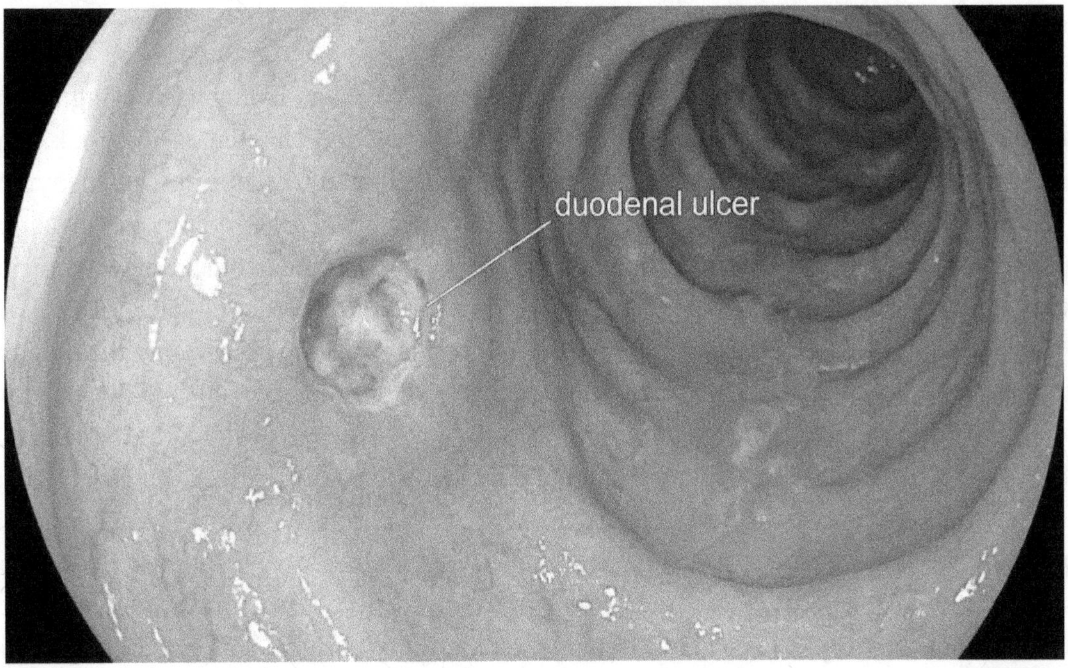


**THE GI THRESHOLD DECISION SYSTEM — Gastric Thresholds — NSAID Gastrointestinal Risk Stratification and Gastroprotection**

**Presentation Signature:** A patient requires ongoing nonsteroidal anti-inflammatory drug therapy for a chronic condition such as osteoarthritis, and the clinician must decide whether gastroprotective co-therapy is warranted.

**Threshold Point:** A prior complicated ulcer, age over 65, or concurrent anticoagulant, corticosteroid, or antiplatelet use each independently raises risk into a category warranting gastroprotection; the presence of two or more such factors defines a high-risk category warranting the most protective strategy available.

**The Call:** Low-risk patients may use a nonselective nonsteroidal anti-inflammatory drug without additional gastroprotection; moderate-risk patients warrant either a cyclooxygenase-2 selective agent or a nonselective agent combined with a proton pump inhibitor; high-risk patients warrant a cyclooxygenase-2 selective agent combined with a proton pump inhibitor, and Helicobacter pylori status should be confirmed and treated if positive in any patient beginning chronic therapy at moderate or higher risk.

**Trap Logic:** Risk factors are frequently assessed individually rather than cumulatively; a patient with two moderate risk factors is not equivalent to a low-risk patient and should not receive a low-risk gastroprotection strategy simply because no single factor appeared severe in isolation.

**Decision Anchor:** Stratify nonsteroidal anti-inflammatory drug gastrointestinal risk cumulatively, not by any single factor in isolation, before selecting an agent and gastroprotective strategy, and confirm Helicobacter pylori status before initiating chronic therapy in at-risk patients.

### Complications: Bleeding, Perforation, and Obstruction

Bleeding is the most common complication of peptic ulcer disease and is managed using the endoscopic risk-stratification and hemostasis principles developed in the second chapter of this book, applying the Forrest classification to guide both endoscopic therapy and inpatient monitoring intensity. Perforation presents with sudden, severe abdominal pain and peritoneal signs, most commonly from an anterior duodenal ulcer perforating into the peritoneal cavity, and is a surgical emergency requiring prompt recognition using the same threshold-based reasoning developed in the first chapter for acute abdominal pain, with free air on upright chest radiograph or cross-sectional imaging confirming the diagnosis before urgent surgical repair. Gastric outlet obstruction, resulting from chronic scarring and edema at the pylorus or duodenal bulb from recurrent ulceration, presents with early satiety, postprandial vomiting of poorly digested food, and weight loss, and its management begins with nasogastric decompression and correction of the metabolic alkalosis and electrolyte derangements that chronic vomiting produces, followed by endoscopic evaluation to distinguish a benign, fibrotic stricture, which may respond to endoscopic balloon dilation, from a malignant cause, which requires an entirely different oncologic management pathway. Coordinating gastroenterology and general or acute care surgery early in a suspected perforation, rather than sequentially after each specialty has independently reached its own conclusion, shortens the interval to definitive repair meaningfully.

### Medical Management and Confirming Healing

Medical management of peptic ulcer disease centers on proton pump inhibitor therapy dosed once daily for a duration determined by ulcer size, complexity, and etiology, generally eight weeks for an uncomplicated duodenal ulcer and somewhat longer for a larger or gastric ulcer, combined with elimination of the causative factor whenever possible, meaning Helicobacter pylori eradication when infection is present and discontinuation or substitution of the causative nonsteroidal anti-inflammatory drug when feasible. Gastric ulcers, unlike duodenal ulcers, require confirmatory follow-up endoscopy to document complete healing, because a gastric ulcer can represent an ulcerated malignancy at initial presentation, and biopsy of the ulcer margin at the index endoscopy, combined with repeat endoscopy to confirm healing after an adequate treatment course, is the standard approach to excluding this possibility; a gastric ulcer that has not healed or has enlarged at follow-up endoscopy requires further evaluation for malignancy rather than simply extending medical therapy further.

### Helicobacter Pylori Eradication and Gastric Cancer Risk Reduction

Population-level and randomized data support Helicobacter pylori eradication as an effective gastric cancer prevention strategy, with the greatest risk reduction observed when eradication is achieved before atrophic gastritis and intestinal metaplasia have already developed, which is the rationale behind population-based test-and-treat and screen-and-treat programs implemented in several high-incidence regions and behind the recommendation to test and treat first-degree relatives of patients with gastric cancer regardless of symptoms. In a patient who already has established atrophic gastritis or intestinal metaplasia at the time of eradication, the risk-reduction benefit, while still present, is attenuated relative to eradication performed before these changes develop, which is why eradicated patients with these findings on biopsy are generally continued on an endoscopic surveillance program rather than considered to have returned to average population risk simply because the infection has been successfully treated. This distinction should be communicated clearly to patients: eradication treats the infection and reduces future risk, but it does not reverse existing atrophic or metaplastic changes, and surveillance recommendations are based on the histologic findings present at the time of diagnosis, not on eradication status alone. Clinicians should frame eradication to patients as risk reduction rather than risk elimination, an important distinction for setting appropriate expectations about ongoing surveillance.

**Reactive and Chemical Gastropathy**

Reactive, or chemical, gastropathy describes mucosal changes distinct from the inflammatory infiltrate that defines true gastritis, characterized instead by foveolar hyperplasia, edema, and smooth muscle proliferation within the lamina propria with relatively little inflammatory cell infiltration, and it most commonly results from chronic bile reflux, particularly in patients who have undergone gastric surgery that disrupts the normal pyloric barrier to duodenal content reflux, or from chronic nonsteroidal anti-inflammatory drug use through a direct chemical irritant effect distinct from the systemic prostaglandin-mediated mechanism discussed earlier in this chapter. The histologic distinction between reactive gastropathy and true gastritis matters clinically because the two conditions, despite some overlapping endoscopic appearance, have different management implications: reactive gastropathy from bile reflux is managed with bile acid sequestrants or, in severe post-surgical cases, surgical revision to restore a more physiologic anatomic configuration, rather than with the acid suppression or antimicrobial therapy that would be directed at Helicobacter pylori-associated gastritis. Because reactive gastropathy lacks the prominent inflammatory infiltrate of true gastritis, its diagnosis depends on histologic review by a pathologist specifically attentive to this distinction rather than on endoscopic appearance alone, which can overlap substantially between the two conditions.

**Portal Hypertensive Gastropathy**

Portal hypertensive gastropathy, a mucosal change distinct from both true gastritis and reactive gastropathy, arises from chronically elevated portal venous pressure in patients with cirrhosis, producing a characteristic mosaic or snakeskin endoscopic appearance from congested, ectatic mucosal and submucosal vessels, and, in severe cases, chronic or acute gastrointestinal blood loss. Unlike the acid- or inflammation-driven gastric conditions discussed elsewhere in this chapter, portal hypertensive gastropathy is managed by addressing the underlying portal hypertension itself, most commonly with nonselective beta-blockade to reduce portal pressure, rather than with acid suppression, antibiotics, or any of the other therapies directed at conventional gastritis, a distinction that becomes clinically important when a cirrhotic patient with chronic, low-grade gastrointestinal blood loss is evaluated, since this entity, and the closely related gastric antral vascular ectasia discussed in a later chapter on cirrhosis and portal hypertension, are common and easily overlooked causes of chronic anemia in this population if the endoscopic findings are not specifically recognized and distinguished from ordinary gastritis. Endoscopic banding or thermal therapy has a limited and generally disappointing role in portal hypertensive gastropathy given its diffuse rather than focal vascular pattern, reinforcing why portal-pressure-directed therapy, not endoscopic hemostasis, is the primary management strategy.

## Gastritis: Classification and Special Forms

### Acute Versus Chronic Gastritis

Acute gastritis, an inflammatory process of rapid onset, is most commonly caused by nonsteroidal anti-inflammatory drug use, alcohol, or acute Helicobacter pylori infection, and it is generally self-limited once the causative exposure is removed, though it can occasionally present with significant erosive bleeding, particularly in the setting of critical illness, discussed further below as stress-related mucosal disease. Chronic gastritis, by contrast, reflects a sustained inflammatory process, most commonly from chronic Helicobacter pylori infection as described earlier in this chapter, and its histologic classification, using a system such as the updated Sydney system, characterizes both the pattern, antral, corpus, or pangastritis, and the degree of atrophy and intestinal metaplasia present, information that carries direct implications for gastric cancer risk stratification and, in some patients, for a decision to pursue endoscopic surveillance. The operative link staging system, which combines histologic scoring of atrophy across multiple standardized biopsy sites into a single stage, further refines this risk stratification and is increasingly used to guide surveillance intervals in patients with confirmed atrophic gastritis, particularly higher stages associated with a meaningfully elevated gastric cancer risk relative to lower stages.

### Autoimmune Gastritis and Pernicious Anemia

Autoimmune gastritis results from immune-mediated destruction of gastric parietal cells, driven by autoantibodies directed against the parietal cell proton pump and against intrinsic factor, and this selective corpus-predominant destruction produces a distinctive clinical and laboratory pattern distinct from Helicobacter pylori-related gastritis: achlorhydria from loss of acid-secreting parietal cells, compensatory hypergastrinemia as the antral G cells respond to the absent acid feedback, and, because intrinsic factor produced by parietal cells is required for vitamin B12 absorption in the terminal ileum, progressive vitamin B12 deficiency culminating in pernicious anemia if the condition remains unrecognized and untreated. The hypergastrinemia in autoimmune gastritis, while a direct physiologic consequence of achlorhydria rather than a primary neuroendocrine process, drives hyperplasia of gastric enterochromaffin-like cells that carries a modestly increased long-term risk of type 1 gastric neuroendocrine tumors, small, usually indolent lesions that are managed with endoscopic surveillance and, when they enlarge or multiply beyond a defined threshold, endoscopic resection, in contrast to the more aggressive behavior of sporadic gastric neuroendocrine tumors arising outside this hypergastrinemic context. Patients with confirmed autoimmune gastritis require lifelong vitamin B12 monitoring and repletion and, given an associated increased risk of gastric adenocarcinoma related to the same atrophic, metaplastic mucosal changes seen in advanced Helicobacter pylori-related chronic gastritis, are generally considered for periodic endoscopic surveillance. Screening for autoimmune gastritis should be considered in a patient with unexplained vitamin B12 deficiency or iron deficiency without an identified gastrointestinal source, since the same corpus-predominant process can impair iron absorption before overt B12 deficiency becomes apparent.

## Stress-Related Mucosal Disease and Prophylaxis

Stress-related mucosal disease describes acute, often multiple, superficial gastric erosions or ulcers arising in critically ill patients, driven by impaired mucosal blood flow and prostaglandin-mediated protection during states of hemodynamic compromise, mechanical ventilation, or severe coagulopathy, and its clinical significance lies primarily in its potential to cause clinically significant bleeding in an already critically ill patient population poorly positioned to tolerate additional hemodynamic stress. Pharmacologic stress ulcer prophylaxis, most commonly with a proton pump inhibitor or histamine-2 receptor antagonist, is indicated in critically ill patients meeting specific risk criteria, most importantly mechanical ventilation anticipated to exceed 48 hours or a significant coagulopathy, rather than applied uniformly to every intensive care unit admission, since indiscriminate prophylaxis in lower-risk patients exposes them to the infectious and other risks of acid suppression discussed in the previous chapter without a proportionate reduction in clinically significant bleeding risk; prophylaxis should also be discontinued once the qualifying risk factor resolves rather than continued through hospital discharge by default, a transition-of-care point at which unnecessary acid suppression is commonly, and avoidably, perpetuated. This targeted, criteria-based approach to prophylaxis mirrors the general principle, developed throughout this book, that a preventive intervention should be matched to a defined risk threshold rather than applied by default.

## Silent Presentation and Special Considerations in Older Adults

Older adults, and particularly those on chronic nonsteroidal anti-inflammatory drug therapy, frequently develop peptic ulcer disease without the typical epigastric pain pattern described earlier in this chapter, a phenomenon attributed to age-related and medication-related blunting of visceral pain perception, meaning that a first presentation with a complication, most commonly bleeding, is disproportionately common in this population relative to younger patients who more often present with symptomatic, uncomplicated disease. This silent presentation pattern reinforces why the cumulative nonsteroidal anti-inflammatory drug risk stratification developed earlier in this chapter must be applied proactively, before symptoms occur, rather than reactively once a patient reports dyspepsia, since a substantial proportion of older, high-risk patients will never report a warning symptom before a complication develops. Polypharmacy further complicates management in this population, since concurrent anticoagulant or antiplatelet therapy, common in older adults with cardiovascular disease, both increases bleeding risk from any ulcer that does form and complicates the timing and safety of any endoscopic intervention that becomes necessary, reinforcing the value of proactive gastroprotection over reactive management after a complication has already occurred. Routine, low-threshold screening for anemia in this population, rather than waiting for a symptomatic presentation, is a reasonable extension of this reasoning.

### Other Causes of Refractory or Atypical Ulcer Disease

Zollinger-Ellison syndrome is the most classically taught cause of refractory ulcer disease, but it is not the only one, and a systematic evaluation of refractory disease should also consider surreptitious or unrecognized nonsteroidal anti-inflammatory drug use, which patients may underreport for the reasons discussed in the first chapter's history-taking section, incomplete Helicobacter pylori eradication that was never confirmed with appropriate follow-up testing, Crohn disease involving the stomach or duodenum, which can produce ulceration with a distinct histologic and endoscopic pattern once biopsied, cytomegalovirus infection in an immunocompromised patient, and, rarely, an underlying malignancy misclassified initially as a benign peptic ulcer, which is precisely why gastric ulcers specifically require the confirmatory healing endoscopy with biopsy described earlier in this chapter. A systematic reassessment of each of these possibilities, rather than an assumption that the original diagnosis and treatment plan must simply need more time, is the appropriate response to any peptic ulcer that fails to behave as expected.

## Management of Zollinger-Ellison Syndrome

Once Zollinger-Ellison syndrome is confirmed and localized, management proceeds along two parallel tracks that should be pursued simultaneously rather than sequentially: acid-related symptom control and oncologic management of the underlying tumor, since a patient can experience ongoing hypersecretory symptoms even while curative or palliative tumor treatment is being arranged, and inadequately controlled acid hypersecretion in the interim carries its own risk of ulcer complications. Clear documentation of which team owns each track prevents either from being neglected.

### Acid Suppression in Zollinger-Ellison Syndrome

Proton pump inhibitor dosing in Zollinger-Ellison syndrome is substantially higher than standard peptic ulcer disease dosing, often requiring two to three times the usual maximum dose divided across multiple daily administrations to adequately control the markedly elevated acid output characteristic of this condition, and dose titration is guided by direct measurement of gastric acid output or, more practically in routine care, by symptom control and endoscopic confirmation of mucosal healing rather than by a fixed, one-size-fits-all dosing regimen. Lifelong acid suppression is required in patients with unresectable or metastatic disease, and even in patients who undergo apparently curative resection, acid suppression is generally continued initially and only carefully weaned under close monitoring, since biochemical cure can take time to confirm definitively and a premature discontinuation of therapy in a patient who is not yet confirmed cured risks a symptomatic and potentially complicated recurrence of hypersecretory disease. This titration is individualized and reassessed periodically rather than fixed at a single starting dose indefinitely.

### Oncologic Management and Surveillance

Surgical resection of a localized, sporadic gastrinoma, performed at a center experienced in pancreaticoduodenal neuroendocrine tumor surgery, offers the best chance of biochemical cure, confirmed postoperatively with a normalized fasting gastrin and, when available, a negative secretin stimulation test, while unresectable, metastatic, or multiple endocrine neoplasia type 1-associated multifocal disease is managed with a combination of long-term acid suppression, somatostatin analogue therapy to control both symptoms and, in some cases, tumor growth, and, for progressive or higher-grade disease, systemic oncologic therapy directed by a multidisciplinary neuroendocrine tumor team. Long-term surveillance, including periodic biochemical testing and imaging, continues indefinitely in all patients given both the possibility of late recurrence after apparently curative resection and the malignant potential, albeit often slow-growing, inherent to this tumor type. This surveillance is lifelong regardless of initial treatment success.

## Zollinger-Ellison Syndrome and Refractory Ulcer Disease

### When to Suspect Gastrinoma

Zollinger-Ellison syndrome, caused by a gastrin-secreting neuroendocrine tumor, most commonly located in the duodenum or pancreas, should be suspected in a patient with peptic ulcer disease that is severe, multiple, located in an atypical distal duodenal or jejunal location, or recurrent or refractory despite adequate acid suppression and confirmed absence of both Helicobacter pylori infection and nonsteroidal anti-inflammatory drug use, since the combination of a negative standard etiologic workup and refractory or atypical disease is precisely the pattern that should redirect diagnostic reasoning toward a hypersecretory cause rather than toward simply escalating standard acid-suppressive therapy further. Diarrhea, resulting from the direct effect of markedly elevated gastric acid delivery overwhelming duodenal and proximal small bowel buffering capacity and inactivating pancreatic enzymes, frequently accompanies the ulcer disease in Zollinger-Ellison syndrome and, when present alongside atypical or refractory peptic ulceration, further strengthens the suspicion for this diagnosis. Zollinger-Ellison syndrome occurs sporadically in the majority of cases but is associated with multiple endocrine neoplasia type 1 in a meaningful minority, which is why a family history of endocrine tumors or the presence of other multiple endocrine neoplasia type 1-associated findings, such as hyperparathyroidism, should be specifically elicited once the diagnosis is being considered. Screening for other multiple endocrine neoplasia type 1-associated tumors, including pituitary and additional pancreatic neuroendocrine lesions, is warranted once this association is suspected or confirmed.

### Diagnostic Evaluation

A fasting serum gastrin level is the initial test when Zollinger-Ellison syndrome is suspected, obtained after proton pump inhibitor therapy has been held for the interval necessary to avoid a false-positive result, since acid suppression itself, through the same negative feedback loop discussed in the autoimmune gastritis section above, elevates serum gastrin, meaning that a markedly elevated gastrin level obtained while a patient remains on standard-dose therapy cannot reliably distinguish medication effect from a true gastrinoma. A markedly elevated fasting gastrin level in the setting of an inappropriately low gastric pH, confirmed by direct gastric pH measurement at the time of testing, is diagnostic, while a borderline elevation requires a secretin stimulation test, which exploits the paradoxical further rise in gastrin produced by secretin administration in a gastrinoma, a paradoxical response not seen in other causes of hypergastrinemia, including the achlorhydria-driven hypergastrinemia of autoimmune gastritis discussed earlier in this chapter, providing the discriminating step between these otherwise overlapping hypergastrinemic states. Once biochemically confirmed, cross-sectional and, increasingly, somatostatin-receptor-based nuclear imaging localize the tumor for surgical planning, since resection of a localized, sporadic gastrinoma offers the possibility of cure, in contrast to the lifelong medical management required for unresectable, metastatic, or multiple endocrine neoplasia type 1-associated multifocal disease. This sequencing avoids an unnecessary additional test in most confirmed cases.

Case Presentation: A 42-year-old woman is referred for a duodenal ulcer identified on endoscopy performed for epigastric pain and diarrhea. Biopsies are negative for Helicobacter pylori, and she denies any nonsteroidal anti-inflammatory drug use. Despite eight weeks of standard-dose proton pump inhibitor therapy, repeat endoscopy shows the ulcer only partially healed, and a second ulcer is now identified in the distal duodenum, an atypical location. Applying the reasoning developed in this chapter, a refractory, atypically located ulcer with confirmed absence of both major identifiable causes, combined with accompanying diarrhea, should prompt evaluation for Zollinger-Ellison syndrome rather than a further empiric increase in acid suppression alone. Proton pump inhibitor therapy is held for the appropriate interval, and a fasting serum gastrin returns markedly elevated at more than ten times the upper limit of normal, with a concurrently low gastric pH, meeting criteria for a biochemically confirmed diagnosis without need for secretin stimulation testing. Cross-sectional imaging identifies a 1.5-centimeter pancreatic head lesion, and somatostatin-receptor imaging confirms a single site of disease without evidence of metastasis. She is referred for surgical resection, with the goal of cure given the localized, apparently sporadic nature of the tumor. This case illustrates the chapter's closing principle: refractory or atypical ulcer disease, once the two dominant causes have been genuinely excluded rather than assumed away, should prompt a specific, threshold-driven evaluation for a hypersecretory cause rather than an open-ended escalation of standard therapy.

Case Presentation: A 78-year-old woman with osteoarthritis on daily ibuprofen for the past two years, atrial fibrillation on apixaban, and a history of a bleeding gastric ulcer eight years earlier presents to the emergency department with dizziness and dark stools noted by her daughter, without any preceding abdominal pain. She has not seen a physician regarding her ibuprofen use since starting it. Applying the cumulative risk-stratification reasoning developed in this chapter, this patient carries multiple independently significant risk factors, a prior complicated ulcer, concurrent anticoagulation, and age over 65, placing her in the highest nonsteroidal anti-inflammatory drug gastrointestinal risk category, and her silent presentation without preceding pain is consistent with the blunted symptom perception discussed above rather than an atypical or unlikely presentation. She is found to have a hemoglobin of 7.1 grams per deciliter and a shock index above 1.0, prompting immediate resuscitation per the threshold reasoning from the first chapter, and apixaban is held while reversal is considered in coordination with cardiology given her ongoing bleeding. Upper endoscopy identifies a Forrest Ib actively oozing gastric ulcer, treated with combination endoscopic hemostatic therapy. Once stabilized, the case is used as an explicit opportunity to review her nonsteroidal anti-inflammatory drug use: given her risk category, ibuprofen is discontinued entirely rather than merely paired with gastroprotection, and alternative analgesic strategies for her osteoarthritis are discussed with her primary care physician. This case illustrates why cumulative risk stratification must be applied proactively rather than only after a complication has already occurred, and why a silent presentation in a high-risk patient should not be treated as reassuring simply because no earlier warning symptom was reported.

| Feature | Helicobacter pylori Ulcer | NSAID-Induced Ulcer | Zollinger-Ellison Syndrome |
|---|---|---|---|
| Typical location | Duodenal bulb or antrum | Anywhere in stomach or duodenum | Distal duodenum or jejunum (atypical) |
| Diagnostic test | Biopsy, urea breath test, stool antigen | Clinical history of NSAID use | Fasting gastrin, secretin stimulation |
| Key associated finding | Chronic gastritis pattern on biopsy | Often asymptomatic until complication | Diarrhea, multiple or refractory ulcers |
| Primary treatment | Antibiotic eradication regimen | Discontinue NSAID, acid suppression | Tumor localization and resection or lifelong PPI |

## THE GI THRESHOLD DECISION SYSTEM — Gastric and Peptic Disease Thresholds

**Presentation Signature:** This chapter's threshold instances addressed dyspepsia pathway selection and cumulative NSAID gastrointestinal risk stratification, two of the highest-volume decisions in general gastroenterology practice.

**Threshold Point:** Age and alarm features determine the dyspepsia pathway; the cumulative count of independent risk factors, not any single factor, determines the NSAID gastroprotection strategy.

**The Call:** Both thresholds convert a common, often low-acuity presentation into a specific, resource-appropriate pathway, avoiding both under-evaluation of a potentially serious process and over-testing of a genuinely low-risk patient.

**Trap Logic:** Treating alarm-feature assessment as optional in a reassuring-seeming dyspepsia presentation, and treating NSAID risk factors individually rather than cumulatively, are the two most common misapplications of this chapter's thresholds.

**Decision Anchor:** Age and alarm features gate the dyspepsia pathway; cumulative risk factor count gates the NSAID gastroprotection strategy. Refractory or atypical disease, once the two dominant causes are genuinely excluded, earns a specific hypersecretory workup rather than open-ended escalation.

## Summary and Key Concepts

Gastric acid secretion converges on the proton pump through three stimulatory pathways, explaining why proton pump inhibitors achieve more complete suppression than agents targeting a single pathway.

Helicobacter pylori testing strategy depends on whether endoscopy is already planned, and results are affected by recent acid suppression or antibiotic use, which must be accounted for before testing.

Bismuth or non-bismuth quadruple therapy for fourteen days has largely supplanted clarithromycin triple therapy given rising resistance, and eradication should be confirmed in every treated patient.

NSAID-induced and Helicobacter pylori-induced ulcers arise through independent, additive mechanisms, and NSAID gastrointestinal risk should be stratified cumulatively across all relevant risk factors before selecting an agent and gastroprotective strategy.

Autoimmune gastritis produces a distinctive pattern of achlorhydria, hypergastrinemia, and vitamin B12 deficiency, and carries increased risk for both gastric neuroendocrine tumors and gastric adenocarcinoma.

Refractory or atypically located peptic ulcer disease, once Helicobacter pylori and NSAID use are genuinely excluded, should prompt evaluation for Zollinger-Ellison syndrome with a fasting gastrin level obtained off acid suppression.

# CHAPTER 6: FUNCTIONAL DYSPEPSIA AND GASTROPARESIS

**Learning Objectives**

1. Apply the Rome IV criteria to diagnose functional dyspepsia and distinguish its postprandial distress and epigastric pain subtypes.
2. Explain the pathophysiologic mechanisms, including impaired gastric accommodation and visceral hypersensitivity, that underlie functional dyspepsia.
3. Identify the major etiologies of gastroparesis and select appropriate diagnostic testing to confirm delayed gastric emptying.
4. Apply a stepwise dietary, pharmacologic, and procedural approach to gastroparesis management.
5. Distinguish functional dyspepsia from gastroparesis and recognize related disorders including rumination syndrome and cyclic vomiting syndrome.

**Chapter Outline**

This chapter addresses the two dominant disorders of gastric symptom generation without a structural or infectious explanation: functional dyspepsia, a disorder of gut-brain interaction defined by the Rome IV criteria and developed here as the expected outcome for most patients whose peptic ulcer and Helicobacter pylori workup, discussed in the previous chapter, is unrevealing, and gastroparesis, a disorder of delayed gastric emptying with a distinct diagnostic and management pathway. The chapter closes with related disorders, rumination syndrome, supragastric belching, and cyclic vomiting syndrome, that share overlapping presentations and are frequently misdiagnosed as one of the two primary conditions.

## Dietary and Complementary Approaches Across Gastric Motility Disorders

Beyond the disease-specific dietary modifications already discussed for gastroparesis, general principles of meal structuring, smaller and more frequent meals, adequate mastication, and avoidance of carbonated beverages, which introduce additional gastric distension, benefit patients across the spectrum of disorders addressed in this chapter, including functional dyspepsia, where a formal trial of a low-fat diet and smaller meal size is a reasonable adjunct to pharmacologic therapy even though the evidence base is less robust than for gastroparesis specifically. Introducing these general measures early, even before a definitive subtype or etiology is established, gives the patient an immediate, actionable starting point while further evaluation proceeds.

**Complementary and Integrative Approaches**

Ginger has modest evidence supporting a prokinetic and antiemetic effect and is a reasonable, low-risk adjunct across several of the conditions discussed in this chapter, though it should be positioned to patients as a complement to, not a replacement for, the evidence-based pharmacologic and behavioral therapies developed throughout this chapter. Acupuncture and gut-directed hypnotherapy have accumulating evidence in functional dyspepsia and related disorders of gut-brain interaction specifically, and referral to practitioners experienced in gastrointestinal applications of these techniques is a reasonable option for patients who prefer to minimize pharmacologic therapy or who have had an incomplete response to the standard sequence developed in this chapter, again positioned as complementary to, rather than a substitute for, the core management pathway. Discussing complementary options openly, rather than dismissing patient interest in them outright, also strengthens the therapeutic relationship and keeps the patient engaged with, rather than seeking outside, the overall care plan.

### Setting Long-Term Expectations

Both functional dyspepsia and gastroparesis are chronic, relapsing-remitting conditions for the majority of affected patients, and setting this expectation explicitly at the time of diagnosis, rather than allowing the patient to assume that a single successful treatment course will produce permanent resolution, supports more realistic long-term engagement with the periodic reassessment and treatment adjustment that these conditions typically require over time. A written summary of the working diagnosis, the current treatment plan, and the specific criteria that would prompt escalation to the next step in the pathway, following the concrete, plan-anchored communication principle emphasized throughout this book, helps patients navigate what can otherwise feel like an open-ended, indefinite course of trial-and-error treatment adjustments. Revisiting this written plan at each follow-up visit, rather than drafting it once and setting it aside, keeps both clinician and patient aligned as the treatment pathway is adjusted over time.

## Overlap With Other Functional Gastrointestinal Disorders

Functional dyspepsia frequently coexists with other disorders of gut-brain interaction, most commonly irritable bowel syndrome, discussed in detail in a later chapter, and this overlap is common enough that clinicians should specifically ask about lower gastrointestinal symptoms, altered bowel habits, and abdominal pain patterns distinct from the upper abdominal symptoms that define functional dyspepsia, in any patient presenting with one of these disorders, since recognizing coexisting conditions changes the overall symptom burden being addressed and can inform a more unified treatment approach, particularly when a single agent, such as a neuromodulator, may address symptoms across multiple regions of the gastrointestinal tract simultaneously rather than requiring an entirely separate treatment plan for each labeled condition. Gastroesophageal reflux disease symptoms also overlap substantially with functional dyspepsia, and the two conditions coexist frequently enough that a patient's reflux symptoms, evaluated using the reasoning developed in the third chapter, should be assessed and, if present, treated as their own entity rather than assumed to be fully explained by a functional dyspepsia diagnosis or vice versa. Documenting all coexisting functional diagnoses together in a single, unified assessment, rather than as a scattered list added over successive visits, helps every subsequent clinician see the full picture at a glance.

### The Broader Concept of Disorders of Gut-Brain Interaction

Functional dyspepsia, gastroparesis in its symptom overlap, irritable bowel syndrome, functional heartburn, and the rumination and belching disorders discussed later in this chapter are increasingly understood not as a collection of unrelated diagnoses but as related expressions of a shared underlying vulnerability in gut-brain signaling, varying in which gut region and which specific mechanism, motor, sensory, or both, predominates in a given patient. This unifying framework has practical value beyond its conceptual elegance: it explains why neuromodulator therapy, a treatment class that might seem mismatched to a gastrointestinal complaint at first glance, has a consistent evidence base across this entire family of disorders, and it supports a management philosophy that treats the whole patient's gut-brain symptom burden holistically rather than pursuing an increasingly narrow, organ-specific diagnostic and therapeutic pathway for each individual symptom in isolation.

### Epidemiology and Impact

Functional dyspepsia affects a substantial proportion of the general population at some point, making it, alongside irritable bowel syndrome, one of the most common disorders encountered in both primary care and gastroenterology practice, and its impact extends well beyond the physical symptoms themselves, with affected patients reporting meaningfully reduced quality of life, work productivity, and, in some studies, healthcare utilization and cost comparable to other chronic gastrointestinal conditions with more visible structural pathology, an impact that is sometimes underappreciated precisely because the condition lacks the structural findings that more readily prompt clinicians and patients alike to take a symptom complex seriously. Recognizing this burden explicitly helps counter the perception, sometimes implicit in how a functional diagnosis is delivered, that a condition without structural findings is inherently less significant or less deserving of a structured, committed treatment approach than a condition with a visible endoscopic or radiologic abnormality. Communicating this burden accurately to colleagues, payers, and patients alike supports appropriate resource allocation for a condition too often deprioritized relative to structurally visible disease.

## Functional Dyspepsia

### Rome IV Diagnostic Criteria and Subtypes

Functional dyspepsia is diagnosed by the Rome IV criteria, which require at least one of four symptoms, bothersome postprandial fullness, early satiation, epigastric pain, or epigastric burning, present for the last three months with symptom onset at least six months before diagnosis, in the absence of structural disease on upper endoscopy that would explain the symptoms, meaning that the diagnosis is one of positive symptom criteria combined with exclusion of an organic cause, not simply a label applied whenever endoscopy is negative. The criteria further divide functional dyspepsia into two overlapping subtypes based on which symptoms predominate: postprandial distress syndrome, characterized by meal-triggered fullness and early satiation, and epigastric pain syndrome, characterized by pain or burning not necessarily related to meals, and this distinction, while imperfect since many patients have features of both, carries treatment relevance because the two subtypes are thought to arise from at least partially distinct underlying mechanisms, developed in the following section, that respond preferentially to different first-line therapies. This exclusion step is not optional.

**Pathophysiology: Gastric Accommodation, Hypersensitivity, and Duodenal Factors**

Impaired gastric accommodation, the normal reflex relaxation of the proximal stomach that allows it to expand and store an ingested meal without a disproportionate rise in intragastric pressure, is a well-documented abnormality in a substantial subset of patients with postprandial distress syndrome, and its failure means that a normal meal volume produces premature, exaggerated fullness because the stomach cannot accommodate it in the physiologically expected way. Visceral hypersensitivity, an exaggerated perception of normal gastric distension, motility, or acid exposure, contributes to both subtypes and parallels the same mechanism discussed in earlier chapters for functional heartburn and functional esophageal disorders, reflecting a broader pattern of disordered gut-brain signaling that spans multiple regions of the gastrointestinal tract rather than being unique to the stomach. Increasing evidence implicates duodenal factors specifically, including low-grade duodenal eosinophilia and increased duodenal mucosal permeability, sometimes following an antecedent enteric infection, as a trigger for the altered sensorimotor signaling that produces symptoms, a post-infectious mechanistic pathway analogous to postinfectious irritable bowel syndrome discussed in a later chapter, and this emerging understanding has begun to inform investigational therapies targeting duodenal eosinophilic inflammation directly rather than gastric motility or acid alone. These mechanisms are not mutually exclusive, and many patients likely have some combination of accommodation failure, hypersensitivity, and duodenal contribution driving their individual symptom pattern.

**Figure 6.1: Gastric Emptying Scintigraphy Time-Activity Curve**

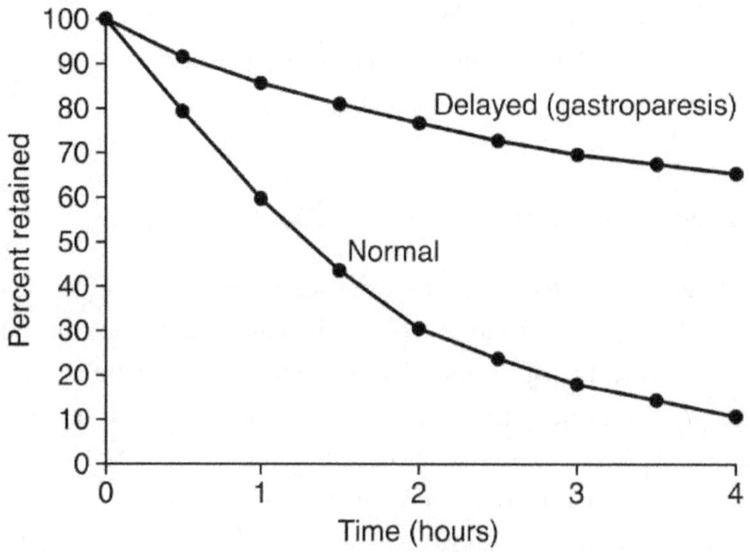

### Diagnostic Evaluation and Exclusion of Organic Disease

The diagnostic evaluation of suspected functional dyspepsia follows directly from the age- and alarm-feature-based reasoning developed in the previous chapter for dyspepsia broadly: a patient under 60 without alarm features may reasonably begin with Helicobacter pylori testing and, if negative or after successful eradication without symptom resolution, a trial of empiric therapy before endoscopy is pursued, while a patient 60 or older, or with any alarm feature, proceeds to upper endoscopy to exclude peptic ulcer disease, malignancy, and other structural causes before a functional diagnosis is assigned. Additional testing beyond endoscopy and Helicobacter pylori assessment is not routinely required to establish the diagnosis, and clinicians should resist the temptation to pursue an escalating series of additional tests, including repeated imaging or gastric emptying studies, in a patient whose presentation is otherwise typical for functional dyspepsia, since this pattern of repeated testing without a clear diagnostic hypothesis to test rarely changes management and can inadvertently reinforce a patient's concern that something serious is being missed. Discipline here avoids both diagnostic delay and diagnostic excess.

### Management: Acid Suppression, Prokinetics, and Neuromodulators

First-line management is guided by the predominant symptom subtype: a trial of proton pump inhibitor therapy is the preferred initial approach for epigastric pain syndrome, reflecting the overlapping role of acid-related hypersensitivity in this subtype even in the absence of demonstrable pathologic reflux, while a prokinetic agent, improving gastric accommodation and emptying, is preferred as initial therapy for postprandial distress syndrome, directly targeting the accommodation defect discussed above. Patients who do not respond adequately to an appropriately matched first-line agent, or who have mixed or refractory symptoms, are candidates for a neuromodulator, most commonly a low-dose tricyclic antidepressant, which reduces visceral hypersensitivity through the same central and peripheral mechanisms discussed in earlier chapters for functional heartburn and functional chest pain, reflecting the shared pathophysiology that links these disorders across different regions of the gastrointestinal tract. Reassess the match between subtype and agent at every follow-up visit.

### THE GI THRESHOLD DECISION SYSTEM — Gastric Motility Thresholds — Sequencing Therapy in Functional Dyspepsia

---

**Presentation Signature:** A patient with confirmed functional dyspepsia, subtyped as postprandial distress or epigastric pain predominant, requires a treatment sequence rather than a single default therapy.

**Threshold Point:** Symptom subtype at diagnosis determines the preferred first-line agent; inadequate response after an adequate trial, generally four to eight weeks, of the subtype-matched first-line agent defines the threshold for adding or switching to a neuromodulator.

**The Call:** Postprandial distress syndrome begins with a prokinetic; epigastric pain syndrome begins with a proton pump inhibitor; inadequate response in either subtype after an adequate trial prompts escalation to a low-dose tricyclic antidepressant or another neuromodulator rather than simply switching between the two first-line agents indefinitely.

**Trap Logic:** Prescribing a proton pump inhibitor and a prokinetic simultaneously as an undifferentiated first step, without regard to which subtype predominates, obscures which agent is actually responsible for any improvement and delays the more targeted, mechanism-based sequencing this threshold describes.

**Decision Anchor:** Match the first-line agent to the predominant symptom subtype, and reserve neuromodulator therapy for genuine first-line failure rather than starting multiple agents together without a plan to isolate what is working.

**PATIENT EDUCATION:** Explain functional dyspepsia as a disorder of gut sensation and movement, not as an absence of a real problem; patients who hear only that endoscopy was normal frequently interpret this as their symptoms being dismissed rather than as the expected, positive step toward a specific, mechanism-based treatment plan.

### The Role of Helicobacter Pylori Eradication in Functional Dyspepsia

Helicobacter pylori testing and eradication, when positive, is recommended as an initial step in the evaluation of dyspepsia broadly, as established in the previous chapter, and a specific subset of patients whose symptoms would otherwise be labeled functional dyspepsia experience durable symptom resolution after successful eradication alone, a response pattern sometimes termed Helicobacter pylori-associated dyspepsia, distinguishing them from patients whose symptoms persist despite eradication and who therefore meet the fuller definition of functional dyspepsia used in this chapter. Current Rome IV methodology specifically requires reassessment at least six months after successful eradication before functional dyspepsia is diagnosed in a previously infected patient, since symptom improvement following eradication can be delayed, and assigning a functional diagnosis prematurely, before this interval has elapsed, risks both an inaccurate diagnosis and premature initiation of neuromodulator or other functional-disease-directed therapy in a patient who might still respond to the infection's resolution alone. This nuance is easy to overlook in a busy practice but meaningfully affects both diagnostic accuracy and the timing of any subsequent therapy.

### Psychological Comorbidity and Integrated Care

Anxiety and depression are more prevalent among patients with functional dyspepsia than in the general population, and this association reflects the same bidirectional gut-brain signaling that underlies the disorder's core pathophysiology rather than implying that the gastrointestinal symptoms are merely psychological in origin or somehow less real, a distinction worth stating explicitly to patients who may otherwise interpret a mention of psychological comorbidity as a dismissal of their physical symptoms. Screening for anxiety and depression using a brief, validated instrument as a routine part of the functional dyspepsia evaluation identifies patients who may benefit from integrated behavioral health involvement, including cognitive behavioral therapy or gut-directed hypnotherapy, both of which have evidence supporting their use in functional gastrointestinal disorders more broadly and can be offered alongside, rather than instead of, the pharmacologic approaches developed in this chapter, particularly in patients whose symptoms remain refractory to an adequately sequenced trial of first-line and neuromodulator therapy. Framing this screening as a routine, universal part of the evaluation, applied to every patient rather than selectively to those who seem visibly distressed, avoids the perception that a mental health inquiry is being triggered by a specific judgment about that individual patient.

## Severity Classification and Its Clinical Use

Gastroparesis severity is commonly graded across a spectrum from mild disease, in which symptoms are intermittent and readily controlled with dietary modification and minimal pharmacotherapy, through compensated disease, in which symptoms are more persistent but nutritional status is maintained through dietary adjustment and medication, to gastroparic crisis or decompensated disease, in which the patient cannot maintain adequate nutrition or hydration by mouth and requires hospitalization for intravenous fluid support, antiemetic therapy, and, in some cases, temporary enteral or parenteral nutrition. This severity framework is clinically useful beyond its descriptive value because it maps directly onto the intensity of intervention warranted at each stage, mirroring the same principle of matching intervention intensity to disease severity that recurs throughout this book, and a patient's severity classification should be reassessed at each visit rather than fixed at the level assigned at initial diagnosis, since gastroparesis severity fluctuates over time, sometimes considerably, in response to glycemic control, medication changes, and other factors discussed throughout this chapter. Documenting the assigned severity level explicitly at each visit, rather than relying on an informal, unrecorded clinical impression, also supports continuity of care when a patient transitions between providers or is evaluated by a different member of a multidisciplinary team.

## Coordinating Care in Complex Gastroparesis

Complex or severe gastroparesis frequently requires coordination across gastroenterology, endocrinology when diabetes is the underlying etiology, nutrition services, and, for patients being evaluated for device-based or surgical intervention, a specialized motility or foregut surgery program, and applying the same explicit, plan-anchored coordination principle developed in earlier chapters prevents the diffusion of responsibility that can otherwise occur when multiple specialties are simultaneously involved in a single patient's care. A written, shared management plan specifying which service is responsible for glycemic optimization, which is responsible for nutritional monitoring and escalation, and which is responsible for reassessing motility-directed therapy, reviewed and updated at a defined interval rather than only when a crisis prompts reassessment, keeps a complex, multidisciplinary gastroparesis case from drifting into reactive, fragmented care. Regular multidisciplinary case conferences, where feasible, further support this coordination for the most complex cases, allowing each involved specialty to hear directly from the others rather than relying solely on written documentation to convey the current status and plan.

## Medication-Induced Delayed Gastric Emptying

Glucagon-like peptide-1 receptor agonists, increasingly prescribed for both type 2 diabetes and weight management, delay gastric emptying as part of their intended pharmacologic mechanism, and this expected, dose-related effect must be distinguished from primary gastroparesis, since the management implications differ substantially: dose adjustment or discontinuation of the causative medication, rather than initiation of gastroparesis-specific prokinetic therapy, is the appropriate first response in a patient whose delayed emptying developed temporally with initiation or dose escalation of one of these agents. Opioid-induced gastrointestinal dysfunction similarly slows gastric emptying as part of a broader pattern of opioid-related gut hypomotility that also affects the small bowel and colon, and in a patient on chronic opioid therapy presenting with symptoms suggestive of gastroparesis, a candid discussion of opioid tapering or rotation, applying the same direct, non-judgmental approach to substance-related history developed in the first chapter, should be part of the management discussion rather than adding prokinetic therapy on top of an unaddressed causative medication. Given the rapidly expanding use of glucagon-like peptide-1 receptor agonists specifically, clinicians should proactively ask about this medication class in any patient newly presenting with upper gastrointestinal symptoms suggestive of delayed emptying, since patients do not always volunteer a relatively new, non-gastrointestinal-labeled medication as relevant to their digestive symptoms. This distinction matters practically as well as diagnostically, since a patient incorrectly labeled with primary gastroparesis may be started on a prokinetic unnecessarily while the actual causative medication continues uninterrupted.

**Figure 6.2: Mechanism of Impaired Gastric Accommodation**

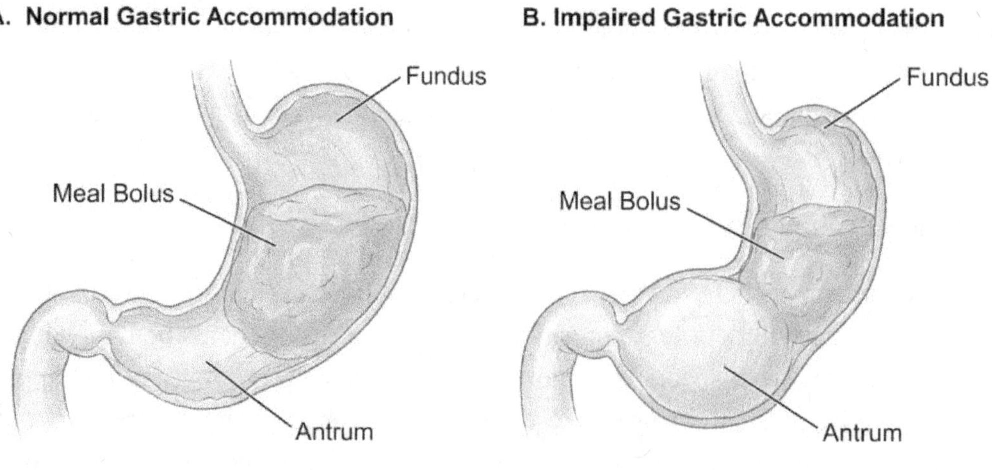


A. Normal Gastric Accommodation B. Impaired Gastric Accommodation

## Gastroparesis in Connective Tissue Disease and Other Systemic Conditions

Scleroderma-spectrum disease produces gastric hypomotility through the same smooth muscle atrophy and fibrosis mechanism discussed in earlier chapters for esophageal involvement, and gastroparesis in this population frequently coexists with the esophageal, small bowel, and colonic manifestations of the same systemic process, meaning that a patient with known scleroderma presenting with new upper gastrointestinal symptoms should be evaluated with an awareness that multiple levels of the gastrointestinal tract may be simultaneously affected rather than assuming an isolated, single-organ process. Amyloidosis, Parkinson disease, and other neurodegenerative and infiltrative conditions are less common but recognized causes of gastroparesis, generally identified through the broader systemic evaluation prompted by the primary underlying condition rather than through a gastroparesis-first diagnostic pathway, and their management follows the same general dietary, pharmacologic, and, when refractory, procedural framework developed in this chapter, adapted to the specific comorbidities and functional status of each affected patient. Coordinating with rheumatology on the overall disease-modifying treatment plan, rather than managing the gastrointestinal manifestations in isolation, reflects the same multidisciplinary coordination principle emphasized throughout this chapter.

## Gastroparesis

### Definition and Etiology

Gastroparesis is defined by objectively confirmed delayed gastric emptying in the absence of mechanical outlet obstruction, and this definition matters clinically because gastroparesis is a diagnosis that requires a positive confirmatory test, not merely a symptom pattern, distinguishing it from functional dyspepsia, in which emptying is typically normal or only mildly delayed and diagnosis rests on symptom criteria rather than an objective emptying threshold. Diabetes mellitus, through chronic hyperglycemia-mediated injury to the vagus nerve and to the interstitial cells of Cajal, the pacemaker cells that coordinate normal gastric motor activity, is among the most common identifiable causes, and postsurgical gastroparesis, following vagal nerve injury during esophageal, gastric, or bariatric surgery, is another well-recognized and clinically important cause; a substantial proportion of cases, however, remain idiopathic despite thorough evaluation, and other recognized causes include connective tissue disease, particularly scleroderma-spectrum disorders sharing the same smooth muscle pathology discussed in earlier chapters for esophageal involvement, certain medications, most notably opioids and glucagon-like peptide-1 receptor agonists, and, less commonly, a paraneoplastic or postviral process. Screening for and quantifying this broader autonomic and peripheral neuropathic burden at the time gastroparesis is diagnosed helps set realistic expectations for treatment response.

### Clinical Presentation and Differential Diagnosis

Nausea, vomiting of partially digested food, often hours after eating, early satiety, postprandial fullness, and bloating characterize gastroparesis, an overlapping symptom profile with postprandial distress syndrome functional dyspepsia that is precisely why objective emptying testing, rather than symptoms alone, is required to distinguish the two conditions. Weight loss and, in more severe or longstanding cases, malnutrition and dehydration from recurrent vomiting reflect a level of physiologic compromise beyond what is typically seen in functional dyspepsia and should prompt more urgent evaluation and more aggressive nutritional support planning, applying the nutritional screening principles introduced earlier in this book. Mechanical gastric outlet obstruction, whether from a peptic or malignant stricture as discussed in the previous chapter or from another structural cause, must be excluded by upper endoscopy before a diagnosis of gastroparesis is assigned, since obstruction and gastroparesis can present with an identical symptom pattern despite requiring entirely different management. A careful review of systems for symptoms suggesting broader diabetic autonomic neuropathy, including orthostatic symptoms, urinary retention, and erectile dysfunction where relevant, can further support the diagnosis when the etiology is presumed diabetic, since gastroparesis rarely occurs as an isolated manifestation of diabetic autonomic dysfunction.

**Diagnostic Evaluation: Gastric Emptying Scintigraphy and Alternatives**

Gastric emptying scintigraphy using a standardized, low-fat solid meal labeled with a radiotracer, with imaging performed at set intervals over four hours, is the reference standard test for confirming delayed gastric emptying, and the four-hour protocol specifically is important, because earlier protocols using shorter imaging durations produced a meaningfully higher false-negative rate by failing to capture delayed emptying that only becomes apparent in the later imaging time points. Medications that independently affect gastric emptying, most importantly opioids and glucagon-like peptide-1 receptor agonists, should be held before testing whenever it is safe to do so, since failing to account for their effect risks misattributing a medication effect to primary gastroparesis, a distinction with direct treatment implications since the management of medication-induced delayed emptying centers on addressing the causative medication rather than on the gastroparesis-specific therapies developed later in this section. The wireless motility capsule, introduced in the second chapter, and a stable isotope breath test using a labeled substrate are alternative methods of assessing gastric emptying, useful particularly when scintigraphy is unavailable or when a broader assessment of whole-gut transit is also desired. Cost and local availability often determine which alternative is used in practice when scintigraphy is not readily obtainable.

**Dietary and Pharmacologic Management**

Dietary modification is first-line therapy for gastroparesis and should be structured rather than generic: small, frequent meals reduce the volume the stomach must process at any one time; a low-fat, low-insoluble-fiber diet reduces the caloric and mechanical load that most slows gastric emptying, since fat delays emptying physiologically even in a normal stomach and indigestible fiber risks bezoar formation in a stomach that already empties poorly; and a shift toward more liquid or blenderized caloric intake in more severe cases exploits the observation that liquid emptying is often relatively preserved even when solid emptying is markedly delayed. Prokinetic pharmacotherapy, most commonly metoclopramide as the primary approved first-line agent in many regions, improves gastric emptying and symptoms, though its use requires explicit counseling about the risk of tardive dyskinesia with prolonged use and a defined plan to use the lowest effective dose for the shortest necessary duration, confirmed against current dosing guidance and periodically reassessed rather than continued indefinitely without reevaluation. Antiemetic therapy addresses symptom control directly and is used adjunctively alongside prokinetic and dietary measures rather than as a substitute for addressing gastric emptying itself, since symptom suppression without improving the underlying delayed emptying leaves the nutritional and metabolic consequences of the disease unaddressed. A registered dietitian with specific experience in gastroparesis is a valuable and often underused resource at this stage, translating these general principles into a concrete, individualized meal plan the patient can actually sustain. Both matter equally in a complete plan.

**Refractory Gastroparesis: Advanced Therapies**

Patients with gastroparesis refractory to dietary and pharmacologic management are candidates for more advanced interventions, selected based on the specific pattern of physiologic dysfunction identified. Gastric electrical stimulation, an implanted device delivering high-frequency, low-energy electrical stimulation to the stomach, improves nausea and vomiting in appropriately selected patients, particularly those with a diabetic etiology, though its effect on the underlying gastric emptying rate itself is more modest than its effect on symptoms, meaning that patient selection and counseling should focus on realistic symptom-control expectations rather than a promise of normalized emptying. Pyloric-directed therapies, including botulinum toxin injection, which despite mixed efficacy data retains a role in carefully selected patients as either a therapeutic or a prognostic trial before a more durable intervention, and per-oral endoscopic pyloromyotomy, a procedure structurally analogous to the esophageal peroral endoscopic myotomy discussed in the fourth chapter but targeting the pylorus instead, are directed specifically at patients whose gastroparesis is thought to be driven substantially by pylorospasm or inadequate pyloric relaxation, a subset increasingly identified using specialized manometric or impedance planimetry assessment of pyloric function. In the most severe, refractory cases with significant nutritional compromise, a venting gastrostomy for symptom palliation combined with a jejunostomy for enteral feeding distal to the poorly emptying stomach provides both symptomatic relief and nutritional support when other measures have failed. Patient selection for gastric electrical stimulation benefits, at some centers, from a period of temporary external stimulation testing to assess likely symptomatic benefit before committing to permanent device implantation, though practice varies regarding how routinely this trial period is used.

## THE GI THRESHOLD DECISION SYSTEM — Gastric Motility Thresholds — Escalating Gastroparesis Therapy by Severity

**Presentation Signature:** A patient with confirmed gastroparesis has already begun dietary modification and a first-line prokinetic, and the clinician must determine whether escalation to a more invasive therapy is warranted.

**Threshold Point:** Persistent, clinically significant symptoms despite an adequate trial of dietary modification and first-line prokinetic therapy, particularly when accompanied by weight loss, recurrent dehydration, or nutritional compromise, defines the threshold for considering advanced, procedural, or device-based therapy.

**The Call:** Patients below this threshold continue optimized dietary and pharmacologic management with close follow-up; patients crossing this threshold are evaluated for gastric electrical stimulation or pyloric-directed therapy based on their specific physiologic pattern, and patients with significant nutritional compromise at any point in this pathway require proactive nutritional support planning rather than waiting for advanced motility therapy to resolve the nutritional deficit first.

**Trap Logic:** Nutritional support is sometimes deferred until motility-directed therapy has been fully escalated, when in a patient with significant weight loss or dehydration, nutritional support should proceed in parallel rather than waiting for a sequential, motility-therapy-first approach that leaves a nutritionally compromised patient unsupported in the interim.

**Decision Anchor:** Escalate gastroparesis therapy based on symptom and nutritional severity despite optimized first-line management, and address nutritional compromise in parallel with, not after, motility-directed escalation.

### Complications of Gastroparesis: Bezoar Formation and Glycemic Interplay

Gastric bezoars, concretions of retained, poorly digested material, most commonly indigestible plant fiber forming a phytobezoar, form in the setting of severely delayed gastric emptying and can themselves worsen symptoms, cause gastric outlet obstruction, or, rarely, embolize distally to cause small bowel obstruction, which is why patients with severe gastroparesis are specifically counseled to avoid high-fiber foods with known bezoar-forming potential, including certain fruits and vegetables, rather than receiving only the general low-fiber dietary counseling discussed earlier in this chapter without this specific warning. Bezoars identified endoscopically are managed with mechanical or enzymatic fragmentation and removal, and recurrent bezoar formation despite adequate dietary counseling should prompt reassessment of both dietary adherence and the adequacy of the current gastroparesis treatment regimen. In patients with diabetic gastroparesis specifically, the relationship between glycemic control and gastric motility runs in both directions: chronic hyperglycemia impairs gastric motility through the mechanisms discussed earlier in this chapter, but acute hyperglycemia at the time of a meal also acutely slows gastric emptying independent of any chronic neuropathic injury, meaning that a diabetic patient with poor day-to-day glycemic control can have gastroparesis symptoms that fluctuate with same-day blood glucose levels, and optimizing glycemic control is therefore both a long-term disease-modifying strategy and a same-day symptom management tool in this population. Patients with a history of prior bezoar formation should carry this information prominently in their medical record, since it materially changes dietary counseling priorities at every subsequent visit, not only the one at which the bezoar was originally diagnosed and treated.

### Postsurgical Gastroparesis: Recognition and Prevention

Postsurgical gastroparesis, following inadvertent or necessary vagal nerve injury during esophageal, gastric, bariatric, or other upper abdominal surgery, should be anticipated and specifically screened for in any postoperative patient with persistent nausea, vomiting, or early satiety extending beyond the expected postoperative recovery window, rather than attributed reflexively to normal postoperative ileus or narcotic-related effects, since normal postoperative ileus is expected to resolve within days while true postsurgical gastroparesis persists and requires the same objective emptying confirmation and structured management approach developed elsewhere in this chapter. Surgeons performing procedures with recognized vagal injury risk, particularly certain bariatric and antireflux procedures, increasingly employ vagal-sparing techniques where oncologically and technically feasible specifically to reduce this risk, and preoperative counseling about this possibility, applying the same precision-in-communication principle emphasized throughout this book, helps set appropriate expectations for a patient who may otherwise interpret postoperative gastroparesis symptoms as an unexpected surgical complication rather than a recognized, if uncommon, risk that was part of the informed consent discussion. Referral to a motility specialist experienced in postsurgical gastroparesis specifically, rather than general gastroenterology follow-up alone, is reasonable for cases that do not respond promptly to initial dietary and pharmacologic measures, given the somewhat distinct natural history and treatment response pattern of this etiology relative to diabetic or idiopathic disease.

## Overlap Syndromes and Differentiation

### Distinguishing Functional Dyspepsia From Gastroparesis

The symptom overlap between postprandial distress syndrome functional dyspepsia and gastroparesis is substantial enough that gastric emptying testing is the practical, decisive differentiator in patients whose presentation could plausibly represent either condition, and clinicians should resist the temptation to assign either label based on symptom pattern alone when the distinction would change management, since prokinetic therapy, dietary structuring, and, in refractory cases, the advanced procedural options developed above are specifically indicated for confirmed delayed emptying and are applied with different intensity and urgency in a patient whose emptying study is normal. It is also worth recognizing explicitly that gastric emptying rate does not correlate tightly with symptom severity in either direction, meaning that a patient with objectively severe delayed emptying can have relatively mild symptoms while a patient with normal or only mildly delayed emptying can have severe, disabling symptoms, a dissociation that reinforces why treatment decisions should integrate both the objective emptying result and the patient's actual symptom burden rather than anchoring on either alone. Ordering a gastric emptying study specifically to resolve this distinction, rather than proceeding empirically with a trial-and-error therapy sequence, is a reasonable and often more efficient use of diagnostic resources whenever the distinction would meaningfully change the treatment plan being considered.

### Cyclic Vomiting Syndrome and Cannabinoid Hyperemesis

Cyclic vomiting syndrome presents with discrete, stereotyped episodes of intense nausea and vomiting separated by symptom-free intervals, a pattern distinct from the more continuous symptom burden of functional dyspepsia or gastroparesis, and its recognition depends on eliciting this specific episodic pattern directly, since a patient may otherwise be repeatedly evaluated for a new, unrelated acute illness each time an episode occurs rather than being recognized as having a single, recurring underlying disorder. Cannabinoid hyperemesis syndrome, a specific and increasingly recognized cause of a cyclic vomiting-like pattern in the setting of chronic, heavy cannabis use, is distinguished by its temporal association with cannabis use and by a characteristic, though not universal, symptomatic relief with hot showers or bathing, a distinctive historical clue that should be specifically elicited, since this diagnosis is often overlooked when a patient does not volunteer cannabis use unprompted, paralleling the underreporting pattern discussed for other substances earlier in this book; sustained cannabis cessation, rather than any pharmacologic intervention, is the only reliably effective long-term treatment. A symptom diary tracking episode timing, potential triggers, and duration over several months can be invaluable in confirming the stereotyped, episodic pattern that defines this syndrome and in distinguishing it from other causes of recurrent nausea and vomiting discussed elsewhere in this chapter. Patients are often reluctant to accept a cannabinoid hyperemesis diagnosis initially, particularly when cannabis use is perceived as therapeutic or benign, and framing the recommendation around the specific, reproducible temporal relationship between use and symptoms, rather than a general anti-cannabis message, improves the likelihood of genuine cessation and symptom resolution.

### Distinguishing Rumination and Belching Disorders From Structural Disease

Because rumination syndrome and supragastric belching present with regurgitant or belching symptoms that overlap superficially with gastroesophageal reflux disease and, in the case of rumination, with gastroparesis-related vomiting, patients are frequently subjected to an extended and ultimately unrevealing structural workup, including repeated endoscopy and cross-sectional imaging, before the correct behavioral diagnosis is finally recognized, a pattern that reflects insufficient attention to the specific historical features, effortlessness and immediate postprandial timing for rumination, and the rapid, high-frequency, largely involuntary pattern for supragastric belching, that distinguish these conditions from their structural mimics rather than a lack of available diagnostic tools. Taking a specifically structured history targeting these distinguishing features at the initial visit, rather than defaulting to a standard reflux or dyspepsia workup, shortens this diagnostic pathway considerably and avoids subjecting the patient to testing that a more targeted initial history would have shown to be unnecessary. A structured, targeted intake questionnaire covering these specific features can help standardize this recognition across a busy practice with variable visit lengths.

## Rumination Syndrome and Belching Disorders

Rumination syndrome and supragastric belching, while classified separately from the primary functional dyspepsia and gastroparesis conditions that dominate this chapter, share the underlying theme that connects every disorder addressed here: a disturbance of normal gastric or esophagogastric motor function that produces genuine, often disabling symptoms without a structural lesion to explain them, and both respond far better to behavioral and physiologic retraining than to any pharmacologic intervention, a therapeutic contrast worth making explicit to patients who may otherwise expect a medication-based solution analogous to the approach used for functional dyspepsia or gastroparesis.

### Rumination Syndrome

Rumination syndrome is characterized by effortless, repetitive regurgitation of recently ingested food into the mouth, typically within minutes of eating, followed by rechewing and either reswallowing or expulsion, a pattern resulting from an involuntary, learned increase in intra-abdominal pressure against a relaxed lower esophageal sphincter rather than from any structural or classic motility abnormality, and its distinction from gastroesophageal reflux disease or gastroparesis-related vomiting is primarily historical, based on the characteristic effortless, non-nauseated, immediately postprandial pattern rather than requiring extensive additional testing in a typical presentation, though high-resolution manometry with impedance can confirm the diagnosis objectively when the history is ambiguous by demonstrating the characteristic simultaneous rise in gastric and intrathoracic pressure that precedes the regurgitation event. Diaphragmatic breathing training, a specific behavioral technique that teaches the patient to consciously counteract the abdominal wall contraction that drives the rumination event, is the primary evidence-based treatment and, unlike gastroparesis or functional dyspepsia, does not center on pharmacologic therapy at all, reflecting the syndrome's fundamentally behavioral, learned mechanism. Patients are often relieved simply to learn that their symptom has a name and a specific, learnable behavioral remedy, since many have previously been told, incorrectly, that they are voluntarily inducing vomiting or have an eating disorder, a misattribution that can be both clinically inaccurate and personally distressing.

**Supragastric Belching**

Supragastric belching results from the rapid, largely unconscious ingestion and immediate expulsion of air into and out of the esophagus without the air ever actually entering the stomach, distinguishing it mechanistically from ordinary gastric belching, in which swallowed air is vented from the stomach itself after a normal physiologic delay, and patients with supragastric belching frequently belch dozens to hundreds of times per day, well beyond the frequency of ordinary physiologic belching, often without full awareness of the behavior's frequency or its voluntary, learned component. As with rumination syndrome, diagnosis rests primarily on recognizing the characteristic clinical pattern, supported when needed by impedance-manometry demonstrating the rapid air influx and efflux without a preceding gastric distension phase, and treatment centers on behavioral therapy directed at the underlying learned behavior rather than on acid suppression or prokinetic pharmacotherapy, which are directed at mechanisms not actually responsible for this particular symptom. As with rumination syndrome, patient education explaining the mechanism in plain, non-judgmental terms is itself a meaningful part of treatment, since patients frequently arrive having been dismissed or misunderstood by prior clinicians unfamiliar with this specific, learnable behavioral pattern.

Case Presentation: A 34-year-old woman with type 1 diabetes and a hemoglobin A1c of 9.2 percent presents with six months of early satiety, postprandial bloating, and intermittent vomiting of undigested food several hours after meals, accompanied by an 11-pound weight loss. Upper endoscopy is normal. Applying the reasoning developed in this chapter, her long-standing, poorly controlled diabetes and the specific pattern of delayed vomiting of undigested food, together with a structurally normal endoscopy, raise suspicion for diabetic gastroparesis rather than functional dyspepsia, and rather than assigning a functional diagnosis based on symptom pattern alone, gastric emptying scintigraphy using the standardized four-hour protocol is obtained, off any opioid or glucagon-like peptide-1 receptor agonist therapy, and confirms markedly delayed gastric emptying. Dietary modification to a low-fat, low-fiber, small-meal pattern and metoclopramide are initiated, alongside close coordination with endocrinology to improve glycemic control, since ongoing hyperglycemia itself further impairs gastric motility and can blunt the response to prokinetic therapy. At three-month follow-up, her symptoms have improved modestly but she has continued to lose weight, now with evidence of mild dehydration on laboratory testing. Given persistent symptoms and nutritional compromise despite optimized first-line therapy, she is referred for evaluation of pyloric-directed therapy and, in parallel rather than sequentially, for dietitian-directed nutritional support planning.

Case Presentation: A 27-year-old woman presents with eighteen months of postprandial fullness, early satiety, and epigastric bloating, without weight loss, vomiting, or alarm features. Helicobacter pylori stool antigen testing is negative, and upper endoscopy performed six months into her symptom course was normal. She was started on omeprazole at that time with minimal improvement. Applying the reasoning developed in this chapter, her symptom pattern, meal-triggered fullness and early satiation predominating over pain, is most consistent with postprandial distress syndrome functional dyspepsia, and her inadequate response to a proton pump inhibitor is expected given that this subtype responds preferentially to prokinetic rather than acid-suppressive therapy; the earlier prescription reflects an undifferentiated approach rather than subtype-matched sequencing. Proton pump inhibitor therapy is discontinued, and a trial of a prokinetic agent is initiated instead, guided explicitly by her predominant symptom subtype. At eight-week follow-up she reports partial but incomplete improvement, with persistent bothersome bloating. Rather than extending the same prokinetic trial indefinitely or empirically adding additional agents, low-dose amitriptyline is added as a neuromodulator, following the threshold developed in this chapter for inadequate response after an adequate subtype-matched first-line trial, with explicit counseling that the medication is being used at a low, pain-modulating dose for a gastrointestinal indication rather than as a psychiatric treatment. At three-month follow-up on the combination regimen, her symptoms have improved substantially.

| Feature | Functional Dyspepsia | Gastroparesis | Rumination Syndrome |
|---|---|---|---|
| Gastric emptying study | Normal or mildly delayed | Objectively delayed | Normal |
| Key symptom pattern | Meal-related fullness or pain | Vomiting of undigested food, hours after eating | Effortless regurgitation within minutes of eating |
| First-line treatment | Subtype-matched PPI or prokinetic | Dietary modification, prokinetic | Diaphragmatic breathing training |
| Confirmatory test | Not required beyond endoscopy | Gastric emptying scintigraphy (4-hour) | Manometry-impedance if history ambiguous |

**THE GI THRESHOLD DECISION SYSTEM — Gastric Motility and Functional Disorder Thresholds**

---

**Presentation Signature:** This chapter's threshold instances addressed subtype-matched sequencing of functional dyspepsia therapy and severity-based escalation of gastroparesis management.

**Threshold Point:** Symptom subtype gates the first-line functional dyspepsia agent; persistent symptoms or nutritional compromise despite optimized first-line gastroparesis therapy gates escalation to advanced procedural options.

**The Call:** Both thresholds convert an overlapping, easily conflated symptom picture into a mechanism-specific pathway, using an objective test, an emptying study, to separate conditions that appear similar but require different management.

**Trap Logic:** Treating symptom pattern as sufficient to distinguish functional dyspepsia from gastroparesis, and sequencing nutritional support after rather than alongside motility-directed escalation, are this chapter's two most consequential threshold misapplications.

**Decision Anchor:** Confirm gastric emptying objectively before committing to a gastroparesis-specific management pathway, match first-line functional dyspepsia therapy to symptom subtype, and address nutritional compromise in parallel with, not after, escalating therapy.

## Summary and Key Concepts

Functional dyspepsia is diagnosed by Rome IV symptom criteria after structural disease is excluded, and its two subtypes, postprandial distress and epigastric pain syndrome, respond preferentially to different first-line agents.

Impaired gastric accommodation, visceral hypersensitivity, and emerging evidence for duodenal eosinophilic inflammation underlie functional dyspepsia's pathophysiology.

Gastroparesis requires objective confirmation of delayed gastric emptying, most reliably by four-hour gastric emptying scintigraphy, and cannot be diagnosed by symptom pattern alone given its overlap with functional dyspepsia.

Dietary modification and prokinetic therapy are first-line for gastroparesis, with gastric electrical stimulation and pyloric-directed therapies reserved for refractory disease with persistent symptoms or nutritional compromise.

Cyclic vomiting syndrome, cannabinoid hyperemesis syndrome, rumination syndrome, and supragastric belching each have a distinctive historical pattern that, once recognized, redirects management away from standard gastroparesis or functional dyspepsia therapy.

Gastric emptying rate does not correlate tightly with symptom severity, reinforcing that treatment decisions should integrate both objective testing and the patient's actual symptom and nutritional burden.

# CHAPTER 7: CELIAC DISEASE AND MALABSORPTIVE DISORDERS

**Learning Objectives**

1. Explain the genetic and immune-mediated pathophysiology of celiac disease and its relationship to gluten exposure.
2. Apply appropriate serologic and histologic testing to diagnose celiac disease, including in seronegative and equivocal cases.
3. Manage celiac disease with a gluten-free diet and structured long-term monitoring, and recognize refractory disease and its complications.
4. Differentiate tropical sprue, Whipple disease, bile acid malabsorption, and protein-losing enteropathy from celiac disease.
5. Apply a structured diagnostic sequence to a patient presenting with chronic malabsorption of unclear cause.

**Chapter Outline**

This chapter develops celiac disease as the prototypical small bowel malabsorptive disorder, covering its genetic and immune pathophysiology, its diagnostic pathway across classic, non-classic, silent, and seronegative presentations, its management through gluten-free diet and structured monitoring, and its complications when refractory. The chapter then surveys other malabsorptive disorders, tropical sprue, Whipple disease, bile acid malabsorption, and protein-losing enteropathy, before closing with a structured diagnostic framework for the patient presenting with chronic malabsorption of unclear cause, connecting each specific finding to a defined next diagnostic step.

**Epidemiology and Screening of At-Risk Populations**

Celiac disease affects a meaningful proportion of the general population in most studied regions, though the majority of affected individuals remain undiagnosed, a gap attributed to the predominance of non-classic and silent presentations discussed later in this section combined with variable clinical awareness of the full range of ways the disease can present. First-degree relatives of an affected patient carry a substantially elevated risk relative to the general population and are reasonable candidates for serologic screening even without symptoms, and several specific associated conditions, including type 1 diabetes mellitus, autoimmune thyroid disease, Down syndrome, Turner syndrome, and selective immunoglobulin A deficiency itself, carry a similarly elevated prevalence of celiac disease that supports at least periodic serologic screening in these populations, applying the same principle of risk-stratified rather than universal screening that has recurred throughout this book. Increasing rates of clinical recognition, rather than a true rise in disease incidence alone, likely account for at least part of the rising diagnosis rates observed in many health systems over recent decades, reflecting improved serologic testing availability and broader clinical awareness of the disease's varied presentations. Repeat screening at intervals in an initially seronegative first-degree relative is reasonable given that celiac disease can develop at any age, meaning a single negative screen does not provide lifelong reassurance in a genuinely high-risk relative.

**Patient Communication at Diagnosis**

A new celiac disease diagnosis carries a substantial lifestyle burden, permanent dietary restriction, that distinguishes it from many other gastrointestinal diagnoses in this book, and framing the diagnosis explicitly around both the seriousness of ongoing gluten exposure, given the complications discussed later in this section, and the genuinely favorable prognosis with strict adherence helps patients engage constructively with a diagnosis that can otherwise feel overwhelming at first presentation. Connecting newly diagnosed patients with celiac-specific patient support organizations and, where available, dietitian-led group education programs, in addition to individual counseling, provides practical, peer-informed strategies for navigating social situations, dining out, and travel that a single clinical encounter cannot fully cover, and this connection should be offered as a standard part of the initial diagnostic conversation rather than left to the patient to discover independently. Scheduling a dedicated follow-up visit specifically to answer questions that arise only after the patient has attempted the diet for several weeks, rather than relying solely on the initial diagnostic visit, further supports this engagement.

## Celiac Disease

**Pathophysiology and Genetic Susceptibility**

Celiac disease is an immune-mediated enteropathy triggered by the ingestion of gluten, a storage protein found in wheat, barley, and rye, in genetically susceptible individuals who carry the human leukocyte antigen DQ2 or DQ8 haplotype, present in the overwhelming majority of confirmed cases, though the presence of either haplotype alone is common in the general population and therefore has high sensitivity but low specificity, meaning that a negative result is genuinely useful for excluding the diagnosis while a positive result confirms only susceptibility rather than disease itself. Gluten-derived peptides, particularly gliadin, resist complete digestion and, upon crossing an intestinal epithelium with increased permeability, are deamidated by tissue transglutaminase, an enzymatic modification that increases their binding affinity for the disease-associated human leukocyte antigen molecules on antigen-presenting cells and triggers a CD4-positive T-cell-mediated immune response directed against the small intestinal mucosa, producing the characteristic villous atrophy, crypt hyperplasia, and intraepithelial lymphocytosis that define the histologic diagnosis. This mechanistic understanding explains two clinically important features of the disease: its strict dependence on continued gluten exposure, such that histologic and symptomatic improvement reliably follows genuine dietary elimination, and its strong familial clustering, since first-degree relatives of an affected patient carry a substantially increased risk and are considered for at least serologic screening even in the absence of symptoms. This is why celiac disease is properly classified as an autoimmune, rather than a simple food allergy, condition, despite its clear external dietary trigger.

## Clinical Presentation: Classic, Non-Classic, and Silent Disease

Classic celiac disease presents with the malabsorptive symptom complex most associated with the condition historically, chronic diarrhea, steatorrhea, weight loss, and, in children, growth failure, reflecting extensive small bowel involvement sufficient to produce overt nutrient malabsorption, but this presentation now represents a minority of newly diagnosed adult cases. Non-classic celiac disease presents with symptoms that do not immediately suggest a malabsorptive process, including isolated iron deficiency anemia, unexplained elevated liver enzymes, osteoporosis or unexplained fracture, infertility or recurrent miscarriage, peripheral neuropathy, and a range of other extraintestinal manifestations, and this presentation pattern is precisely why celiac serology has become part of the standard evaluation for unexplained iron deficiency anemia introduced in the first chapter, alongside the endoscopic evaluation for occult bleeding. Silent celiac disease describes patients with confirmed serologic and histologic disease who report no symptoms at all, typically identified through screening of a high-risk group such as a first-degree relative or a patient with an associated autoimmune condition, and the clinical significance of silent disease lies in its association with the same long-term complications, discussed later in this chapter, as symptomatic disease, meaning that the absence of symptoms should not be interpreted as a reason to defer treatment once the diagnosis is confirmed. Recognizing this shift in presentation pattern over time is itself clinically important, since a clinician anchored on the classic malabsorptive picture may fail to consider celiac disease in a patient whose presentation looks nothing like the textbook description. Recognizing this broad list as a single unifying diagnostic possibility, rather than pursuing each symptom through an entirely separate specialty workup, can shorten a diagnostic odyssey considerably. Explaining this reasoning directly to an asymptomatic, screening-identified patient is often necessary, since the absence of any felt illness can make a lifelong dietary commitment feel disproportionate without a clear rationale.

## Serologic and Histologic Diagnosis

Tissue transglutaminase immunoglobulin A antibody testing, paired with a total immunoglobulin A level to exclude selective immunoglobulin A deficiency, a condition disproportionately prevalent in celiac disease and one that produces a false-negative tissue transglutaminase result if unrecognized, is the preferred initial serologic test given its high sensitivity and specificity in an adequately gluten-exposed patient. Deamidated gliadin peptide immunoglobulin G testing is used preferentially in patients with confirmed immunoglobulin A deficiency, substituting for the immunoglobulin A-based test that would otherwise be unreliable in this population, and endomysial antibody testing, while highly specific, is used more selectively given its greater cost and operator-dependent interpretation relative to the standardized, automated tissue transglutaminase assay. Regardless of which serologic test is used, testing must be performed while the patient is on a gluten-containing diet, since even a brief period of gluten restriction before testing can produce a false-negative result by allowing partial immunologic and histologic recovery, a timing consideration that parallels the acid-suppression timing issue affecting Helicobacter pylori testing discussed in an earlier chapter and that should be specifically confirmed with the patient before testing is ordered. Point-of-care rapid antibody tests exist but are generally reserved for settings where laboratory-based testing is not readily accessible, given their somewhat lower accuracy relative to standardized laboratory assays.

## The Marsh Classification and Biopsy Technique

Duodenal biopsy remains required to confirm the diagnosis in essentially all adult patients with positive serology, since serology alone, despite its high accuracy, is not considered sufficient for a diagnosis carrying lifelong dietary implications, and biopsies should be obtained from both the duodenal bulb and the more distal duodenum, using multiple samples, typically four to six, because histologic changes can be patchy and a limited or poorly distributed biopsy sampling can produce a false-negative result even in a patient with genuine, serologically confirmed disease. The Marsh classification grades the histologic severity of enteropathy from Marsh 0, normal mucosa, through Marsh 1, isolated intraepithelial lymphocytosis without architectural distortion, to Marsh 3, the villous atrophy with crypt hyperplasia that defines classic celiac enteropathy, and this staging is clinically useful both for confirming the diagnosis, since a positive serology with Marsh 3 histology is considered definitive, and for interpreting an equivocal case, since Marsh 1 changes alone are nonspecific and can be seen in a range of other conditions, including Helicobacter pylori infection and nonsteroidal anti-inflammatory drug use, and require correlation with serology and the broader clinical picture rather than being treated as diagnostic of celiac disease in isolation. Communicating this multi-biopsy requirement to the endoscopist performing the procedure, rather than assuming a single sample will suffice, is a straightforward step that prevents an inadequate biopsy from prolonging the diagnostic pathway unnecessarily. Pathologists reporting Marsh 1 changes alone should explicitly note this correlation requirement, prompting the ordering clinician to revisit the serology and clinical context rather than treating the histology report in isolation.

Figure 7.1: Marsh Classification of Celiac Enteropathy

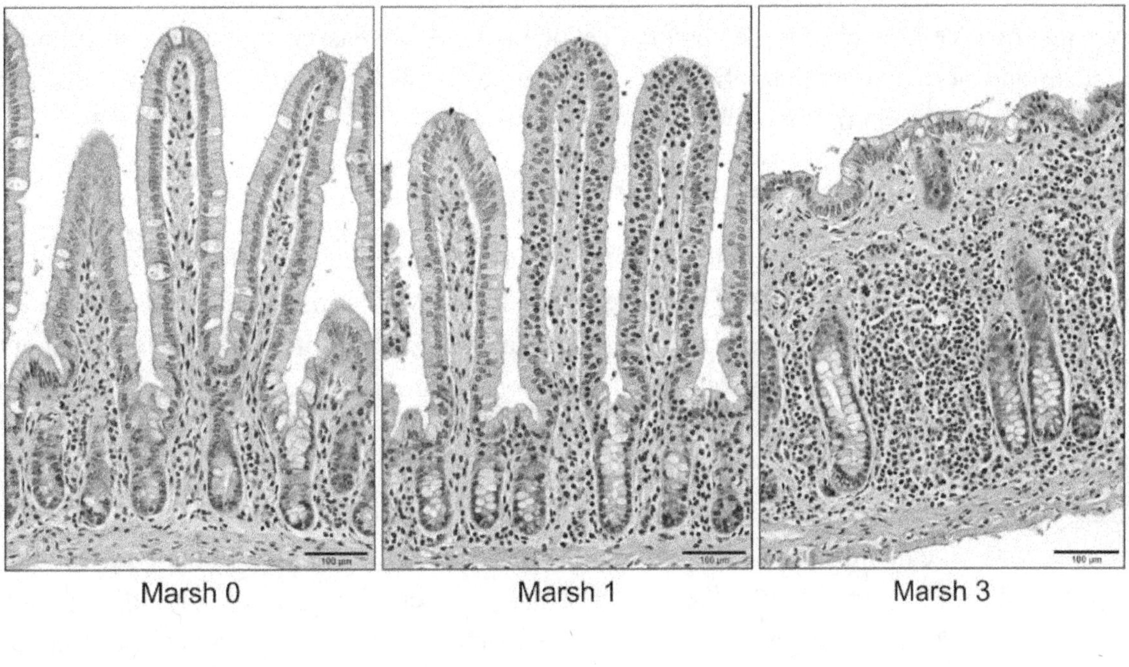

**THE GI THRESHOLD DECISION SYSTEM — Small Bowel Thresholds — Diagnosing Celiac Disease in the Seronegative or Equivocal Patient**

**Presentation Signature:** A patient with a clinical presentation suggestive of celiac disease has negative or equivocal serology, or has already reduced gluten intake before testing was performed, complicating straightforward interpretation.

**Threshold Point:** A negative tissue transglutaminase result in a patient with normal total immunoglobulin A and adequate ongoing gluten intake has a high negative predictive value; a negative result in a patient with reduced gluten intake before testing, or with unrecognized immunoglobulin A deficiency, cannot be interpreted as reliably excluding the diagnosis.

**The Call:** In a patient with genuinely negative serology on an adequate gluten-containing diet with normal immunoglobulin A, celiac disease is unlikely and duodenal biopsy is not routinely required; in a patient with a compelling clinical presentation, high genetic risk, or an inadequate gluten challenge or unrecognized immunoglobulin A deficiency at the time of testing, duodenal biopsy or a supervised gluten challenge followed by repeat serology and biopsy should be pursued despite the negative initial serology.

**Trap Logic:** A patient who has already self-initiated a gluten-free diet before evaluation, common given widespread public awareness of the diet, presents the most common and most consequential trap: testing performed in this setting can be falsely reassuring, and the correct response is a structured, supervised gluten reintroduction protocol before retesting, not acceptance of a falsely negative result obtained during self-directed dietary restriction.

**Decision Anchor:** Before accepting a negative celiac serology as reassuring, confirm adequate ongoing gluten intake and normal immunoglobulin A; when either is uncertain, pursue biopsy or a supervised gluten challenge rather than the negative serologic result alone.

### Management: Gluten-Free Diet and Structured Monitoring

Strict, lifelong avoidance of gluten-containing grains is the only established effective treatment for celiac disease, and effective dietary counseling requires more than a verbal instruction to avoid wheat, barley, and rye: referral to a dietitian experienced specifically in celiac disease, education about cross-contamination risk in shared kitchen equipment and processing facilities, and guidance on reading food labels for hidden gluten sources together determine whether a patient achieves genuine, sustained dietary adherence rather than partial avoidance that permits ongoing low-level mucosal injury. Structured monitoring after diagnosis includes reassessment of celiac serology, expected to normalize over the following six to twelve months with successful dietary adherence, and this declining antibody titer serves as a practical, noninvasive marker of adherence that should be checked periodically rather than assumed based on the patient's self-report alone, since normalized serology despite reported strict adherence is reassuring while persistently elevated serology should prompt a more detailed dietary review, ideally with dietitian involvement, to identify an unrecognized source of ongoing gluten exposure. Some centers also incorporate a follow-up duodenal biopsy at an appropriate interval to directly confirm mucosal healing, particularly in patients whose presentation was severe or whose adherence is uncertain, complementing rather than replacing serologic monitoring.

### Refractory Celiac Disease and Complications

Refractory celiac disease, persistent or recurrent villous atrophy and symptoms despite at least twelve months of confirmed strict dietary adherence, is an uncommon but important diagnosis to consider once ongoing gluten exposure has been genuinely excluded, since it carries distinct management and prognostic implications; type 1 refractory disease, without an aberrant, clonal intraepithelial lymphocyte population, is managed with immunosuppressive therapy and carries a more favorable prognosis than type 2 refractory disease, in which an aberrant lymphocyte population is identified and which carries a substantially elevated risk of progression to enteropathy-associated T-cell lymphoma, a rare but aggressive malignancy that represents the most feared long-term complication of poorly controlled celiac disease. Other recognized complications of longstanding, inadequately treated celiac disease include osteoporosis, from chronic calcium and vitamin D malabsorption, hyposplenism, which increases susceptibility to encapsulated organism infection and warrants consideration of specific vaccination and infection-prevention counseling, and an increased risk of other gastrointestinal malignancies, reinforcing why the structured monitoring and adherence-reinforcement approach developed above is not merely a matter of symptom control but a strategy for preventing serious downstream complications. Distinguishing genuine refractory disease from ongoing, unrecognized gluten exposure is the essential first step before this diagnosis is entertained, since the latter is far more common and is managed entirely differently, through more intensive dietary review rather than immunosuppression. Frame these consistently as preventable outcomes. Always.

### Dermatitis Herpetiformis and Other Extraintestinal Manifestations

Dermatitis herpetiformis, an intensely pruritic, symmetric vesiculobullous rash typically distributed over the extensor surfaces of the elbows, knees, and buttocks, is considered the specific cutaneous manifestation of celiac disease, arising from immunoglobulin A deposition at the dermal papillary tips, and its presence is sufficiently specific that a confirmed diagnosis by skin biopsy demonstrating this granular immunoglobulin A deposition pattern is considered diagnostic of underlying celiac disease even without independent duodenal biopsy confirmation, though most patients undergo both evaluations given the informational and monitoring value of documenting the degree of enteropathy directly. Beyond dermatitis herpetiformis, other extraintestinal manifestations, including elevated transaminases from celiac hepatitis, which resolves with dietary treatment and should prompt celiac testing in any patient with unexplained mild transaminase elevation, and neurologic manifestations, including peripheral neuropathy and, less commonly, gluten ataxia, an immune-mediated cerebellar process, further illustrate why celiac disease functions as a multisystem disorder rather than one confined to the gastrointestinal tract, and why the serologic screening threshold developed earlier in this chapter should be applied liberally across this broad range of otherwise unexplained presentations. Treatment of the skin manifestation itself, when needed for symptom control while dietary treatment takes effect over the following months, typically involves dapsone, which requires screening for glucose-6-phosphate dehydrogenase deficiency before initiation given the risk of dapsone-induced hemolysis in affected individuals.

### Non-Celiac Gluten Sensitivity

Non-celiac gluten sensitivity describes patients who report symptomatic improvement with gluten avoidance despite negative celiac serology and normal duodenal histology on a gluten-containing diet, and its existence as a distinct clinical entity remains an area of active investigation, since blinded challenge studies have shown that a substantial proportion of self-identified gluten-sensitive individuals do not reliably distinguish gluten-containing from gluten-free challenge material when neither they nor the investigator knows which is being administered, suggesting that a nocebo effect or sensitivity to another wheat component, such as fermentable oligosaccharide, disaccharide, monosaccharide, and polyol content discussed in a later chapter on irritable bowel syndrome, may explain symptoms in at least some affected individuals. Regardless of the precise underlying mechanism, celiac disease must be genuinely excluded before a diagnosis of non-celiac gluten sensitivity is assigned, using the same adequately gluten-exposed serologic and, where indicated, histologic evaluation developed earlier in this chapter, since a patient who empirically adopts a gluten-free diet without this evaluation forecloses the opportunity for accurate celiac testing later, exactly as illustrated in this chapter's case presentation. Whatever the precise mechanism ultimately proves to be, patients who genuinely benefit symptomatically from gluten avoidance after appropriate celiac exclusion should not be denied that management strategy simply because the underlying pathophysiology remains incompletely characterized, provided they understand that their condition, unlike celiac disease, does not carry the same risk of silent mucosal injury or long-term complication from inadvertent gluten exposure.

### Autoimmune Enteropathy and Other Rare Mucosal Causes

Autoimmune enteropathy, a rare disorder producing severe, often refractory diarrhea and villous atrophy resembling celiac disease histologically but occurring in a patient without the genetic susceptibility markers or serologic response to a gluten-free diet that would confirm celiac disease, should be considered when a patient with a celiac-like presentation fails to respond to strict dietary gluten elimination and has negative or atypical celiac serology, particularly in the presence of other autoimmune conditions or, in children, a broader immune dysregulation syndrome. Anti-enterocyte antibodies, when present, support the diagnosis, though their absence does not exclude it, and management centers on immunosuppressive therapy directed at the underlying autoimmune process rather than dietary modification, a fundamentally different treatment strategy from celiac disease that underscores the clinical importance of distinguishing the two conditions correctly rather than assuming an atypical or nonresponsive presentation simply represents unusually severe or refractory celiac disease. Given its rarity and the specialized immunosuppressive management it requires, referral to a center with specific expertise in this diagnosis is reasonable once it is seriously suspected, rather than attempting an extended trial-and-error management approach in a general gastroenterology practice. Early referral avoids a prolonged, ineffective trial of dietary measures alone. Prompt referral matters here.

### Common Variable Immunodeficiency and Malabsorption

Common variable immunodeficiency, a primary immunodeficiency characterized by impaired antibody production, is associated with a celiac-like enteropathy and chronic diarrhea in a subset of affected patients, and its recognition matters because the malabsorptive component may respond only partially to gluten restriction, if at all, since the underlying mechanism differs from classic celiac disease, and because affected patients require immunoglobulin replacement therapy and heightened surveillance for recurrent sinopulmonary infection, gastrointestinal infection, particularly with Giardia, and lymphoproliferative and autoimmune complications that extend well beyond the gastrointestinal manifestations alone. A low or absent immunoglobulin level identified incidentally during the celiac serology workup described earlier in this chapter, rather than the expected normal or elevated total immunoglobulin A used to validate tissue transglutaminase testing, should prompt consideration of this underlying immunodeficiency rather than being treated only as a technical limitation of the celiac testing itself. Coordination with immunology or allergy-immunology specialists experienced in primary immunodeficiency is essential once this diagnosis is confirmed, since the gastrointestinal manifestations are only one component of a condition requiring comprehensive, multisystem monitoring and treatment. This coordination should begin promptly once the diagnosis is confirmed. Delay is costly here.

## Other Malabsorptive Disorders

### Tropical Sprue and Whipple Disease

Tropical sprue, a malabsorptive small bowel disease occurring in residents of or travelers to specific tropical and subtropical regions, is thought to result from a persistent, abnormal small bowel bacterial colonization following an acute enteric infection, producing chronic diarrhea, malabsorption, and folate and vitamin B12 deficiency, and its diagnosis requires both a compatible geographic exposure history, without which the diagnosis should not be entertained, and small bowel biopsy demonstrating partial villous blunting distinct from, though sometimes difficult to distinguish histologically from, celiac disease; response to prolonged antibiotic therapy, typically several months, combined with folate repletion, both confirms the diagnosis retrospectively and constitutes definitive treatment. Whipple disease, caused by infection with the actinomycete Tropheryma whipplei, produces a distinctive multisystem illness combining malabsorption and weight loss with migratory arthralgia, which frequently precedes the gastrointestinal manifestations by years and is easily misattributed to a primary rheumatologic process, along with neurologic and cardiac involvement in more advanced cases; diagnosis rests on small bowel biopsy demonstrating periodic acid-Schiff-positive macrophages within the lamina propria, and prolonged antibiotic therapy with an agent that achieves adequate central nervous system penetration is required given the disease's propensity for neurologic involvement and relapse if treatment is inadequate. Empiric treatment is sometimes initiated based on compatible history and biopsy findings alone when confirmatory testing is not readily available, given the relatively low risk and potential benefit of a prolonged antibiotic and folate repletion trial in a patient with a genuinely compatible exposure history. Relapse after Whipple disease treatment, sometimes presenting predominantly with neurologic symptoms even when the initial presentation was gastrointestinal, underscores the importance of long-term follow-up rather than considering the disease definitively cured once initial symptoms resolve.

### Bile Acid Malabsorption

Bile acid malabsorption results from impaired ileal reabsorption of bile acids, whether from primary ileal disease such as Crohn disease or ileal resection, or, in its more common primary or idiopathic form, from an intrinsic dysregulation of bile acid synthesis and enterohepatic circulation without identifiable ileal pathology, and the excess bile acids reaching the colon stimulate colonic secretion and motility, producing a chronic, often urgent, watery diarrhea that is frequently and, for the reasons developed below, consequentially misdiagnosed as diarrhea-predominant irritable bowel syndrome. Diagnosis, where available, uses a nuclear medicine test measuring retention of an orally administered radiolabeled bile acid analog at one week, with low retention confirming excessive bile acid loss, though this test is not universally available, making an empiric therapeutic trial of a bile acid sequestrant a reasonable and commonly used pragmatic diagnostic and therapeutic strategy in practice; a robust response to sequestrant therapy both treats the condition and retrospectively supports the diagnosis in a setting where the specific nuclear medicine test cannot be obtained. Recognizing this condition specifically prevents patients from being managed indefinitely with the fiber-based and antispasmodic therapies typically used for irritable bowel syndrome, agents that do not target the underlying mechanism and that a substantial proportion of bile acid malabsorption patients will find inadequate, as illustrated in this chapter's second case.

### Protein-Losing Enteropathy

Protein-losing enteropathy describes excessive gastrointestinal loss of serum proteins, most clinically apparent as hypoalbuminemia disproportionate to any identified hepatic or renal cause, and it arises from one of several distinct mechanisms: mucosal erosion or ulceration, as can occur in severe inflammatory bowel disease; a primary lymphatic abnormality, as in intestinal lymphangiectasia, in which dilated, disrupted lymphatic channels leak protein-rich lymph directly into the bowel lumen; or a nonspecific increase in mucosal permeability seen in a range of inflammatory and infiltrative small bowel conditions. Diagnosis is confirmed by measuring fecal alpha-1 antitrypsin clearance, a protein resistant to intestinal digestion whose fecal concentration, when elevated relative to its serum concentration, directly quantifies enteric protein loss, and management addresses the specific underlying cause identified through further endoscopic, histologic, or imaging evaluation directed by the clinical context, since protein-losing enteropathy is a laboratory and physiologic finding requiring an underlying explanation rather than a standalone diagnosis with its own dedicated treatment. In children specifically, protein-losing enteropathy following certain congenital cardiac surgeries, related to altered lymphatic and venous pressure dynamics, is a recognized and distinct clinical scenario requiring coordination with cardiology alongside the gastroenterology-directed evaluation described here.

### Secondary Lactose Intolerance in Active Malabsorptive Disease

Secondary lactose intolerance, resulting from loss of the brush-border enzyme lactase in the setting of active villous injury from celiac disease or another small bowel process, commonly accompanies the malabsorptive disorders discussed in this chapter and can persist temporarily even after the underlying disease is otherwise treated, since brush-border enzyme recovery can lag behind the resolution of villous architecture more broadly. Distinguishing secondary, disease-related lactose intolerance from primary, genetically determined lactase nonpersistence matters for patient counseling, since secondary lactose intolerance is expected to improve as the underlying small bowel disease heals and dairy can often be reintroduced gradually over time, whereas primary lactase nonpersistence represents a fixed, lifelong trait; conflating the two can lead a patient to avoid dairy unnecessarily and permanently once their underlying disease has actually resolved, adding an avoidable and nutritionally significant dietary restriction on top of the gluten avoidance already required. A time-limited trial of dairy reintroduction several months into treatment, once mucosal healing is reasonably expected, gives a concrete way to test whether the restriction is still needed rather than leaving it in place indefinitely by default. This point is worth stating plainly to patients. Say this plainly.

## Nutritional Deficiencies and Repletion in Malabsorptive Disease

Celiac disease and the other malabsorptive disorders discussed in this chapter each characteristically deplete a specific set of nutrients, and screening for the specific pattern relevant to the confirmed or suspected diagnosis, rather than a generic panel applied uniformly, produces more efficient and clinically meaningful repletion. Iron, folate, and vitamin D deficiency are common in celiac disease given the proximal small bowel's role in their absorption, while vitamin B12 deficiency is less consistently present given its more distal ileal absorption site, and its presence in a patient with celiac disease should specifically prompt consideration of coexisting autoimmune gastritis, discussed in an earlier chapter, or, if the small bowel disease is extensive enough to involve the terminal ileum, direct malabsorption from the celiac process itself. A single, comprehensive nutritional panel obtained at diagnosis, rather than an incremental, symptom-triggered series of individual tests ordered over successive visits, is generally more efficient and gives both clinician and patient a complete baseline picture from which to plan repletion. A full nutritional panel at diagnosis, rather than only the two or three most commonly checked values, captures this fuller pattern from the outset.

### Fat-Soluble Vitamins and Trace Elements

Vitamins A, D, E, and K, requiring adequate fat absorption for uptake, are preferentially depleted in any condition producing significant steatorrhea, including extensive celiac disease, tropical sprue, and pancreatic exocrine insufficiency, and vitamin K deficiency specifically can present with an elevated prothrombin time or unexpected bruising or bleeding that, if not connected back to the underlying malabsorptive process, can be misattributed to a primary coagulopathy rather than recognized as a nutritional consequence of the gastrointestinal disease. Zinc deficiency, less routinely screened for than the vitamins discussed above, contributes to impaired wound healing, altered taste, and, in more severe cases, a distinctive acrodermatitis-like skin eruption, and copper deficiency, while less common, has been increasingly recognized as a cause of a myeloneuropathy that can mimic vitamin B12 deficiency both clinically and, to some degree, in its laboratory findings, reinforcing the value of a directed, disease-specific nutritional evaluation rather than assuming that correcting the more commonly screened deficiencies addresses the full nutritional burden of significant malabsorptive disease. A targeted history for symptoms of fat-soluble vitamin deficiency, including night blindness, easy bruising, and peripheral neuropathy, can prompt more focused testing than a generic panel would in a resource-constrained setting where broad screening is not readily available. Both zinc and copper deficiency should be considered specifically in a patient with persistent neurologic or dermatologic findings despite adequate correction of the more commonly measured vitamin levels.

## Small Intestinal Bacterial Overgrowth as a Malabsorptive Contributor

Small intestinal bacterial overgrowth, developed in full mechanistic and diagnostic detail in the following chapter, deserves mention here specifically because it frequently coexists with and can masquerade as, complicate, or be misattributed as the sole explanation for the malabsorptive disorders discussed throughout this chapter. Untreated celiac disease, through the small bowel dysmotility and structural changes chronic inflammation can produce, is itself a recognized risk factor for secondary small intestinal bacterial overgrowth, meaning that a celiac patient whose diarrhea and bloating do not fully resolve despite confirmed strict dietary adherence and normalized serology should be evaluated for coexisting bacterial overgrowth rather than assumed to have ongoing gluten exposure or refractory disease by default. This overlap is a specific, recurring example of a broader diagnostic principle that applies throughout gastroenterology: response to treatment of the presumed primary diagnosis should be verified rather than assumed, and incomplete response should prompt evaluation for a coexisting or alternative process rather than an automatic escalation of therapy directed at the original diagnosis alone. Empiric breath testing or a therapeutic antibiotic trial, detailed fully in the next chapter, is a reasonable next step in a treated celiac patient with this specific pattern of incomplete response, rather than repeat duodenal biopsy alone, which would primarily assess mucosal healing rather than evaluate for coexisting bacterial overgrowth. This overlap is discussed further in the next chapter. More detail follows.

## Celiac Disease in Pregnancy and Special Populations

Untreated or inadequately controlled celiac disease is associated with adverse reproductive outcomes, including infertility, recurrent miscarriage, and intrauterine growth restriction, mechanistically linked to the same chronic nutrient malabsorption and low-grade systemic inflammation discussed throughout this chapter, and this association is part of why celiac serology is a reasonable component of the evaluation for otherwise unexplained infertility or recurrent pregnancy loss, paralleling its inclusion in the evaluation of other non-classic presentations discussed earlier. A patient with confirmed celiac disease who becomes pregnant should be reassured that strict dietary adherence, rather than any special modification of the standard gluten-free diet during pregnancy, is the appropriate approach, alongside heightened attention to the nutritional repletion discussed later in this chapter, given the increased demand for iron, folate, and other micronutrients that pregnancy itself imposes on top of any pre-existing malabsorptive deficit. Preconception counseling for a woman with known celiac disease planning pregnancy is a reasonable opportunity to confirm dietary adherence and nutritional status proactively, rather than addressing these issues for the first time only after pregnancy has already begun. This reassurance is often welcome, since many pregnant patients worry unnecessarily that their existing dietary restriction requires further modification during pregnancy. Discuss this proactively. Every time.

**Pediatric-Onset and Transition to Adult Care**

Celiac disease diagnosed in childhood presents a distinct set of considerations at the transition to adult gastroenterology care, since long-term dietary adherence and disease monitoring, initially managed largely by parents, must be transferred to the young adult patient's own responsibility, a transition associated in some studies with a temporary decline in adherence and follow-up engagement during adolescence and young adulthood. Adult gastroenterologists receiving a young adult patient with a pediatric-onset celiac diagnosis should specifically reassess adherence, repeat serology to confirm current disease control, and take the transition visit itself as an opportunity to re-engage the patient directly in their own long-term management plan, applying the same explicit, plan-anchored communication principle developed throughout this book rather than assuming continuity of care and understanding that may not, in practice, have been fully maintained through the pediatric-to-adult transition. A structured transition checklist, covering current adherence status, most recent serology and bone density results, and any outstanding nutritional concerns, handed off explicitly from the pediatric to the adult team, reduces the likelihood that important elements of the patient's history are lost during this handoff. Treating this visit as a genuine restart of engagement, not merely a records transfer, improves long-term outcomes. This step matters. Truly.

**Bone Health Assessment in Malabsorptive Disease**

Chronic malabsorption of calcium and vitamin D, common to celiac disease, tropical sprue, and extensive small bowel disease of any cause, produces a measurably elevated risk of osteopenia and osteoporosis independent of the traditional age- and sex-based risk factors used to guide bone density screening in the general population, and current guidance supports bone density screening at or shortly after diagnosis in adults with celiac disease, rather than deferring to the standard age-based screening interval, given this disease-specific risk elevation. Repletion of calcium and vitamin D to guideline-directed targets, confirmed with periodic laboratory monitoring rather than assumed adequate based on supplementation alone, since malabsorption can blunt the expected response to standard oral repletion doses, is a core component of long-term celiac disease management that is easy to deprioritize relative to the more immediately symptomatic aspects of the disease but that carries substantial long-term consequences, including fragility fracture, if neglected. Weight-bearing exercise, where feasible given the patient's overall clinical status, and smoking and alcohol reduction where relevant further support the bone health strategy alongside the nutritional and pharmacologic measures already discussed, mirroring the standard, multi-pronged approach to osteoporosis prevention used outside the context of malabsorptive disease.

### Infection Prevention in Hyposplenic Celiac Disease

Functional hyposplenism, an acquired reduction in splenic function without anatomic splenectomy, occurs in a subset of patients with longstanding, poorly controlled celiac disease, thought to result from chronic immune activation affecting splenic tissue over time, and its clinical significance lies in an increased susceptibility to infection with encapsulated organisms, most importantly Streptococcus pneumoniae, Haemophilus influenzae type b, and Neisseria meningitidis, the same organisms of particular concern in a patient who has undergone surgical splenectomy for another reason. Screening for functional hyposplenism, using either a peripheral blood smear looking for Howell-Jolly bodies, red blood cell inclusions normally cleared by a functioning spleen, or splenic imaging, is a reasonable consideration in a patient with longstanding, poorly controlled disease, and confirmed hyposplenism supports consideration of the same vaccination strategy, including pneumococcal, Haemophilus influenzae type b, and meningococcal vaccination, used for patients with anatomic asplenia, a connection that is easily overlooked since the patient has not undergone any surgical procedure that would typically prompt this vaccination discussion. Patients identified with confirmed hyposplenism also benefit from explicit counseling about seeking prompt medical attention for febrile illness, given their elevated risk of rapidly progressive bacteremia relative to the general population, a counseling point that parallels standard practice for patients with anatomic asplenia. This vaccination discussion should be documented explicitly in the chart so it is not repeated unnecessarily or, conversely, overlooked at a future visit. Note it clearly.

## Emerging and Investigational Approaches

Several pharmacologic strategies are under active investigation as adjuncts to, though not replacements for, the gluten-free diet in celiac disease, including enzymatic approaches designed to degrade immunogenic gluten peptides before they can trigger the immune cascade described earlier in this chapter, and agents targeting the tight junction permeability that allows gluten peptides to cross the intestinal epithelium in the first place. None of these investigational approaches has yet reached a level of evidence supporting routine clinical use as of this writing, and patients should be counseled accurately that the gluten-free diet remains the only established, evidence-based treatment, while also being made aware, particularly if they express frustration with the diet's social and practical burden, that active research toward pharmacologic adjuncts is ongoing, since this awareness can support engagement with dietary treatment in the interim rather than premature adoption of an unproven alternative therapy. Enrollment in a clinical trial is a reasonable option to discuss with appropriately interested and eligible patients, both for the potential individual benefit and for the broader contribution to advancing the evidence base in this area. This field continues to evolve rapidly. Watch this space.

## Diagnostic Approach to Chronic Malabsorption

### Distinguishing Malabsorption From Maldigestion

Malabsorption, a failure of the intestinal mucosa to absorb nutrients that have been adequately digested, is mechanistically distinct from maldigestion, a failure to adequately break down nutrients before absorption can occur, most commonly from pancreatic exocrine insufficiency, and this distinction, while sometimes producing an overlapping clinical picture of steatorrhea and weight loss, guides the diagnostic pathway meaningfully: a fecal elastase level, a marker of pancreatic exocrine function, screens efficiently for maldigestion from pancreatic insufficiency, while the small bowel-directed serologic and histologic evaluation developed throughout this chapter targets true mucosal malabsorption, and a workup that fails to consider both categories in parallel risks an incomplete or delayed diagnosis in a patient whose presentation does not clearly favor one over the other from the outset. Reviewing this distinction explicitly with a patient, rather than allowing them to assume all chronic diarrhea and weight loss reflects a single unified process, also helps set realistic expectations for how many discrete test results may be needed before a specific explanation is reached.

Figure 7.2: Mechanism of Bile Acid Malabsorption

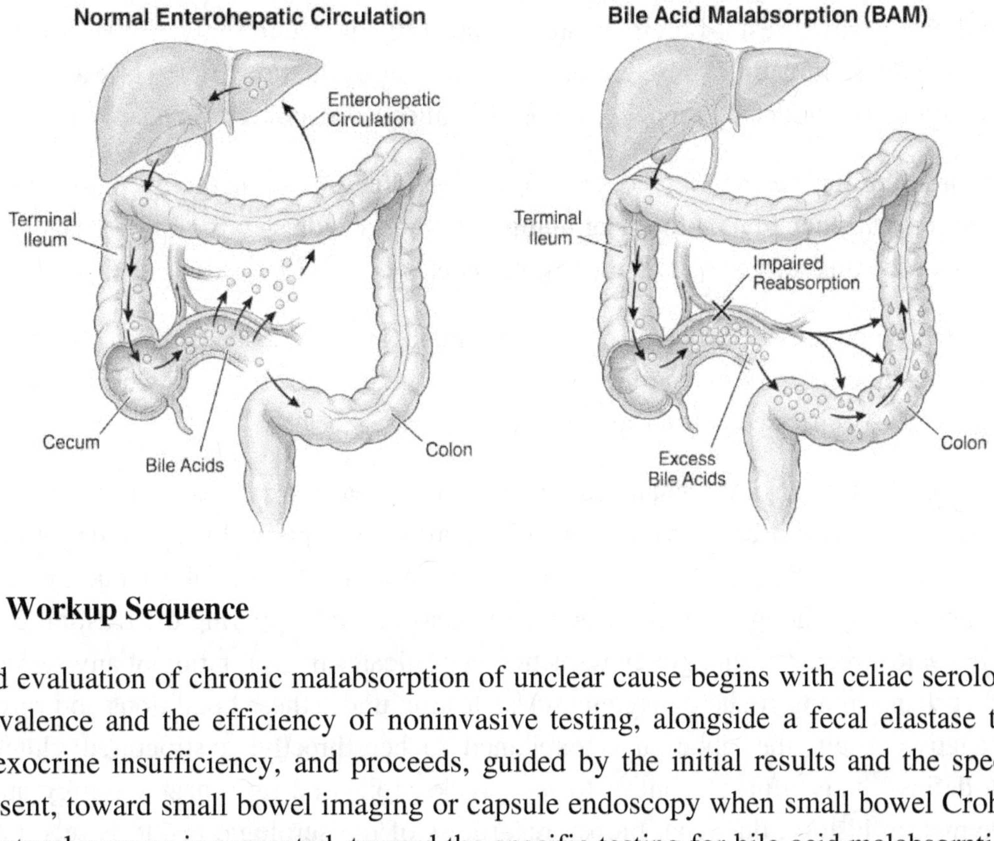


### Structured Workup Sequence

A structured evaluation of chronic malabsorption of unclear cause begins with celiac serology, given its relative prevalence and the efficiency of noninvasive testing, alongside a fecal elastase to screen for pancreatic exocrine insufficiency, and proceeds, guided by the initial results and the specific clinical features present, toward small bowel imaging or capsule endoscopy when small bowel Crohn disease or another structural process is suspected, toward the specific testing for bile acid malabsorption described above when the predominant symptom is watery, urgent diarrhea without other malabsorptive features, and toward duodenal biopsy, which may identify Whipple disease, tropical sprue, or other specific mucosal pathology even when celiac serology is negative, particularly when the clinical picture remains unexplained after the initial round of testing. Documenting the results of each step as they return, rather than waiting until the full sequence is complete to review the case, allows the pathway to be adjusted promptly if an early result already points clearly toward a specific diagnosis. No single fixed order applies universally; the specific presenting features should determine which second-tier test is prioritized first.

## THE GI THRESHOLD DECISION SYSTEM — Small Bowel Thresholds — Sequencing the Malabsorption Workup

**Presentation Signature:** A patient presents with chronic diarrhea, weight loss, or laboratory evidence of a specific nutrient deficiency, and the underlying mechanism, malabsorptive, maldigestive, or another process entirely, has not yet been established.

**Threshold Point:** The presence or absence of steatorrhea and other classic malabsorptive features, together with the fecal elastase result, separates the initial workup into a pancreatic-insufficiency-directed pathway and a small bowel mucosal-disease-directed pathway; a normal fecal elastase and negative celiac serology in a patient with predominantly watery, non-fatty diarrhea shifts the threshold toward bile acid malabsorption and other secretory or motility-related causes.

**The Call:** Order celiac serology and fecal elastase together as an efficient initial parallel screen rather than sequentially; a positive result on either directs the pathway accordingly, while negative results on both, in a patient with a compatible presentation, direct further evaluation toward bile acid malabsorption, small bowel imaging, or duodenal biopsy for a specific mucosal pathology such as Whipple disease.

**Trap Logic:** Ordering the pancreatic and small bowel evaluations sequentially rather than in parallel, waiting for one to return negative before beginning the other, needlessly prolongs a diagnostic pathway that can be efficiently run simultaneously in most patients.

**Decision Anchor:** Screen for both malabsorptive and maldigestive mechanisms in parallel at the outset of a chronic malabsorption workup, and let the pattern of the initial results, not an assumed hierarchy of likelihood, direct the specific second-tier testing that follows.

Case Presentation: A 46-year-old woman presents with two years of intermittent bloating, loose stools, and fatigue, previously diagnosed as irritable bowel syndrome by a prior clinician without further testing. She mentions, when asked directly, that she reduced her bread and pasta intake about a year ago because she felt it seemed to help, though she still eats gluten occasionally. Applying the reasoning developed in this chapter, her self-directed partial gluten reduction complicates interpretation of any serology obtained now, and rather than sending tissue transglutaminase testing under these conditions and risking a falsely reassuring negative result, the situation is explained to her directly: a structured gluten challenge, consuming a defined daily gluten quantity for six weeks, followed by repeat serology and, given her compelling symptom history, duodenal biopsy regardless of the serologic result, is recommended. She completes the challenge, and serology returns positive with Marsh 3 histology on biopsy, confirming celiac disease. She is referred to a dietitian experienced in celiac disease, and her symptoms improve substantially over the following months, with normalization of her tissue transglutaminase titer confirmed at six-month follow-up. This case illustrates the chapter's central diagnostic principle: a patient's self-directed dietary modification before evaluation is a common and easily overlooked source of false-negative celiac testing, and recognizing this pattern, rather than accepting a negative result obtained under these conditions, is what allowed the correct diagnosis to be reached.

Case Presentation: A 51-year-old man, six years after laparoscopic cholecystectomy, presents with two years of urgent, watery diarrhea occurring multiple times daily, worse after meals, without weight loss, blood, or nocturnal symptoms. He was diagnosed with diarrhea-predominant irritable bowel syndrome by a prior clinician and tried multiple antispasmodic and fiber-based therapies without benefit. Applying the reasoning developed in this chapter, the specific combination of postprandial urgency, a temporal relationship to cholecystectomy, which removes the gallbladder's buffering effect on bile acid delivery to the intestine and can unmask or worsen bile acid malabsorption, and a normal malabsorptive picture otherwise, raises suspicion for bile acid malabsorption rather than primary irritable bowel syndrome. Because the specific nuclear medicine retention test is not available at the treating institution, an empiric trial of cholestyramine, a bile acid sequestrant, is initiated as a pragmatic diagnostic and therapeutic strategy. Within two weeks, his diarrhea frequency and urgency improve substantially, a response supporting the diagnosis retrospectively. Celiac serology, sent at the same visit given the overlapping presentation, is negative, and fecal elastase is normal, further supporting bile acid malabsorption as the primary explanation rather than a small bowel mucosal or pancreatic process. This case illustrates a recurring theme from this chapter: a specific historical detail, in this case a prior cholecystectomy and the postprandial timing of symptoms, redirected the diagnostic reasoning toward a specific, treatable mechanism after a nonspecific label had left the patient without adequate symptom control for two years.

| Disorder | Key Diagnostic Test | Distinguishing Clinical Clue |
|---|---|---|
| Celiac disease | tTG-IgA with total IgA; duodenal biopsy | Response to gluten-free diet; family history |
| Tropical sprue | Compatible travel history; biopsy; antibiotic response | Geographic exposure is required for diagnosis |
| Whipple disease | Duodenal biopsy, PAS-positive macrophages | Migratory arthralgia preceding GI symptoms |
| Bile acid malabsorption | SeHCAT retention test or sequestrant trial | Urgent watery diarrhea, often post-cholecystectomy |
| Protein-losing enteropathy | Fecal alpha-1 antitrypsin clearance | Hypoalbuminemia without hepatic or renal cause |

**Presentation Signature:** This chapter's threshold instances addressed interpreting celiac serology in the seronegative or dietary-confounded patient and sequencing the broader malabsorption workup efficiently.

**Threshold Point:** Confirmed adequate gluten intake and normal immunoglobulin A validate a negative celiac serology; fecal elastase and celiac serology run in parallel, not sequentially, separate the pancreatic and small bowel mucosal diagnostic pathways.

**The Call:** Both thresholds prevent a common source of diagnostic delay: accepting a confounded negative test at face value, and testing sequentially when parallel testing would reach the answer faster.

**Trap Logic:** Self-directed dietary gluten reduction before testing is the single most common reason celiac serology is misinterpreted, and it requires active elicitation, since patients rarely volunteer this history unprompted.

**Decision Anchor:** Confirm gluten exposure and immunoglobulin A status before trusting a negative celiac serology, and screen for pancreatic and small bowel mucosal causes of malabsorption in parallel rather than sequentially.

## Summary and Key Concepts

Celiac disease is an immune-mediated enteropathy triggered by gluten in HLA-DQ2/DQ8-susceptible individuals, and its presentation spans classic malabsorptive, non-classic, and silent phenotypes.

Tissue transglutaminase IgA with total IgA is the preferred initial serologic test, but results are only interpretable when gluten intake has been adequate and ongoing at the time of testing.

Duodenal biopsy with Marsh classification remains required to confirm the diagnosis in adults, and self-directed pre-testing gluten reduction is a common, underrecognized cause of false-negative results.

Refractory celiac disease, type 1 versus type 2, carries markedly different prognoses, with type 2 disease carrying a substantial risk of progression to enteropathy-associated T-cell lymphoma.

Tropical sprue, Whipple disease, bile acid malabsorption, and protein-losing enteropathy each have a distinguishing clinical clue and confirmatory test that separates them from celiac disease and from each other.

A structured malabsorption workup screens for malabsorptive and maldigestive mechanisms in parallel using celiac serology and fecal elastase, letting the pattern of results direct subsequent, more targeted testing.

# CHAPTER 8: SMALL INTESTINAL BACTERIAL OVERGROWTH, SHORT BOWEL SYNDROME, AND SMALL BOWEL MOTILITY DISORDERS

**Learning Objectives**

1. Explain the pathophysiology and risk factors for small intestinal bacterial overgrowth and select appropriate diagnostic testing.
2. Apply an antibiotic treatment strategy for small intestinal bacterial overgrowth and manage recurrent disease.
3. Describe the phases of intestinal adaptation after major small bowel resection and apply a stepwise nutritional and pharmacologic management strategy for short bowel syndrome.
4. Recognize the indications for intestinal rehabilitation and transplantation in severe short bowel syndrome.
5. Evaluate and manage chronic intestinal pseudo-obstruction and other small bowel motility disorders.

**Chapter Outline**

This chapter addresses three related small bowel disorders unified by their shared consequence, impaired nutrient absorption and altered luminal physiology: small intestinal bacterial overgrowth, in which excessive or abnormally located colonic-type bacteria in the small bowel disrupt digestion and absorption; short bowel syndrome, in which insufficient small bowel length after resection produces a spectrum of malabsorption requiring structured nutritional rehabilitation; and chronic intestinal pseudo-obstruction, in which a primary motility disorder produces obstructive symptoms without a mechanical lesion. Each section connects a specific diagnostic or severity threshold to a defined management pathway, continuing this book's recurring approach.

## Small Intestinal Bacterial Overgrowth

### Pathophysiology and Risk Factors

The proximal small bowel normally harbors a relatively sparse bacterial population, maintained by a combination of gastric acid, which limits the survival of ingested organisms; the migrating motor complex, a cyclical pattern of propulsive contractions that sweeps bacteria distally during the fasting state; an intact ileocecal valve, which limits retrograde translocation of the much denser colonic bacterial population; and normal small bowel anatomy, without blind loops or strictures that create a stagnant reservoir. Small intestinal bacterial overgrowth develops when one or more of these protective mechanisms fails: profound or prolonged acid suppression reduces the gastric barrier; any condition impairing small bowel motility, including diabetic autonomic neuropathy, scleroderma-spectrum disease, and the chronic intestinal pseudo-obstruction discussed later in this chapter, disables the migrating motor complex's sweeping function; surgically altered anatomy, including a blind afferent limb after certain gastric surgeries or a surgically bypassed or absent ileocecal valve, creates a stagnant reservoir; and structural abnormalities, including strictures, diverticula, or adhesions, similarly create pockets where normal luminal flow is disrupted. Once excessive bacterial colonization is established, the bacteria themselves cause disease through several converging mechanisms: premature carbohydrate fermentation producing the gas responsible for bloating and distension, bacterial deconjugation of bile acids impairing fat digestion and producing the bile-acid-related diarrhea mechanism discussed in the previous chapter, and, in more severe or longstanding cases, direct bacterial competition for and consumption of nutrients, particularly vitamin B12, alongside bacterial overproduction of certain other nutrients, such as folate, producing a distinctive combined pattern of low B12 with normal or elevated folate that can itself be a diagnostic clue. Each of these mechanisms operates largely independently, which is why more than one predisposing factor can coexist in the same patient, and why a thorough evaluation should not stop once a single plausible explanation, such as chronic proton pump inhibitor use, has been identified, if a second, more mechanistically significant factor, such as an underlying motility disorder, remains unexamined.

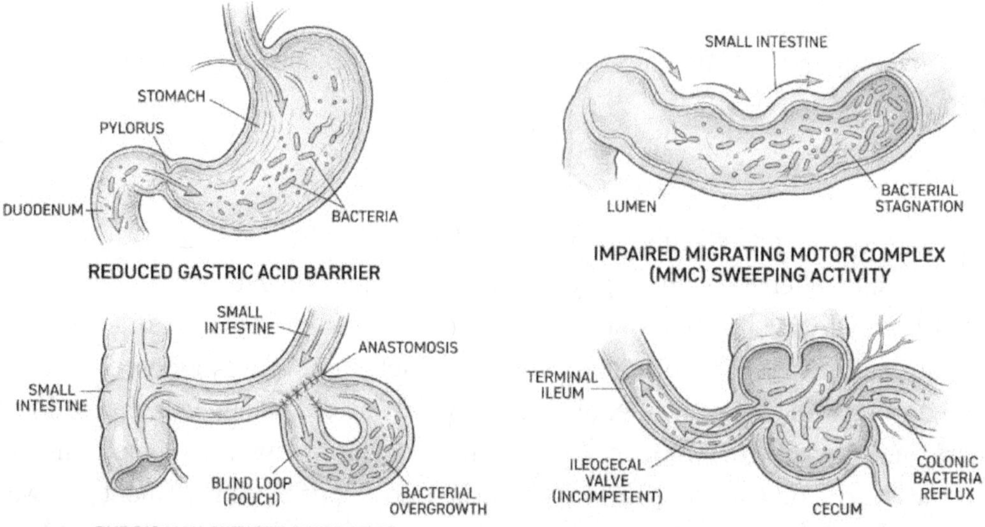

FIGURE 8.1: MECHANISMS PREDISPOSING TO SMALL INTESTINAL BACTERIAL OVERGROWTH

## Clinical Presentation

Bloating, abdominal distension, excessive flatulence, and diarrhea, sometimes alternating with constipation, constitute the core symptom complex, and this overlap with irritable bowel syndrome, discussed in a later chapter, is substantial enough that small intestinal bacterial overgrowth is increasingly recognized as an underlying or contributing mechanism in a meaningful subset of patients carrying an irritable bowel syndrome label, particularly the diarrhea-predominant subtype. Weight loss and overt evidence of malabsorption, including steatorrhea and specific nutrient deficiencies, occur in more severe or longstanding cases and should prompt more urgent evaluation and treatment, while the vitamin B12 and folate pattern described above, when present, offers a specific, actionable diagnostic clue that distinguishes bacterial overgrowth from many of its symptomatic mimics. Because bacterial overgrowth so often develops as a secondary consequence of another underlying condition, evaluation should always include a search for the specific predisposing factor, a motility disorder, surgically altered anatomy, or a structural lesion, since treating the overgrowth alone without addressing its underlying cause typically produces only temporary improvement before recurrence, a pattern developed further in the treatment discussion below. Directly asking about the specific temporal pattern of symptoms relative to meals, and about the presence or absence of the specific predisposing risk factors catalogued in the preceding section, helps distinguish a presentation more likely to represent true bacterial overgrowth from one more likely to represent an alternative functional or structural process.

**Diagnostic Testing: Breath Testing and Alternatives**

Breath testing, using either lactulose or glucose as the ingested substrate with serial measurement of exhaled hydrogen and methane, is the most widely available and practical diagnostic approach, and its interpretation, introduced briefly in the second chapter, depends on identifying a rise in breath gas concentration that occurs too early to represent normal colonic fermentation of the substrate, adjusted for the individual patient's estimated small bowel transit time. Methane measurement specifically identifies a distinct clinical entity, intestinal methanogen overgrowth, in which methane-producing archaea rather than hydrogen-producing bacteria predominate, and this distinction matters because methane itself is known to slow intestinal transit directly, producing a presentation weighted toward constipation rather than diarrhea, and because the antibiotic regimen most effective against methanogen overgrowth differs somewhat from the standard regimen used for hydrogen-predominant bacterial overgrowth, discussed in the treatment section below. Jejunal aspirate culture, historically considered the diagnostic reference standard, quantifying bacterial colony counts directly from small bowel fluid obtained at the time of upper endoscopy, is used less commonly in current practice given its invasiveness, the technical variability in aspirate collection, and the comparable practical utility of noninvasive breath testing in most clinical scenarios, though it retains a role in research settings and in selected complex cases where breath testing has been inconclusive. Selecting an experienced laboratory with standardized testing protocols and clear reporting of the raw gas concentration curve, rather than only a binary positive-or-negative summary result, allows the ordering clinician to apply the interpretive nuances discussed throughout this section rather than relying solely on an automated threshold determination.

**THE GI THRESHOLD DECISION SYSTEM — Small Bowel Thresholds — Interpreting Breath Testing and Selecting Antibiotic Therapy**

---

**Presentation Signature:** A patient with bloating, distension, and altered bowel habits, often previously labeled with irritable bowel syndrome, undergoes breath testing for suspected small intestinal bacterial overgrowth.

**Threshold Point:** A rise in hydrogen of a defined magnitude within the early testing window, adjusted for estimated small bowel transit time, defines a positive hydrogen-predominant test; a rise in methane above a separate defined threshold at any point during testing defines methane-predominant overgrowth, or intestinal methanogen overgrowth, regardless of the hydrogen pattern.

**The Call:** Hydrogen-predominant overgrowth is treated with an antibiotic regimen targeting predominantly gram-negative and anaerobic small bowel flora; methane-predominant overgrowth is treated with a regimen that adds or substitutes an agent with activity against methanogenic archaea, since standard hydrogen-directed therapy alone is less reliably effective against this specific pattern.

**The Call:** A negative breath test in a patient with a strong clinical suspicion and a clear predisposing risk factor should prompt consideration of jejunal aspirate culture or an empiric antibiotic trial rather than immediate abandonment of the diagnosis, given breath testing's imperfect sensitivity.

**Trap Logic:** Treating every positive breath test identically, without distinguishing the hydrogen- from the methane-predominant pattern, risks under-treating methane-predominant disease with a regimen not adequately directed at the organisms actually responsible.

**Decision Anchor:** Match antibiotic selection to the specific gas pattern identified on breath testing, and pursue further evaluation in a breath-test-negative patient with a compelling clinical picture rather than accepting a single negative result as definitive.

### Treatment: Antibiotics and Recurrence Management

Rifaximin, a minimally systemically absorbed antibiotic with broad activity against small bowel flora and a favorable safety profile suited to repeated courses, is the most extensively studied and generally preferred first-line agent for hydrogen-predominant small intestinal bacterial overgrowth, while methane-predominant disease typically requires the addition of a second agent, most commonly neomycin, given evidence that combination therapy achieves substantially higher methane normalization rates than rifaximin alone in this specific pattern. Symptomatic and, where retested, breath-test improvement following an appropriate antibiotic course supports the diagnosis retrospectively, paralleling the pragmatic, response-based diagnostic confirmation strategy already introduced in this book for bile acid malabsorption in the previous chapter. A typical treatment course runs ten to fourteen days, and clinical improvement is generally assessed within one to two weeks of completion rather than during the antibiotic course itself, since a brief interval is needed for the reduced bacterial burden to translate into measurable symptomatic change.

### Recurrence and the Underlying Predisposing Condition

Recurrence after successful initial treatment is common, particularly in patients whose underlying predisposing condition, whether a motility disorder, surgically altered anatomy, or a structural lesion, cannot itself be corrected, and repeated antibiotic courses, sometimes cycled at defined intervals rather than only in response to symptom recurrence, are a reasonable and commonly used long-term strategy in this population, alongside dietary approaches, such as reduced intake of readily fermentable carbohydrates, that may extend the symptom-free interval between courses even when they do not eradicate the underlying colonization pattern. Prokinetic therapy, when a motility disorder is the identified predisposing condition, addresses the underlying mechanism directly by restoring more effective migrating motor complex activity, and its use as maintenance therapy between antibiotic courses, rather than only during active gastroparesis or dysmotility symptom flares, is a reasonable strategy specifically aimed at reducing bacterial overgrowth recurrence frequency in this population. Discussing this recurrence pattern candidly with the patient at the time of initial diagnosis, rather than only after a first recurrence has already caused frustration, sets realistic long-term expectations for a condition that, in the setting of an unmodifiable predisposing factor, functions more like a chronic disease requiring periodic management than an acute infection cured once and permanently resolved. Plan for this from the start.

## Short Bowel Syndrome

### Definition and Anatomic Considerations

Short bowel syndrome describes the malabsorptive state that follows extensive small bowel resection, most commonly from mesenteric ischemia, Crohn disease requiring repeated resection, radiation enteritis, or a complicated abdominal surgical catastrophe, and its severity depends not only on the absolute length of remaining small bowel but critically on which specific segments remain and whether the colon remains in continuity. The jejunum and ileum, despite performing broadly overlapping absorptive functions for most macronutrients, differ in specialized capacity: the terminal ileum is the sole site of vitamin B12 and bile acid active reabsorption, meaning that ileal loss, even when jejunal length is preserved, produces the bile acid malabsorption pattern discussed in the previous chapter and requires lifelong vitamin B12 repletion, while extensive jejunal loss with a preserved ileum and colon is generally better tolerated, since the ileum can adapt over time to assume many of the jejunum's absorptive functions, an adaptive capacity the jejunum does not reciprocally have for the ileum's specialized functions. Colonic continuity matters substantially for a related reason: an intact colon salvages additional calories through bacterial fermentation of otherwise unabsorbed carbohydrate into short-chain fatty acids and slows overall transit, meaningfully reducing the parenteral nutrition dependence of a patient with a given length of remaining small bowel compared to an anatomically identical patient whose colon has also been resected or is not in continuity. Reviewing the operative report in detail, as discussed further below, is an essential first step in evaluating any patient with short bowel syndrome, since the specific segments resected and remaining, not total length alone, drive this severity assessment. Length alone is insufficient.

### Phases of Intestinal Adaptation

Intestinal adaptation after major resection proceeds through three recognized phases that should shape both prognostic counseling and the pace of nutritional advancement. The acute phase, in the days to weeks immediately following resection, is characterized by large-volume fluid and electrolyte losses and requires primarily intravenous fluid and electrolyte support with cautious, gradual introduction of enteral intake. The adaptation phase, extending over the following one to two years, is characterized by structural and functional intestinal adaptation, including villous hyperplasia and increased absorptive surface area in the remaining bowel, a process that can be further supported pharmacologically as discussed below, during which enteral and oral intake are progressively advanced as tolerated while parenteral support is titrated down in parallel rather than withdrawn abruptly. The maintenance, or stabilization, phase reflects the patient's eventual, relatively stable long-term nutritional status, which for some patients means successful weaning from parenteral nutrition entirely and for others means a stable requirement for long-term partial or complete parenteral support, a distinction that becomes reasonably clear only after the adaptation phase has been given adequate time to run its course, generally at least one to two years, before being considered a fixed, long-term outcome. Setting this multi-year timeline explicitly with the patient at the outset, rather than allowing them to expect rapid resolution, supports more realistic engagement with what is often a slow, incremental process punctuated by both progress and setbacks.

## Nutritional and Fluid Management

Oral rehydration solution formulated specifically for high-output states, with a sodium concentration substantially higher than standard commercial sports drinks or diluted juice, is essential in patients with significant ongoing fluid losses, particularly those with a jejunostomy or high-output stoma, because standard oral fluids with inadequate sodium concentration are poorly absorbed across the remaining bowel and can paradoxically worsen net fluid losses rather than correct them, a counterintuitive point that requires explicit patient education since the instinctive response to fluid loss, drinking more of an ordinary beverage, is often the wrong one in this specific population. Enteral nutrition, advanced gradually and preferentially over parenteral nutrition whenever the remaining bowel can tolerate it, is preferred because enteral nutrients themselves are a primary stimulus for the structural adaptation described above, meaning that even partial enteral intake alongside parenteral support serves an adaptation-promoting purpose beyond its direct caloric contribution, and small, frequent meals with separation of solid food from liquid intake, rather than combined consumption, is a specific, practical strategy that reduces the osmotic load delivered to the remaining bowel at any one time and is a common source of preventable symptom exacerbation when overlooked. Providing the patient with the specific recipe or a reliable commercial source for an appropriately concentrated solution, rather than a general instruction to drink an oral rehydration product, ensures the sodium concentration actually delivered matches what the remaining bowel requires for effective absorption.

## Pharmacologic Therapy

Antimotility agents, including loperamide and, in more severe cases, codeine or diphenoxylate-atropine, slow transit and increase contact time between luminal contents and the remaining absorptive surface, and dosing in short bowel syndrome is frequently higher than standard dosing used for ordinary diarrhea, reflecting both reduced absorptive surface for the medication itself and the greater degree of hypermotility being targeted. Antisecretory therapy, including proton pump inhibitors to reduce the secretory hypergastrinemia that commonly accompanies extensive small bowel resection in its early phases, and, in refractory high-output states, somatostatin analogues, which reduce a range of gastrointestinal secretions simultaneously, reduce the fluid volume the remaining bowel must process. Glucagon-like peptide-2 analogue therapy, a more recently developed class specifically targeting the trophic, adaptation-promoting signaling pathway that glucagon-like peptide-2 mediates physiologically, has demonstrated the ability to reduce parenteral nutrition volume requirements in appropriately selected patients with short bowel syndrome, representing a therapy that, unlike the symptomatic approaches above, is specifically designed to enhance the structural adaptation process itself rather than only manage its downstream consequences. Dosing decisions should be individualized and reassessed regularly as the patient's remaining absorptive capacity and adaptation status evolve over the phases described above, rather than fixed at whatever dose was initially effective in the acute postoperative period. Patient selection and ongoing monitoring for glucagon-like peptide-2 analogue therapy specifically are typically managed in coordination with a specialized intestinal rehabilitation program given the expertise required.

### Complications of Long-Term Parenteral Nutrition

Catheter-related bloodstream infection is among the most consequential complications of long-term parenteral nutrition dependence, given both its acute morbidity and the risk of losing venous access sites over a patient's lifetime with recurrent catheter infections, and meticulous catheter care education, along with prompt evaluation of any fever in a parenteral-nutrition-dependent patient for catheter infection specifically, applying the same threshold-based urgency reasoning developed throughout this book, is a critical component of long-term management. Parenteral-nutrition-associated liver disease, ranging from simple steatosis to progressive fibrosis and, in severe cases, liver failure, results from a combination of the parenteral lipid formulation used, particularly older soy-based lipid emulsions now increasingly replaced by fish-oil-containing or mixed-lipid formulations with a more favorable hepatic safety profile, and the absence of enteral stimulation itself, reinforcing why maximizing enteral intake whenever tolerated, discussed above, serves a hepatoprotective as well as an adaptation-promoting purpose. Metabolic bone disease, from a combination of mineral and vitamin D deficits, chronic metabolic acidosis in some patients, and certain components of long-term parenteral formulations, requires the same periodic bone density monitoring and repletion approach developed in the previous chapter for malabsorptive disease more broadly. A written, patient-accessible protocol for catheter care and for recognizing early signs of infection empowers the patient to act as an active partner in preventing this complication rather than relying solely on periodic clinic visits to catch problems. Serial liver enzyme and bilirubin monitoring at regular intervals allows early detection of parenteral-nutrition-associated liver disease before it progresses to a more advanced, less reversible stage. Combining bone density monitoring with the broader nutritional laboratory panel already being drawn periodically avoids adding a separate, easily forgotten testing schedule.

### THE GI THRESHOLD DECISION SYSTEM — Small Bowel Thresholds — When Intestinal Rehabilitation or Transplant Referral Is Warranted

**Presentation Signature:** A patient with short bowel syndrome remains dependent on parenteral nutrition well into or beyond the expected adaptation phase, and the clinician must determine whether continued medical optimization or referral to a specialized intestinal rehabilitation program is appropriate.

**Threshold Point:** Persistent, significant parenteral nutrition dependence beyond the one- to two-year adaptation window, particularly when accompanied by recurrent catheter infections, progressive parenteral-nutrition-associated liver disease, or loss of usable venous access sites, defines the threshold for referral to a specialized intestinal rehabilitation program.

**The Call:** Patients below this threshold continue optimized medical, nutritional, and pharmacologic management, including glucagon-like peptide-2 analogue therapy where appropriate, with periodic reassessment of weaning potential; patients crossing this threshold, especially with progressive liver disease or loss of vascular access, are referred for comprehensive intestinal rehabilitation evaluation, which may include advanced surgical lengthening procedures or, in the most severe cases, evaluation for intestinal transplantation.

**Trap Logic:** Delaying rehabilitation referral until parenteral-nutrition-associated liver disease has become advanced or venous access has been substantially exhausted meaningfully worsens transplant candidacy and outcomes; referral should occur proactively once the threshold criteria are met, not only after these complications have already become severe.

**Decision Anchor:** Reassess parenteral nutrition dependence formally at the one- to two-year mark, and refer for specialized intestinal rehabilitation evaluation proactively once dependence persists with any of the complicating features above, rather than waiting for a crisis to prompt the referral.

### Intestinal Rehabilitation and Transplantation

Specialized intestinal rehabilitation programs, combining nutritional, medical, and surgical expertise, offer bowel-lengthening procedures, such as serial transverse enteroplasty, that surgically increase the functional absorptive surface of dilated, poorly functioning remaining bowel without further sacrificing bowel length, and these procedures can, in appropriately selected patients, meaningfully reduce or eliminate parenteral nutrition dependence. Intestinal transplantation, whether isolated or combined with liver transplantation in patients with advanced parenteral-nutrition-associated liver disease, is reserved for patients with irreversible intestinal failure and either life-threatening complications of parenteral nutrition, including recurrent catheter sepsis or progressive liver disease, or loss of adequate venous access, and outcomes, while historically more limited than for other solid organ transplants, have improved substantially with advances in immunosuppression and surgical technique, making timely referral, per the threshold developed above, an important determinant of eventual candidacy and outcome. Not every patient with persistent parenteral nutrition dependence is a candidate for bowel-lengthening surgery, and careful patient selection by a center with specific expertise in these procedures is essential to achieving the outcomes described here rather than exposing an unsuitable candidate to added surgical risk without a reasonable expectation of benefit. Patients and families should understand that transplant referral, once initiated, is itself a lengthy evaluation process, reinforcing why timely referral matters well before a crisis forces an urgent decision.

## Nutrient-Specific Deficiencies and Surgical Considerations in Short Bowel Syndrome

Beyond the general fluid, electrolyte, and macronutrient management already discussed, short bowel syndrome produces a predictable pattern of specific micronutrient deficiencies that mirrors, but often exceeds in severity, the pattern discussed in the previous chapter for celiac disease and other malabsorptive conditions, since the absorptive surface loss in short bowel syndrome is typically more extensive and anatomically defined. Magnesium deficiency deserves particular emphasis, since it is both extremely common in this population, driven by direct malabsorption and by excessive fecal or stomal losses, and clinically consequential, contributing to muscle cramping, cardiac arrhythmia risk, and, notably, impaired parathyroid hormone secretion that can worsen the calcium and bone metabolism derangements also common in this population, meaning that a low calcium level in a short bowel patient should always prompt a concurrent magnesium check rather than calcium repletion alone. Oral magnesium repletion is often poorly tolerated because magnesium salts themselves have a cathartic, diarrhea-promoting effect that is particularly problematic in a population whose primary management challenge is already excessive fluid loss, and topical or, in more severe cases, intravenous repletion strategies are frequently required as a practical alternative to oral supplementation in this specific population. Zinc deficiency is also common in this population given both direct malabsorption and increased losses through high-output stool or stoma output, and it should be assessed and repleted alongside the more routinely checked electrolytes and fat-soluble vitamins discussed in the previous chapter. Periodic magnesium monitoring should continue even after apparent initial correction, since ongoing losses can rapidly re-establish deficiency without sustained repletion. Discussing this oral-tolerability trade-off directly with the patient prevents frustration when a supplement recommended for a different condition proves poorly tolerated in this specific context.

### Surgical Considerations at the Time of Resection

The surgical decisions made at the time of the index resection meaningfully shape a patient's subsequent short bowel syndrome course, and involving a surgeon with specific experience in intestinal failure, where feasible even in an emergent setting, to preserve every centimeter of viable bowel and to document precisely which segments were resected and which remain, provides essential information that shapes every subsequent management decision developed throughout this chapter. Preservation of the ileocecal valve specifically, when oncologically or otherwise clinically appropriate to do so, meaningfully slows transit and reduces the risk of secondary bacterial overgrowth from colonic reflux, reinforcing why this anatomic detail, discussed earlier in this chapter as a key determinant of bacterial overgrowth risk, should be a specific consideration in surgical planning whenever an alternative exists that does not compromise the primary indication for surgery, whether oncologic resection margins or control of the underlying inflammatory or ischemic process. Precise documentation of resected and remaining bowel length in the operative report, rather than a vague description, is a small documentation practice with outsized downstream value, since this measurement directly informs every subsequent prognostic and management discussion covered in this chapter. Involving the gastroenterology or nutrition support team early, even during the initial hospitalization, allows this longer-term management perspective to inform surgical decision-making from the outset rather than being applied only after the patient has already been discharged. This anatomic preservation decision, made in the operating room, has consequences felt by the patient and care team for years afterward. This single line of documentation is easy to overlook amid the many other priorities of an emergent operative report.

## SIBO Testing Pitfalls and Diagnostic Confounders

Breath testing accuracy depends on several practical factors that, when overlooked, produce misleading results in either direction. A fermentable-carbohydrate-restricted diet for the 24 hours preceding testing and an overnight fast immediately before the test are both required to establish an appropriate low baseline against which the ingested substrate's effect can be distinguished, and recent antibiotic use, which can suppress small bowel flora enough to produce a false-negative result for a period of several weeks afterward, should be specifically elicited before testing is scheduled, paralleling the medication-timing considerations already emphasized for Helicobacter pylori and celiac disease testing elsewhere in this book. Rapid small bowel transit, whether from an underlying motility disorder or simply individual physiologic variation, can cause the ingested substrate to reach the colon and begin normal fermentation earlier than the standard interpretive thresholds assume, producing a false-positive result that mimics small intestinal bacterial overgrowth, which is why some testing protocols incorporate a transit marker or use glucose, which is more completely absorbed in the proximal small bowel under normal circumstances, as an alternative substrate specifically to reduce this source of false-positive interpretation relative to lactulose, which is not absorbed and is more susceptible to this transit-related confounding. Providing the patient with clear, written pre-test instructions covering diet, fasting, and medication timing, rather than a brief verbal reminder easily forgotten before the scheduled test date, meaningfully reduces the rate of technically inadequate or misleading results. These preparation steps are simple but frequently overlooked in practice.

### Distinguishing SIBO From Its Symptomatic Mimics

The bloating, gas, and altered bowel habit symptom complex of small intestinal bacterial overgrowth overlaps substantially with irritable bowel syndrome, functional dyspepsia when upper abdominal symptoms predominate, and, as discussed in the previous chapter, bile acid malabsorption and celiac disease, and clinicians should resist anchoring on bacterial overgrowth as the default explanation simply because breath testing is a familiar and accessible test to order, particularly when a compelling predisposing risk factor for bacterial overgrowth, such as those catalogued earlier in this chapter, is absent. A negative, technically adequate breath test in a patient without an identifiable predisposing condition should prompt genuine reconsideration of these alternative diagnoses rather than repeated bacterial overgrowth testing or empiric antibiotic trials pursued indefinitely in search of a positive result. Ordering breath testing as a first-line, undifferentiated screen for any patient with bloating, without first considering whether a plausible predisposing factor exists, both lowers the pretest probability of a true positive result and increases the likelihood of a confounded or misleading test outcome. Context always matters more than a familiar test order.

## Postoperative Ileus and Its Distinction From Chronic Pseudo-obstruction

Postoperative ileus, a transient, expected reduction in bowel motility following abdominal surgery, must be distinguished from the chronic intestinal pseudo-obstruction discussed later in this chapter, since the two conditions, while sharing a superficially similar obstructive symptom picture, differ fundamentally in expected duration, underlying mechanism, and management, and conflating them can lead either to premature, unnecessary escalation of workup for a self-limited postoperative process or, conversely, to underappreciation of a genuine chronic motility disorder misattributed indefinitely to prolonged postoperative recovery. Standard postoperative ileus typically resolves within three to five days of abdominal surgery, and a range of perioperative strategies, including minimizing opioid use through multimodal analgesia, early postoperative mobilization, and, where appropriate, early initiation of a limited oral diet rather than the traditional practice of prolonged nil-by-mouth status until flatus is passed, have been shown to shorten its duration meaningfully as part of enhanced recovery after surgery protocols now widely adopted across many surgical specialties. Consulting gastroenterology for straightforward, expected postoperative ileus within its normal resolution window is generally unnecessary and can be reserved for cases that are prolonged or atypical, applying the same triage discipline emphasized throughout this book. Reserve escalation for atypical cases.

### Prolonged Postoperative Ileus

Postoperative ileus persisting beyond the expected window, generally considered prolonged beyond five days, should prompt evaluation for a specific contributing factor rather than continued observation alone: mechanical obstruction from an early postoperative complication such as an internal hernia or adhesive band, electrolyte derangements, particularly hypokalemia, which directly impairs smooth muscle contractility, ongoing opioid use, which independently and substantially delays motility recovery through direct effects on enteric opioid receptors, and, less commonly, an evolving intra-abdominal process such as an anastomotic leak or abscess that itself impairs motility as a secondary inflammatory phenomenon. Systematically working through this differential, rather than reflexively extending nil-by-mouth status and continued observation indefinitely, applies the same active diagnostic reasoning emphasized throughout this book to a scenario that is easy to manage passively simply because some degree of ileus is expected after every abdominal operation. A structured checklist covering these possibilities, reviewed explicitly whenever ileus extends past the expected window, standardizes this evaluation across a busy surgical or medical service.

## Psychosocial Impact and Multidisciplinary Support in Chronic Small Bowel Disease

Living with short bowel syndrome, chronic intestinal pseudo-obstruction, or recurrent small intestinal bacterial overgrowth imposes a substantial and often underrecognized psychosocial burden, including anxiety around eating, social isolation related to dietary restriction and the practical demands of parenteral nutrition administration, and, for patients dependent on home parenteral nutrition, a considerable daily time commitment and disruption to employment and travel, and screening for this burden using the same brief, validated instruments discussed in earlier chapters for other chronic gastrointestinal conditions is an appropriate standard component of ongoing management rather than an optional addition reserved for patients who volunteer distress unprompted. Home parenteral nutrition, in particular, requires substantial patient and caregiver education and ongoing support, ideally delivered through a dedicated nutrition support team including pharmacy, nursing, and social work expertise alongside the medical management developed throughout this chapter, since the technical demands of safe catheter care and infusion administration are considerable and errors carry serious consequences, including the catheter infections discussed earlier in this chapter. Connecting patients with peer support communities specific to home parenteral nutrition or short bowel syndrome, where available, provides practical, lived-experience guidance that a clinical encounter alone cannot fully replicate. This screening is quick.

**Coordinating Long-Term, Multidisciplinary Care**

The conditions addressed in this chapter, more than perhaps any other topic in this book, require sustained coordination across gastroenterology, surgery, nutrition support services, and, for the most complex cases, specialized intestinal rehabilitation and transplant programs, and applying the explicit, plan-anchored coordination principle emphasized throughout this book is essential given both the number of involved specialties and the years-long duration over which this coordination typically must be sustained. A single identified point of contact, generally the gastroenterologist or the nutrition support team managing the patient's primary long-term care, who maintains an updated, comprehensive summary of the current management plan and actively coordinates input from other involved specialties, prevents the fragmentation that a purely reactive, specialty-siloed approach to this patient population tends to produce over time. Scheduled, proactive check-ins from this coordinating contact, rather than only reactive contact triggered by a crisis, further supports continuity across this typically years-long care relationship. This matters over years.

**Considerations in Pediatric-Onset Intestinal Failure**

Short bowel syndrome arising in infancy, most commonly following necrotizing enterocolitis, intestinal atresia, or gastroschisis, differs from adult-onset disease in an important respect: the pediatric intestine retains a greater capacity for both structural and functional adaptation over time, meaning that a degree of intestinal failure that might appear permanent based on remaining length alone can improve substantially over years of growth and continued adaptation in a way less consistently seen in adults, which shapes both prognostic counseling and the threshold for pursuing aggressive rehabilitation versus earlier transplant referral in this population. Adult gastroenterologists who inherit a pediatric-onset short bowel syndrome patient at the transition to adult care should specifically review the detailed history of the patient's adaptation trajectory over childhood, since this longitudinal pattern provides prognostic information that a single snapshot of the patient's current anatomy and status alone cannot fully convey, echoing the transition-of-care principle already developed in the previous chapter for pediatric-onset celiac disease. This distinction should be discussed explicitly with families early in the course of pediatric intestinal failure, since it materially affects both the emotional experience of the diagnosis and the treatment intensity pursued during the extended pediatric adaptation window. Always.

## Medication-Related and Other Secondary Causes of Small Bowel Dysmotility

Beyond the scleroderma-spectrum disease, diabetic autonomic neuropathy, and paraneoplastic causes already discussed, several medication classes produce clinically significant small bowel hypomotility as an on-target or off-target effect, most importantly opioids, which slow transit throughout the entire gastrointestinal tract via direct effects on enteric mu-opioid receptors, and certain anticholinergic and antipsychotic medications, whose motility-slowing effect is frequently underrecognized as contributing to a patient's symptoms because it is not the primary indication for which the medication was prescribed. A careful, comprehensive medication review, applying the same direct, systematic approach to medication history developed in the first chapter, is therefore an essential early step in evaluating any patient with symptoms suggestive of small bowel dysmotility, since a medication-related cause, once identified, is addressed through dose adjustment, discontinuation, or substitution rather than through the more invasive manometric and secondary-cause evaluation that would otherwise be pursued for suspected primary chronic intestinal pseudo-obstruction. Maintaining an updated, complete medication list at every visit, rather than relying on the patient to spontaneously report every medication they take, is the practical foundation that makes this review possible. Simple habit.

## Amyloidosis and Other Infiltrative Causes

Amyloidosis, whether primary or secondary to a chronic inflammatory or plasma cell dyscrasia-related process, infiltrates the intestinal wall and autonomic nerves, producing a small bowel dysmotility pattern that can closely resemble diabetic or scleroderma-related disease, and its recognition depends on maintaining a specific index of suspicion in a patient with an unexplained dysmotility pattern who does not have one of the more commonly encountered predisposing conditions already discussed, particularly when accompanied by other systemic features suggestive of amyloid involvement, such as unexplained proteinuria, cardiomyopathy, or peripheral neuropathy affecting other organ systems beyond the gastrointestinal tract. Tissue biopsy demonstrating amyloid deposition, obtained either from the gastrointestinal tract itself or from a more accessible site such as abdominal fat pad aspiration, confirms the diagnosis, and management addresses the underlying plasma cell or inflammatory process driving amyloid production, since the intestinal manifestations themselves are a downstream consequence of a systemic process rather than a primary, independently treatable gastrointestinal disease. Hematology or rheumatology co-management, depending on the underlying driver identified, is essential once this diagnosis is confirmed, mirroring the multidisciplinary coordination already emphasized for the other secondary causes discussed in this chapter. Every time.

## Small Bowel Motility Disorders

### Chronic Intestinal Pseudo-obstruction

Chronic intestinal pseudo-obstruction produces the clinical picture of mechanical bowel obstruction, including distension, pain, nausea, and vomiting, without an identifiable mechanical lesion, arising instead from a primary disorder of the intestinal smooth muscle, myopathic pseudo-obstruction, or the enteric neurons and interstitial cells of Cajal that coordinate its contraction, neuropathic pseudo-obstruction, and it may be primary or idiopathic, or secondary to an identifiable systemic cause, including scleroderma-spectrum disease, mitochondrial disorders, paraneoplastic syndromes, most classically associated with small cell lung cancer, and certain medications. The distinction between myopathic and neuropathic forms, while not always possible to establish definitively without specialized full-thickness intestinal biopsy obtained at a center with specific expertise in this evaluation, carries some prognostic and management relevance, and secondary causes should always be actively sought, since identifying and treating an underlying paraneoplastic process, for example, changes management fundamentally from the symptomatic, motility-directed approach used for primary or idiopathic disease. Episodes are frequently intermittent, with periods of relative symptomatic quiescence interrupted by acute exacerbations resembling a true bowel obstruction, and this pattern, once recognized, should prompt maintenance of a longitudinal symptom record so that exacerbation frequency and severity, rather than the clinician's most recent single encounter, guide escalation decisions.

### Evaluation of Suspected Dysmotility

Evaluation begins, as with any suspected obstructive process, by excluding a true mechanical obstruction through cross-sectional imaging and, where indicated, endoscopic evaluation, since mistaking chronic intestinal pseudo-obstruction for the diagnosis in a patient who in fact has a mechanical lesion, or the reverse, subjecting a patient with true pseudo-obstruction to repeated unnecessary surgery in a mistaken search for a mechanical cause that does not exist, are both consequential and avoidable errors. Once mechanical obstruction is excluded, small bowel manometry, obtained at a specialized motility center, characterizes the specific pattern of dysmotility and can help distinguish myopathic from neuropathic disease based on the amplitude and coordination of the pressure waves recorded, while a directed evaluation for the secondary causes listed above, including autoimmune and paraneoplastic antibody panels and, where clinically indicated, age-appropriate malignancy screening, should proceed in parallel rather than only after an exhaustive primary motility workup has been completed. A prior, well-documented history of extensive workup already excluding mechanical causes should be actively sought and reviewed before repeating imaging that has already been performed, both to avoid unnecessary radiation exposure and to prevent the diagnostic fatigue that repeated, redundant testing can produce in a patient already navigating a chronic, difficult-to-diagnose condition. This exclusion step is not optional.

## Management of Chronic Intestinal Pseudo-obstruction

Management follows a similarly staged approach to the gastroparesis framework developed in an earlier chapter: dietary modification toward smaller, lower-residue, more easily transited meals; prokinetic pharmacotherapy, though with generally more modest efficacy in this population than in gastroparesis given the frequently more severe and diffuse nature of the underlying motility disorder; and, in more severe cases, nutritional support ranging from enteral access placed distal to the most severely affected bowel segment through parenteral nutrition when enteral tolerance is inadequate, applying the same short bowel syndrome nutritional principles developed earlier in this chapter even though the underlying mechanism, a motility disorder rather than reduced bowel length, differs. Small intestinal bacterial overgrowth, given the impaired migrating motor complex activity intrinsic to this condition, is a near-universal complicating feature in chronic intestinal pseudo-obstruction and should be anticipated and treated proactively using the antibiotic strategies developed earlier in this chapter, applied cyclically given the essentially unmodifiable underlying motility abnormality driving recurrent overgrowth in this population. Surgical intervention, including venting procedures to relieve symptomatic distension or, in the most severe and refractory cases, intestinal transplantation following the same threshold reasoning developed for short bowel syndrome above, is reserved for patients who fail maximal medical and nutritional management. Setting realistic expectations from the outset, that management aims to reduce symptom burden and maintain adequate nutrition rather than to cure an underlying, generally irreversible motility abnormality, supports more sustainable long-term engagement with what is typically a lifelong condition.

FIGURE 8.2: SMALL BOWEL ANATOMY AND SHORT BOWEL SYNDROME SEVERITY

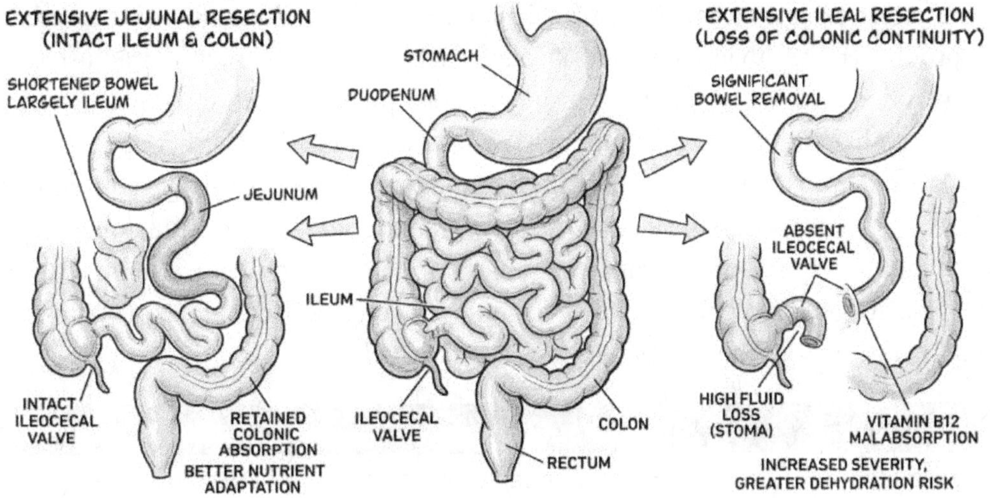


Case Presentation: A 58-year-old woman with limited cutaneous systemic sclerosis presents with progressive bloating, early satiety, and intermittent diarrhea alternating with constipation over the past year, alongside a 14-pound weight loss. She has known esophageal hypomotility, previously discussed in this book's chapters on esophageal disease, managed with aggressive acid suppression. Applying the reasoning developed in this chapter, her scleroderma-spectrum disease is a well-recognized cause of small bowel hypomotility through the same smooth muscle pathology affecting her esophagus, and this hypomotility is a specific, well-documented risk factor for small intestinal bacterial overgrowth via impaired migrating motor complex function; her alternating bowel pattern and weight loss are consistent with this diagnosis rather than a primary irritable bowel process. Glucose breath testing demonstrates an early, exaggerated rise in both hydrogen and methane, confirming combined-pattern bacterial overgrowth. She is treated with rifaximin plus neomycin, given the methane-predominant component, with substantial symptomatic improvement. Given the underlying, unmodifiable motility disorder, she is counseled that recurrence is likely and started on a low-dose prokinetic agent as maintenance therapy between anticipated future antibiotic courses, with a plan for scheduled, proactive retreatment rather than waiting for symptoms to recur severely each time. This case illustrates the chapter's recurring theme connecting its three major topics: an underlying motility disorder predisposes to bacterial overgrowth, and durable management requires addressing the underlying predisposing condition, not only the overgrowth itself, in each recurrence.

Case Presentation: A 44-year-old man underwent extensive small bowel resection eighteen months ago for mesenteric ischemia, leaving 90 centimeters of jejunum in continuity with an intact colon, and has remained dependent on parenteral nutrition five nights weekly since surgery. He reports gradual improvement in oral tolerance over the past six months and asks whether weaning from parenteral nutrition is realistic. Applying the reasoning developed in this chapter, he is now at the boundary between the adaptation and maintenance phases, and his preserved colonic continuity, despite extensive jejunal loss, is a favorable anatomic factor supporting continued weaning attempts given the colon's capacity to salvage additional calories through fermentation. A structured trial of advancing oral and enteral intake, with close monitoring of stool output, weight, and nutritional laboratory markers, alongside optimized antimotility and antisecretory pharmacotherapy, is undertaken in coordination with a dedicated intestinal rehabilitation program rather than attempted through incremental, unstructured adjustment in a general gastroenterology clinic alone. Given his reasonably preserved remaining bowel length and colonic continuity, glucagon-like peptide-2 analogue therapy is also initiated to further support adaptation. Over the following four months, his parenteral nutrition requirement is successfully reduced to twice weekly, with a plan for continued reassessment toward further weaning. This case illustrates the chapter's core prognostic principle for short bowel syndrome: anatomic factors, remaining segment type and colonic continuity, not resected length alone, should shape both the realistic weaning expectations discussed with the patient and the intensity of the rehabilitation effort pursued.

| Condition | Key Diagnostic Test | First-Line Management |
|---|---|---|
| SIBO, hydrogen-predominant | Glucose or lactulose breath test | Rifaximin |
| SIBO, methane-predominant | Breath test with methane measurement | Rifaximin plus neomycin |
| Short bowel syndrome | Documented resected length and remaining anatomy | Oral rehydration, enteral advancement, antimotility agents |

| | | |
|---|---|---|
| Chronic intestinal pseudo-obstruction | Exclude mechanical cause; small bowel manometry | Dietary modification, prokinetics, nutritional support |

**THE GI THRESHOLD DECISION SYSTEM — Small Bowel Motility and Nutritional Failure Thresholds**

**Presentation Signature:** This chapter's threshold instances addressed matching antibiotic therapy to breath test gas pattern and determining when parenteral-nutrition-dependent short bowel syndrome warrants specialized rehabilitation referral.

**Threshold Point:** Hydrogen versus methane predominance on breath testing determines antibiotic selection; persistent parenteral nutrition dependence beyond the one- to two-year adaptation window, especially with complications, determines rehabilitation referral timing.

**The Call:** Both thresholds prevent a generic, one-size-fits-all response, either treating all bacterial overgrowth identically regardless of gas pattern, or delaying specialized referral until a preventable complication has already become severe.

**Trap Logic:** Treating bacterial overgrowth in isolation without addressing its underlying predisposing motility or anatomic cause, and delaying intestinal rehabilitation referral until vascular access or liver function has already been substantially compromised, are this chapter's most consequential threshold misapplications.

**Decision Anchor:** Match antibiotic therapy to breath test gas pattern, treat the underlying predisposing condition alongside any overgrowth episode, and refer proactively for intestinal rehabilitation once the adaptation-phase threshold is crossed, rather than reactively after complications accumulate.

## Summary and Key Concepts

Small intestinal bacterial overgrowth develops when gastric acid, migrating motor complex activity, the ileocecal valve, or normal anatomy fails to limit small bowel bacterial colonization, and its symptom overlap with irritable bowel syndrome is substantial.

Breath testing gas pattern, hydrogen versus methane predominant, determines antibiotic selection, and recurrence is common when the underlying predisposing condition cannot be corrected.

Short bowel syndrome severity depends on which small bowel segments remain and whether colonic continuity is preserved, not on remaining length alone, and management proceeds through defined acute, adaptation, and maintenance phases.

Oral rehydration with high-sodium solutions, enteral advancement, and targeted pharmacotherapy including glucagon-like peptide-2 analogues form the core of short bowel syndrome management, with intestinal rehabilitation referral warranted for persistent parenteral nutrition dependence with complications.

Chronic intestinal pseudo-obstruction mimics mechanical obstruction without a structural lesion and requires careful exclusion of true obstruction before pursuing manometric and secondary-cause evaluation.

Small intestinal bacterial overgrowth is a near-universal complicating feature of chronic intestinal pseudo-obstruction and should be anticipated and treated proactively and cyclically given the underlying, generally unmodifiable motility abnormality.

# CHAPTER 9: INFLAMMATORY BOWEL DISEASE: ULCERATIVE COLITIS AND CROHN DISEASE

**Learning Objectives**

1. Explain the immune, genetic, and environmental factors contributing to inflammatory bowel disease and distinguish ulcerative colitis from Crohn disease mechanistically and clinically.
2. Classify ulcerative colitis by extent and severity and apply a stepwise medical management approach, including recognition of acute severe disease.
3. Classify Crohn disease by location and behavior and apply an appropriate treatment strategy, including early biologic therapy in high-risk patients.
4. Recognize and manage perianal Crohn disease and the major extraintestinal manifestations of inflammatory bowel disease.
5. Apply colorectal cancer surveillance guidelines and manage pregnancy, infection risk, and nutrition in patients with inflammatory bowel disease.

**Chapter Outline**

This chapter develops inflammatory bowel disease from its shared immune pathophysiology through the distinguishing features of ulcerative colitis and Crohn disease, disease-specific classification and severity assessment, stepwise medical management including biologic and small-molecule therapy, colectomy and perianal disease management, and the extraintestinal manifestations, cancer surveillance, pregnancy, infection risk, and nutritional considerations that apply across both conditions. Each section links a specific classification or severity threshold to a defined management pathway.

## Pathophysiology and Classification of Inflammatory Bowel Disease

### Immune Dysregulation and Genetic and Environmental Factors

Inflammatory bowel disease arises from a dysregulated mucosal immune response to the intestinal microbiota in a genetically susceptible host, and rather than reflecting a single causal defect, current understanding implicates a convergence of genetic susceptibility, more than two hundred loci identified through genome-wide association studies, including genes governing epithelial barrier function, autophagy, and innate immune recognition of microbial products, with environmental factors, including tobacco smoking, which paradoxically worsens Crohn disease while appearing protective against ulcerative colitis, early-life antibiotic exposure, and a Westernized diet and living environment associated with rising incidence in newly industrializing regions. The intestinal epithelial barrier and its overlying mucus layer normally maintain a controlled separation between luminal microbiota and the underlying immune system, and a breach in this barrier, whether from a primary genetic defect in barrier proteins or from microbiota-driven injury, permits an inappropriate, sustained immune activation against commensal organisms that would not otherwise provoke this response, a mechanism that explains why therapies targeting several different points in this inflammatory cascade, developed later in this chapter, can each achieve meaningful clinical benefit despite acting through distinct molecular mechanisms.

**Distinguishing Ulcerative Colitis From Crohn Disease**

Ulcerative colitis and Crohn disease, while sharing the broad immune-mediated mechanism described above, differ in anatomic distribution, depth of inflammation, and histologic pattern in ways that carry direct management consequences. Ulcerative colitis produces continuous, superficial, mucosal-predominant inflammation beginning in the rectum and extending proximally to a variable degree without skip areas, confined to the colon, while Crohn disease can affect any segment of the gastrointestinal tract from mouth to anus, characteristically in a discontinuous, skip-lesion pattern, with inflammation extending transmurally through the full thickness of the bowel wall rather than remaining confined to the mucosa, a distinction that directly explains why Crohn disease, but not ulcerative colitis, produces the fistulizing and stricturing complications discussed later in this chapter, since only transmural inflammation can erode through the full bowel wall to form a fistula tract or mature into a fibrotic stricture.

**Figure 9.1:** Anatomic and Histologic Comparison of Ulcerative Colitis and Crohn Disease

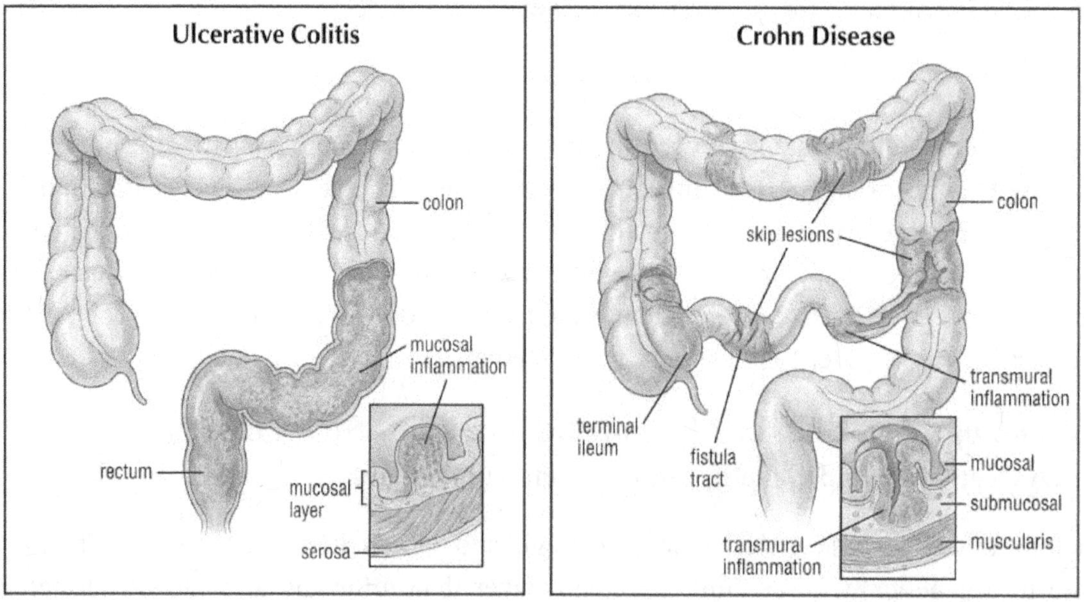


Histologically, both conditions demonstrate chronic inflammatory changes including crypt architectural distortion and basal plasmacytosis, but granuloma formation, when present, is specific to Crohn disease and, when identified on biopsy, is considered strong supportive evidence for that diagnosis over ulcerative colitis, though its absence does not exclude Crohn disease given its inconsistent presence even in confirmed cases. A meaningful minority of patients present with features that do not cleanly fit either classic pattern, termed indeterminate colitis or inflammatory bowel disease unclassified, and this diagnostic uncertainty, while sometimes frustrating for both clinician and patient, should be communicated honestly rather than forced into a premature, potentially inaccurate binary classification, since the specific diagnosis carries real implications, particularly for the colectomy and pouch surgery discussed later in this chapter.

## Ulcerative Colitis

### Clinical Presentation and Extent Classification

Bloody diarrhea, rectal urgency, and tenesmus constitute the core presenting symptom complex of ulcerative colitis, directly reflecting its rectal-predominant, mucosal inflammatory pattern, and the Montreal classification documents disease extent, using colonoscopic assessment of the proximal margin of inflammation, as proctitis, confined to the rectum, left-sided colitis, extending to the splenic flexure, or extensive colitis, extending beyond the splenic flexure, a classification that directly informs both treatment route selection, discussed below, and colorectal cancer surveillance intensity, discussed later in this chapter, since surveillance requirements differ meaningfully between proctitis alone and more extensive disease given their different associated cancer risk. Documenting extent explicitly at every colonoscopy, rather than only at initial diagnosis, matters because disease extent can change over time, either extending proximally or regressing with effective treatment, and current extent, not the extent recorded at diagnosis, should guide ongoing management decisions. Extent drives everything.

### Disease Severity Assessment

The Truelove and Witts criteria, despite their age, remain the most widely used framework for classifying ulcerative colitis flare severity, incorporating stool frequency, the presence and degree of visible blood, fever, tachycardia, anemia, and elevated inflammatory markers into mild, moderate, and severe categories, and this classification carries direct, urgent management implications developed in the rhythm instance below, since acute severe ulcerative colitis meeting these criteria requires hospitalization and a structured, time-bound treatment algorithm rather than outpatient management. The Mayo endoscopic subscore, introduced in the second chapter, provides an objective, endoscopy-based measure of mucosal inflammation that complements clinical severity scoring, and the growing emphasis in current practice on confirming endoscopic remission, mucosal healing visible at colonoscopy, rather than relying on symptomatic improvement alone, reflects accumulating evidence that endoscopic healing, more than symptom resolution alone, predicts durable long-term outcomes including reduced colectomy and hospitalization risk.

### Medical Management: Aminosalicylates, Corticosteroids, Biologics, and Small Molecules

Aminosalicylates, delivered orally, rectally, or both depending on disease extent, remain first-line therapy for mild to moderate ulcerative colitis, particularly proctitis and left-sided disease where rectal formulations achieve high local drug concentration directly at the site of inflammation, and combination oral plus rectal therapy achieves higher remission rates than either route alone in appropriately selected patients with disease extending proximal to the rectum. Corticosteroids induce remission effectively in moderate to severe flares but are not appropriate for long-term maintenance therapy given their well-documented toxicity profile, and a corticosteroid-dependent or corticosteroid-refractory disease course, rather than prompting an extended or repeated steroid course, should prompt escalation to a steroid-sparing maintenance strategy, most commonly a biologic agent. Biologic therapy, including anti-tumor necrosis factor agents, anti-integrin agents that block leukocyte trafficking into the intestinal mucosa, and anti-interleukin-23 agents, alongside small-molecule oral therapies including Janus kinase inhibitors and sphingosine-1-phosphate receptor modulators, has transformed moderate to severe ulcerative colitis management, and selection among this expanding therapeutic armamentarium is guided by disease severity and extent, prior treatment exposure and response, comorbidities including cardiovascular and thromboembolic risk factors that affect the safety profile of certain small-molecule agents, and patient preference regarding route of administration.

**THE GI THRESHOLD DECISION SYSTEM — Colitis Thresholds — Acute Severe Ulcerative Colitis and the Day-Three Decision**

---

**Presentation Signature:** A hospitalized patient with ulcerative colitis meets Truelove and Witts criteria for acute severe disease and has been started on intravenous corticosteroids.

**Threshold Point:** Response to intravenous corticosteroids is formally reassessed at 72 hours using a validated predictive index incorporating stool frequency and C-reactive protein; failure to meet response criteria at this point defines the threshold for medical rescue therapy or surgery, and continuing intravenous steroids beyond this window without response is not an appropriate default.

**The Call:** Patients meeting response criteria at 72 hours continue and are transitioned to oral corticosteroids with a steroid-sparing maintenance agent initiated; patients not meeting response criteria proceed to medical rescue therapy, most commonly infliximab or a calcineurin inhibitor, with colorectal surgery consulted concurrently rather than only after rescue therapy has also failed, given the risk of continued clinical deterioration during any further trial of medical therapy.

**Trap Logic:** Extending intravenous corticosteroid therapy beyond 72 hours in a nonresponding patient, hoping for delayed improvement, delays definitive rescue therapy and is associated with worse outcomes than timely escalation; the 72-hour assessment is a hard checkpoint, not a suggested guideline to be extended at clinical discretion.

**Decision Anchor:** Formally reassess corticosteroid response at 72 hours using an objective, validated index, and escalate to medical rescue therapy or surgery immediately upon meeting nonresponse criteria, with surgical consultation obtained concurrently rather than sequentially.

**Colectomy Indications**

Colectomy is curative for ulcerative colitis, since the disease is anatomically confined to the colon and rectum, and this curative potential distinguishes surgical decision-making in ulcerative colitis fundamentally from Crohn disease, where surgery, discussed later in this chapter, is never curative given the disease's potential to recur anywhere along the gastrointestinal tract. Indications for colectomy include the acute severe disease refractory to medical rescue therapy described above, colonic perforation or toxic megacolon, medically refractory chronic disease substantially impairing quality of life despite optimized therapy, and the confirmation of colorectal neoplasia or high-grade dysplasia on surveillance, discussed later in this chapter. Restorative proctocolectomy with ileal pouch-anal anastomosis, constructing a neorectal reservoir from the terminal ileum, is the preferred surgical approach in appropriately selected patients, preserving continence and avoiding a permanent ostomy, though it carries its own long-term complication profile, including pouchitis, an inflammatory condition of the pouch itself managed initially with antibiotic therapy, that patients should be counseled about explicitly before proceeding with this surgical approach rather than only after a complication has already developed. Discussing the curative nature of colectomy explicitly with patients facing this decision can reframe surgery as a definitive treatment option rather than only a last-resort failure of medical therapy, which is how it is sometimes perceived. Setting this expectation explicitly avoids surprise later. Cure is real here.

Figure 9.2: Endoscopic Mayo Subscore in Ulcerative Colitis

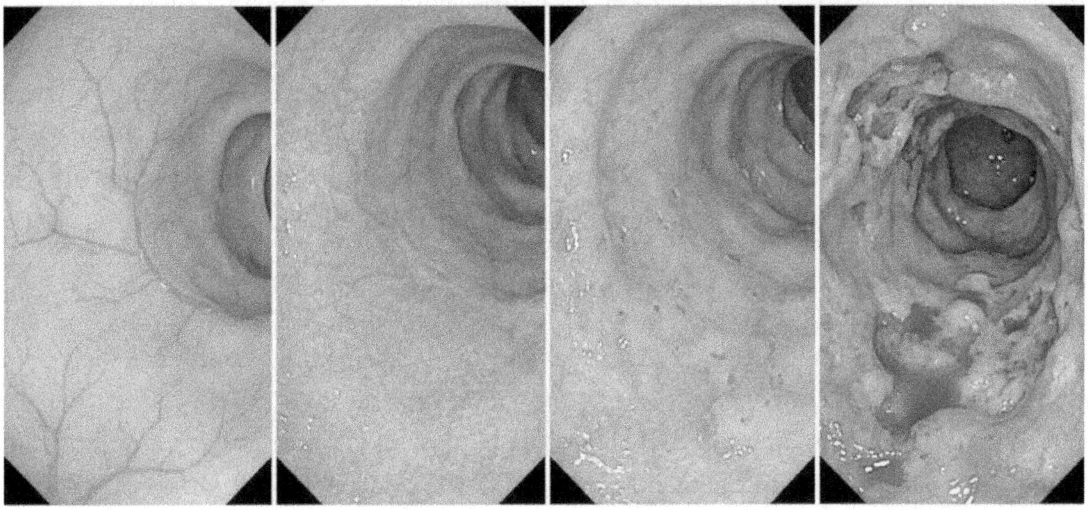

Mayo 0 Mayo 1 Mayo 2 Mayo 3

## Crohn Disease

### Clinical Presentation and Montreal Classification

Crohn disease presents with a symptom pattern determined substantially by disease location: ileal or ileocolonic disease, the most common distribution, produces abdominal pain, often right lower quadrant given the predilection for terminal ileal involvement, diarrhea, and weight loss, while isolated colonic disease can present similarly to ulcerative colitis with bloody diarrhea and urgency, and upper gastrointestinal involvement, though less common, can produce dysphagia, epigastric pain, or nausea depending on the specific segment affected. The Montreal classification documents age at diagnosis, disease location, ileal, colonic, ileocolonic, or isolated upper gastrointestinal, and disease behavior, inflammatory, stricturing, or penetrating, or fistulizing, and this behavioral classification specifically carries significant prognostic and treatment implications, since stricturing and penetrating disease behaviors are associated with a substantially higher risk of surgery and generally warrant earlier, more aggressive medical therapy than inflammatory-only disease, a distinction developed further in the treatment strategy discussion below. Perianal symptoms, discussed in detail later in this chapter, can also be the presenting feature in some patients and should be specifically asked about even when the primary complaint appears to be luminal.

**Diagnostic Evaluation and Disease Monitoring**

Ileocolonoscopy with biopsy remains the primary diagnostic tool, but because Crohn disease can affect small bowel segments beyond endoscopic reach, cross-sectional enterography, introduced in the second chapter, is essential for complete disease mapping, distinguishing active inflammatory disease, characterized by mural hyperenhancement and stratification, from chronic fibrostenotic change, a distinction that directly determines whether escalating anti-inflammatory therapy or a mechanical, endoscopic or surgical, intervention is the appropriate response to a stricture. Fecal calprotectin, introduced in the first chapter as a marker supporting the distinction between organic and functional bowel disease, has an expanded role in Crohn disease specifically as a noninvasive marker for longitudinal disease activity monitoring, allowing more frequent assessment of inflammatory status between periodic endoscopic or radiologic reassessments, and a rising calprotectin trend in a clinically quiescent patient should prompt reassessment rather than reassurance, since biochemical activity frequently precedes clinically apparent relapse. Repeating enterography at defined intervals, rather than only when new symptoms arise, allows subclinical progression to be caught before it becomes clinically apparent.

**Medical Management: Treatment Strategy and Sequencing**

Treatment strategy in Crohn disease has shifted substantially from a traditional step-up approach, beginning with less potent therapy and escalating only after treatment failure, toward earlier introduction of biologic therapy in patients identified at diagnosis as having risk factors for a complicated disease course, including younger age at diagnosis, extensive disease, deep ulceration on endoscopy, perianal disease, and stricturing or penetrating behavior at presentation, since accumulating evidence indicates that earlier, more effective disease control in this higher-risk population reduces the cumulative risk of bowel damage, surgery, and disability over time relative to a step-up approach that allows ongoing subclinical inflammation to accumulate irreversible bowel damage before more effective therapy is introduced. Treat-to-target management, setting a specific, objective treatment goal, generally endoscopic healing or, where available, biomarker normalization, rather than symptom control alone, and adjusting therapy systematically until that target is achieved, mirrors the endoscopic-healing emphasis already discussed for ulcerative colitis and reflects the same underlying evidence that objective disease control, not symptom resolution alone, predicts durable long-term outcomes across both conditions. Communicating this treat-to-target framework to the patient, including the specific objective markers being tracked and what would prompt a change in therapy, gives them a concrete way to understand why treatment might be adjusted even when they feel subjectively well.

**THE GI THRESHOLD DECISION SYSTEM — Crohn Disease Thresholds — Risk Stratification and Early Biologic Therapy**

**Presentation Signature:** A patient newly diagnosed with Crohn disease requires an initial treatment strategy, and the clinician must decide between a conventional step-up approach and early biologic therapy.

**Threshold Point:** The presence of one or more high-risk features at diagnosis, younger age, extensive small bowel involvement, deep ulceration, perianal disease, or stricturing or penetrating behavior, defines the threshold favoring early biologic therapy over a conventional step-up approach.

**The Call:** Patients with high-risk features at diagnosis are offered early biologic therapy, typically an anti-tumor necrosis factor agent given the most extensive long-term outcome data in this specific early, high-risk population, rather than starting with corticosteroids and aminosalicylates alone; patients without high-risk features may reasonably begin with a more conventional, stepwise approach with close monitoring for treatment failure or emergence of high-risk features over time.

**Trap Logic:** Applying a uniform step-up approach to every newly diagnosed patient regardless of risk profile exposes high-risk patients to a period of undertreated inflammation during which irreversible bowel damage can accumulate before more effective therapy is eventually introduced.

**Decision Anchor:** Stratify risk at diagnosis using the specific high-risk features identified above, and offer early biologic therapy to high-risk patients rather than defaulting to a uniform step-up sequence for every newly diagnosed patient.

**Perianal Crohn Disease**

Perianal fistulizing disease, resulting from transmural inflammation eroding through the bowel wall to form a tract connecting the intestinal lumen to the perianal skin or adjacent structures, affects a substantial proportion of Crohn disease patients over the disease course and requires a combined medical and surgical approach rather than either alone, since medical therapy, most effectively anti-tumor necrosis factor biologic therapy, addresses the underlying inflammatory drive while surgical intervention, including seton placement to maintain fistula tract drainage and prevent abscess formation while medical therapy takes effect, addresses the mechanical and infectious complications that medical therapy alone cannot resolve. Pelvic magnetic resonance imaging, providing detailed delineation of fistula tract anatomy relative to the anal sphincter complex as introduced in the second chapter, should be obtained before definitive surgical planning in complex perianal disease, since fistula anatomy directly determines which surgical approach can be pursued without compromising continence, and combined medical-surgical management, ideally coordinated explicitly between gastroenterology and a colorectal surgeon experienced in Crohn-related perianal disease specifically, produces better outcomes than either specialty managing the condition in isolation. Patients should be counseled that fistula healing, unlike luminal symptom control, often takes many months even with optimal therapy, setting realistic expectations for this specific complication.

Figure 9.3: Perianal Fistula Anatomy on Pelvic MRI

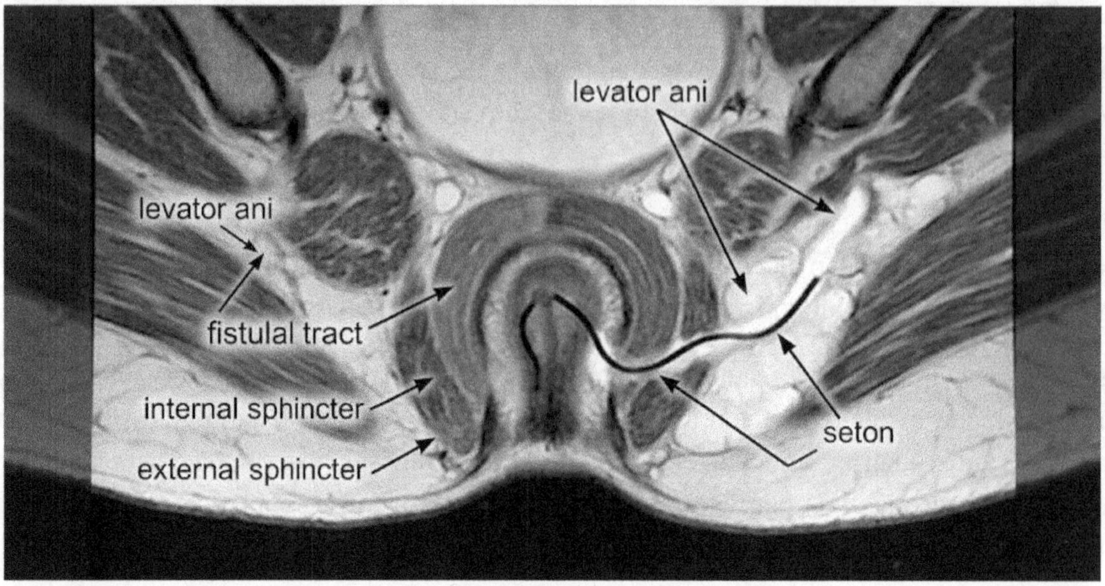


## Small Bowel Strictures and Surgical Management in Crohn Disease

Fibrostenotic strictures, the end result of chronic transmural inflammation and repeated injury-repair cycles, present with obstructive symptoms, cramping abdominal pain, distension, and, in severe cases, overt obstruction, and management depends on distinguishing an inflammatory component amenable to escalated medical therapy from a predominantly fibrotic stricture, which will not respond to anti-inflammatory therapy regardless of its intensity, a distinction made using the mural enhancement and stratification criteria on cross-sectional enterography introduced earlier in this chapter. Short, endoscopically accessible strictures, most commonly at the ileocecal anastomosis in a patient with prior resection, are amenable to endoscopic balloon dilation, applying the same incremental, cautious approach to stricture dilation developed in the fourth chapter, while longer or endoscopically inaccessible strictures require surgical management, either strictureplasty, which widens the stenotic segment without removing bowel length, or segmental resection, and the choice between these surgical approaches is guided by stricture length, number, and location, with strictureplasty specifically favored when preserving bowel length is a priority, such as in a patient who has already undergone multiple prior resections and is at risk for the short bowel syndrome discussed in the previous chapter. A stricture that has remained stable and asymptomatic on serial imaging does not necessarily require intervention, and the decision to dilate or resect should be driven by symptom burden and obstruction risk rather than by the mere radiographic presence of narrowing. Repeat dilation over time is common and should be discussed as an expected part of managing this complication, similar to the counseling already established for benign esophageal strictures in an earlier chapter. Always confirm first.

### Postoperative Recurrence and Prophylaxis

Crohn disease recurs after surgical resection in a substantial proportion of patients within years, typically beginning at the neoterminal ileum immediately proximal to the surgical anastomosis, and this predictable recurrence pattern is the basis for postoperative endoscopic surveillance, generally performed within six to twelve months of surgery regardless of symptoms, since endoscopic recurrence reliably precedes symptomatic recurrence and early identification allows medical therapy to be escalated before clinical relapse and further bowel damage occur. Risk-stratified postoperative prophylactic therapy, more intensive in patients with recognized risk factors for recurrence including smoking, prior multiple resections, and penetrating disease behavior at the time of surgery, applies the same risk-based treatment intensity principle developed earlier in this chapter for initial treatment strategy selection, extending it specifically to the postoperative period rather than treating surgery as having reset the disease course to a low-risk baseline. Discussing this planned surveillance colonoscopy with the patient before hospital discharge after surgery, rather than only at a later outpatient visit, improves the likelihood it is actually completed within the recommended window. Explicit counseling about the recurrence-reducing benefit of sustained smoking cessation specifically, beyond its general health benefits, gives postoperative patients an additional, concrete motivation tied directly to their surgical outcome. Worth it.

## Extraintestinal Manifestations and Complications

### Extraintestinal Manifestations

Extraintestinal manifestations affect a substantial proportion of inflammatory bowel disease patients and are broadly categorized by their relationship to intestinal disease activity: manifestations that generally parallel bowel inflammation, including peripheral arthritis, episcleritis, and erythema nodosum, which typically improve as intestinal inflammation is controlled, and manifestations that follow an independent course unrelated to bowel disease activity, including axial spondyloarthritis, primary sclerosing cholangitis, discussed further in a later chapter on cholestatic liver disease, uveitis, and pyoderma gangrenosum, which may require independent, targeted treatment even when intestinal disease is well controlled. Recognizing this distinction changes clinical reasoning meaningfully: a patient with new joint pain and well-controlled bowel disease should not automatically have their intestinal therapy escalated on the assumption that the joint symptom reflects undertreated bowel inflammation, since an independent-course manifestation requires its own targeted evaluation and treatment, often in coordination with rheumatology, ophthalmology, or dermatology depending on the specific manifestation. Osteoporosis and osteopenia, resulting from a combination of chronic inflammation, corticosteroid exposure, and malabsorption in small bowel Crohn disease, warrant the same periodic bone density monitoring and repletion approach already developed in earlier chapters for other malabsorptive and chronic inflammatory conditions, and this monitoring should not be deferred simply because a patient's intestinal disease itself is well controlled, since cumulative corticosteroid exposure from prior flares often persists as an ongoing risk factor even after steroids are discontinued. Involving the relevant specialist early, rather than after intestinal therapy has already been escalated unnecessarily, saves time and avoids exposing the patient to added medication risk without benefit.

## Colorectal Cancer Surveillance in Inflammatory Bowel Disease

Chronic colonic inflammation, whether from ulcerative colitis or colonic Crohn disease, carries an increased colorectal cancer risk that rises with disease duration and extent, and surveillance colonoscopy, generally beginning eight to ten years after diagnosis of extensive disease and continuing at intervals determined by ongoing risk factors, including disease activity, primary sclerosing cholangitis co-diagnosis, which substantially elevates risk and prompts earlier and more frequent surveillance, and family history of colorectal cancer, differs from average-risk population screening in both timing and technique, employing chromoendoscopy or high-definition white-light examination with targeted biopsy of any visible lesion, applying the enhanced detection principles introduced in the second chapter, given the frequently subtle, flat morphology of dysplasia arising in a background of chronic colitis. Dysplasia identified on surveillance, whether associated with a visible lesion or found on random biopsy, requires expert gastrointestinal pathology confirmation, paralleling the same confirmation principle established for Barrett esophagus dysplasia earlier in this book, before a management decision, endoscopic resection, intensified surveillance, or colectomy, is finalized. Patients should understand this surveillance requirement as a specific, disease-related recommendation distinct from average-risk population colorectal cancer screening, since confusion between the two can lead a patient to mistakenly believe a recent average-risk screening colonoscopy satisfies their IBD-specific surveillance needs when it was neither timed nor technically performed to meet that different standard.

## Inflammatory Bowel Disease in Pregnancy

Active inflammatory bowel disease at the time of conception and during pregnancy is a stronger risk factor for adverse pregnancy outcomes, including preterm birth and low birth weight, than continued medication use, a point that requires explicit, repeated counseling given the common and understandable instinct among pregnant or conception-planning patients to discontinue medication out of concern for fetal safety, when in fact achieving and maintaining disease remission before and throughout pregnancy is the single most protective step available. Most inflammatory bowel disease medications, including aminosalicylates and anti-tumor necrosis factor biologic agents, are considered compatible with pregnancy and continued use, with some agents transitioned in timing near delivery to limit fetal and neonatal drug exposure, while a smaller number of agents, including methotrexate, are contraindicated and require a structured transition to an alternative therapy well before conception is attempted, reinforcing the value of proactive, ideally preconception, counseling for any patient of reproductive age with inflammatory bowel disease. Coordinated care between gastroenterology and maternal-fetal medicine throughout pregnancy, rather than each specialty managing their respective domain independently, ensures that medication decisions account for both disease control and pregnancy-specific safety considerations simultaneously. This preconception planning should be revisited periodically, not treated as a single conversation completed once and never revisited as circumstances change.

## Therapeutic Drug Monitoring and Biologic Failure

Loss of response to a previously effective biologic agent, whether presenting as a symptomatic flare, rising inflammatory markers, or endoscopic recurrence, should prompt a structured evaluation before the agent is abandoned or a new drug class is started, since a substantial proportion of apparent treatment failures reflect inadequate drug exposure, either from accelerated drug clearance or from the development of anti-drug antibodies, rather than a genuine lack of efficacy of the mechanism itself. Therapeutic drug monitoring, measuring serum drug trough levels and, where relevant, anti-drug antibody titers, distinguishes several distinct failure patterns that each warrant a different response: a low trough level without significant antibodies supports dose escalation or interval shortening of the same agent; a low trough level with high-titer antibodies supports switching to a different agent within the same class only if the antibody response is not expected to cross-react, or more commonly switching out of class entirely; and an adequate trough level despite clinical or endoscopic activity indicates a genuine mechanistic failure warranting a switch to an agent with a different mechanism of action rather than dose adjustment of the current one. Applying this structured approach, rather than empirically escalating dose or switching agents without this diagnostic step, prevents both under-treatment, when a genuine mechanistic failure is instead met with a dose increase that cannot help, and unnecessary loss of an otherwise salvageable therapy, when inadequate drug exposure is instead met with a premature switch to a new drug class. Ordering trough and antibody levels together, rather than trough alone, provides the complete picture needed to correctly classify the failure pattern in a single test rather than requiring a second round of testing after an ambiguous initial result.

### Proactive Versus Reactive Monitoring

Reactive therapeutic drug monitoring, performed at the time of apparent treatment failure as described above, is the most widely used and best-evidenced application of this testing, while proactive monitoring, checking trough levels at defined intervals in patients who are currently doing well, is used more selectively, generally to confirm adequate drug exposure has been achieved after treatment initiation or dose adjustment, or in specific higher-risk clinical scenarios such as perianal fistulizing disease, discussed earlier in this chapter, where the drug exposure required for fistula healing is known to exceed that required for luminal disease control alone, making confirmation of adequate levels valuable even in an apparently well-controlled patient. Insurance coverage and cost of trough level testing vary by setting and should be considered when deciding how liberally to apply proactive monitoring in a given practice environment. Weigh this locally.

## Microscopic Colitis and Its Distinction From Inflammatory Bowel Disease

Microscopic colitis, encompassing collagenous and lymphocytic colitis, produces chronic, nonbloody, watery diarrhea with a grossly and radiographically normal-appearing colon, distinguishing it sharply from the endoscopically visible inflammation that defines ulcerative colitis and Crohn colitis, and diagnosis depends entirely on histologic examination of random colonic biopsies, since the endoscopic appearance provides no diagnostic clue and biopsies must be obtained even from a completely normal-appearing mucosa whenever this diagnosis is being considered. Collagenous colitis is distinguished histologically by a thickened subepithelial collagen band, while lymphocytic colitis is distinguished by increased intraepithelial lymphocytes without this collagen thickening, though the clinical presentation and management of both subtypes are similar enough that the distinction carries limited independent treatment implication. Microscopic colitis is strongly associated with specific medication exposures, particularly proton pump inhibitors, nonsteroidal anti-inflammatory drugs, and selective serotonin reuptake inhibitors, and a careful medication review, applying the same systematic approach emphasized throughout this book, identifying and discontinuing a potentially causative agent where clinically feasible, is a reasonable first step before pharmacologic treatment, most commonly budesonide, which has the strongest evidence base for inducing and maintaining remission in this specific condition. Distinguishing microscopic colitis from diarrhea-predominant irritable bowel syndrome and from the bile acid malabsorption discussed in the seventh chapter can be genuinely difficult on clinical grounds alone, since all three produce chronic watery diarrhea with an unremarkable gross endoscopic appearance, which is precisely why random biopsy during colonoscopy for chronic diarrhea evaluation, rather than proceeding only if the mucosa looks abnormal, is essential.

## Pouchitis and Other Long-Term Complications of Ileal Pouch-Anal Anastomosis

Pouchitis, nonspecific inflammation of the constructed ileal pouch reservoir, is the most common long-term complication after restorative proctocolectomy, affecting a substantial proportion of patients at some point after surgery, and it presents with increased stool frequency, urgency, and pelvic discomfort that patients may initially attribute to normal pouch function rather than recognizing as a treatable complication, making clear pre- and postoperative counseling about expected versus concerning pouch symptoms an important component of long-term surgical follow-up. Antibiotic therapy, most commonly ciprofloxacin or metronidazole, induces remission in the large majority of acute pouchitis episodes, and chronic or relapsing pouchitis, occurring in a smaller subset of patients, may require maintenance antibiotic therapy, probiotic therapy, which has specific evidence supporting its use in this exact clinical scenario, or, in refractory cases, the same biologic therapies used for luminal Crohn and ulcerative colitis. A subset of patients with chronic, antibiotic-refractory pouchitis are ultimately found to have Crohn disease of the pouch, an important distinction since it changes management toward the biologic-forward strategies discussed earlier in this chapter and carries different long-term prognostic implications for pouch survival than antibiotic-responsive pouchitis alone. Structured patient education materials describing the expected range of normal pouch function versus symptoms warranting evaluation, provided proactively after surgery rather than only in response to a worried phone call, help patients calibrate this distinction more confidently on their own. Recognizing this subset promptly avoids a prolonged, ineffective cycle of repeated antibiotic courses for what is, in fact, a distinct disease process.

## Specific Opportunistic Infections and Malignancy Risk in IBD Therapy

Beyond the general infection screening already discussed, certain therapeutic classes carry distinct, recognized infection and malignancy risks that warrant specific counseling and monitoring. Thiopurine therapy is associated with an increased risk of non-melanoma skin cancer and, in young male patients with concurrent or sequential Epstein-Barr virus infection and thiopurine exposure, a rare but serious hepatosplenic T-cell lymphoma, which has led many practices to favor combination strategies with lower cumulative thiopurine exposure or to avoid thiopurine monotherapy altogether in young male patients when a suitable alternative exists. Anti-tumor necrosis factor therapy carries an increased risk of reactivation of latent tuberculosis and hepatitis B, as discussed earlier in this chapter, and a modestly increased risk of serious infection more broadly, while Janus kinase inhibitors carry a specific, labeled risk of herpes zoster reactivation, which has led to a specific recommendation for zoster vaccination, using the recombinant, nonlive formulation appropriate for immunosuppressed patients, before or during therapy with this drug class specifically. These risks should be weighed against, not used to categorically avoid, an otherwise appropriate therapy, since untreated or undertreated inflammatory bowel disease itself carries its own serious complications, and the goal of this counseling is informed, shared decision-making rather than default avoidance of effective treatment options. This vaccination step is easy to overlook.

### Sun Protection and Dermatologic Surveillance

Given the skin cancer risk associated with thiopurine therapy and, to a lesser degree, other immunosuppressive agents used in inflammatory bowel disease, routine sun protection counseling and annual dermatologic skin examination are reasonable standard components of long-term management for patients on these therapies, applying the same proactive screening philosophy already emphasized for bone health, infection risk, and nutritional status throughout this book, rather than addressing skin findings only after a patient or their primary care physician happens to notice something concerning. These counseling points, though seemingly small compared to the primary disease management discussed throughout this chapter, meaningfully reduce long-term morbidity when applied consistently across a large population of patients on chronic immunosuppressive therapy. Small effort, real payoff.

## Medication Adherence and Communicating Treatment Plans

Nonadherence to maintenance therapy is a common and significant driver of disease relapse in inflammatory bowel disease, and it is frequently underrecognized because patients, out of a desire to avoid disappointing their clinician or out of genuine underestimation of missed doses, often overreport their own adherence when asked directly, making an open, nonjudgmental discussion of the practical barriers to adherence, cost, complexity of the regimen, injection anxiety for self-administered biologics, and simple forgetfulness, more productive than a direct adherence question alone. Applying the same precise, concrete communication principle emphasized throughout this book, explaining not just what medication to take but specifically why disease remission matters beyond symptom control, including the bowel-damage-prevention rationale developed earlier in this chapter, helps patients understand the stakes of adherence during periods when they may feel well and be tempted to reduce or skip a maintenance therapy that no longer seems necessary. Screening for these specific practical barriers at every visit, not only at treatment initiation, catches adherence problems that emerge later in the treatment course, such as a new financial hardship or a change in insurance coverage affecting medication access. Small habits, sustained, matter most.

### Shared Decision-Making in Treatment Selection

With multiple biologic and small-molecule options now available across several distinct mechanisms of action, treatment selection increasingly involves genuine shared decision-making rather than a single algorithmically determined choice, and presenting the patient with the specific trade-offs between reasonable options, route and frequency of administration, monitoring requirements, and the specific risk profile relevant to that individual patient's comorbidities and preferences, supports both informed consent and, by extension, the long-term adherence discussed above, since a patient who participated meaningfully in selecting their therapy is generally more invested in continuing it than one who was simply told which medication to take. Decision aids summarizing the key differentiating features of available options in accessible, plain-language terms can support this conversation, particularly for patients navigating this choice for the first time. This process takes time and repetition.

### Transition From Pediatric to Adult IBD Care

Inflammatory bowel disease diagnosed in childhood or adolescence carries distinct considerations at the transition to adult gastroenterology care, paralleling the transition principles already developed in earlier chapters for pediatric-onset celiac disease and short bowel syndrome, and adult gastroenterologists inheriting a pediatric-onset IBD patient should specifically review growth trajectory, since growth failure can be an underrecognized marker of inadequately controlled disease activity in a growing child, pubertal development history, since active inflammatory disease can delay puberty independent of nutritional status, and the specific treatment history and response pattern over the pediatric course, which provides prognostic context that a single adult-clinic snapshot cannot convey. A structured transition visit, ideally with some overlap or joint communication between the pediatric and adult teams rather than an abrupt handoff, supports continuity of both the medical management and the patient's own increasing self-management responsibility as they move into adult care. Family involvement should shift gradually and explicitly across the transition period, from parents managing the disease on the child's behalf to the young adult managing it themselves with family in a supportive rather than primary role, a shift that benefits from being planned deliberately over a series of visits rather than occurring abruptly at a single appointment. This overlap matters practically.

## Psychosocial Impact and Mental Health Screening in IBD

Anxiety and depression are more prevalent in inflammatory bowel disease patients than in the general population, driven by a combination of the direct psychosocial burden of a chronic, sometimes unpredictable and socially sensitive illness and, increasingly recognized, a bidirectional gut-brain relationship in which psychological stress can itself influence disease activity through neuroimmune pathways, paralleling the shared gut-brain mechanism discussed in an earlier chapter for functional gastrointestinal disorders, though inflammatory bowel disease, unlike those functional conditions, also carries objective, structural inflammatory pathology requiring its own independent treatment. Routine screening for anxiety and depression using a brief, validated instrument, applying the same standard already established in this book for other chronic gastrointestinal conditions, identifies patients who may benefit from integrated behavioral health support, and this screening carries particular importance in inflammatory bowel disease given evidence that untreated psychological distress is associated with reduced medication adherence, discussed earlier in this chapter, and, in some studies, higher rates of disease flare, meaning that mental health support functions not only as an independent quality-of-life intervention but as a component of comprehensive disease management. Coordinating with a mental health professional experienced in chronic illness or, specifically, gastrointestinal disease, where available, provides more targeted support than a general referral, given the specific ways a visible, unpredictable, and at times socially stigmatizing illness like IBD shapes a patient's psychological experience. This referral matters.

## Infection Risk, Vaccination, and Nutrition in Inflammatory Bowel Disease

### Infection Risk and Vaccination in Immunosuppressed Patients

Immunosuppressive and biologic therapy for inflammatory bowel disease increases susceptibility to a range of infections, and pre-treatment screening, including for latent tuberculosis and chronic hepatitis B infection, both of which can reactivate under immunosuppression with serious consequences, should be completed before initiating biologic therapy rather than after, applying the same proactive-rather-than-reactive principle emphasized throughout this book for other predictable complications. Vaccination status should be reviewed and, where indicated, updated before immunosuppressive therapy begins whenever possible, since live vaccines are generally contraindicated once a patient is immunosuppressed, meaning that any needed live vaccination, such as varicella or measles-mumps-rubella in a nonimmune patient, must be completed before therapy starts or deferred indefinitely, while inactivated vaccines, including seasonal influenza and age-appropriate pneumococcal vaccination, remain appropriate and recommended throughout the course of immunosuppressive therapy and should not be withheld. A dedicated pre-biologic screening checklist, applied consistently to every patient before a first biologic dose, prevents this screening step from being inadvertently skipped in the course of a busy clinic visit focused primarily on disease activity assessment. Documenting the specific vaccines reviewed and their status at the time immunosuppression begins creates a clear record later clinicians can reference without reconstructing this history from scratch.

### Nutrition in Inflammatory Bowel Disease

Malnutrition and specific micronutrient deficiencies are common in inflammatory bowel disease, particularly Crohn disease involving the small bowel, through a combination of reduced intake during active symptomatic flares, malabsorption from diseased or resected bowel segments, applying the small bowel principles developed in earlier chapters, and increased metabolic demand from chronic inflammation itself, and proactive nutritional screening, applying the principles introduced in the first chapter, should be a routine component of inflammatory bowel disease management rather than reserved for patients with overt weight loss. Exclusive enteral nutrition, providing complete nutritional intake through a formula diet with exclusion of regular food, has evidence supporting its use as a primary induction therapy specifically in pediatric Crohn disease, achieving remission rates comparable to corticosteroids while additionally supporting the growth that corticosteroid therapy can impair, and while its use in adult patients is more limited by tolerability and adherence challenges, it retains a role as an adjunctive or bridging strategy in appropriately motivated adult patients, particularly ahead of surgery to optimize nutritional status preoperatively. Vitamin B12 deficiency specifically should be anticipated in any patient with terminal ileal resection or extensive ileal disease, applying the same anatomic reasoning developed in the previous chapter for short bowel syndrome, and repleted with parenteral rather than oral therapy when ileal absorption is significantly compromised. Dietitian involvement throughout this process, both in pediatric induction and in adult adjunctive or preoperative use, improves both tolerability and the likelihood the full intended course is completed successfully. Consistency here pays off.

Case Presentation: A 26-year-old woman with known extensive ulcerative colitis is admitted with eight bloody stools daily, fever to 38.6 degrees Celsius, heart rate of 108 beats per minute, and a hemoglobin of 9.8 grams per deciliter, meeting Truelove and Witts criteria for acute severe disease. Stool studies exclude superimposed infection, and abdominal imaging excludes toxic megacolon. Applying the reasoning developed in this chapter, she is admitted, intravenous corticosteroids are started, and colorectal surgery is consulted at the time of admission rather than only if medical therapy fails, ensuring surgical evaluation has already occurred should rescue therapy become necessary. At 72 hours, formal reassessment using the validated predictive index shows she has not met response criteria, with persistent stool frequency and an elevated C-reactive protein. Rather than extending intravenous steroids further, she proceeds to medical rescue therapy with infliximab, and surgery remains involved throughout in case of continued deterioration. She responds to rescue therapy over the following days and is discharged on a maintenance biologic regimen with close outpatient follow-up. This case illustrates the chapter's central acute-severity threshold: the 72-hour reassessment is a fixed checkpoint that triggers immediate escalation, not a milestone to be extended when a patient has not yet, but might still, respond.

Case Presentation: A 31-year-old man with ileocolonic Crohn disease, diagnosed three years ago with deep ulceration on his index colonoscopy and treated with an anti-tumor necrosis factor biologic from diagnosis given this high-risk feature, presents with a new perianal abscess and drainage. Examination confirms a perianal fistula, and pelvic MRI demonstrates a single transsphincteric tract without a horseshoe configuration or associated abscess after incision and drainage. Applying the reasoning developed in this chapter, combined medical and surgical management is pursued rather than either alone: a seton is placed by colorectal surgery to maintain drainage and prevent recurrent abscess formation, while his biologic therapy is optimized, including consideration of dose escalation or therapeutic drug monitoring to confirm adequate drug exposure, since perianal fistula healing often requires higher sustained drug levels than luminal disease control alone. Coordinated follow-up between gastroenterology and colorectal surgery is scheduled explicitly, with a shared plan for eventual seton removal once sustained fistula healing is confirmed. This case illustrates the chapter's combined-modality principle for perianal Crohn disease: neither medical therapy alone, which cannot resolve the mechanical and infectious complications of an active fistula tract, nor surgery alone, which does not address the underlying inflammatory drive, is sufficient in isolation.

| Feature | Ulcerative Colitis | Crohn Disease |
|---|---|---|
| Distribution | Continuous, rectum-predominant | Discontinuous, skip lesions, any GI segment |
| Depth of inflammation | Mucosal | Transmural |
| Characteristic complications | Toxic megacolon, colectomy is curative | Strictures, fistulas, abscesses; surgery not curative |
| Smoking effect | Appears protective | Worsens disease course |
| Granulomas on biopsy | Absent | Supportive when present, not required |

**THE GI THRESHOLD DECISION SYSTEM — Inflammatory Bowel Disease Thresholds**

**Presentation Signature:** This chapter's threshold instances addressed the fixed 72-hour reassessment in acute severe ulcerative colitis and risk-based selection of early biologic therapy in newly diagnosed Crohn disease.

**Threshold Point:** Formal, objective response criteria at 72 hours of intravenous corticosteroids gate escalation in acute severe colitis; specific high-risk features at Crohn disease diagnosis gate the choice between step-up and early biologic therapy.

**The Call:** Both thresholds replace open-ended, reactive management with a scheduled or criteria-based decision point, converting disease severity and risk profile into a specific, time-bound treatment pathway.

**Trap Logic:** Extending steroid therapy past the 72-hour checkpoint in hope of delayed response, and applying a uniform step-up strategy regardless of Crohn disease risk profile, are this chapter's most consequential threshold misapplications.

**Decision Anchor:** Reassess acute severe colitis objectively at 72 hours and escalate immediately upon nonresponse; stratify Crohn disease risk at diagnosis and offer early biologic therapy to high-risk patients rather than a uniform step-up default.

## Summary and Key Concepts

Inflammatory bowel disease arises from dysregulated mucosal immune activation against intestinal microbiota in a genetically susceptible host, modulated by environmental factors including smoking, which has opposite effects on the two conditions.

Ulcerative colitis produces continuous, mucosal, rectum-predominant inflammation confined to the colon, while Crohn disease produces discontinuous, transmural inflammation anywhere in the GI tract, explaining their distinct complication profiles.

Acute severe ulcerative colitis requires hospitalization, intravenous corticosteroids, and a fixed 72-hour objective reassessment that triggers immediate escalation to rescue therapy or surgery upon nonresponse.

Newly diagnosed Crohn disease with high-risk features, younger age, extensive disease, deep ulceration, perianal involvement, or stricturing or penetrating behavior, warrants early biologic therapy rather than a conventional step-up approach.

Perianal fistulizing Crohn disease requires combined medical and surgical management, and extraintestinal manifestations should be classified as bowel-activity-parallel or independent-course before treatment escalation decisions are made.

Colorectal cancer surveillance in IBD uses enhanced detection technique and begins earlier than average-risk screening, and disease remission before and during pregnancy is more protective than medication discontinuation for most IBD therapies.

# CHAPTER 10: IRRITABLE BOWEL SYNDROME AND DISORDERS OF GUT-BRAIN INTERACTION

**Learning Objectives**

1. Apply the Rome IV criteria to diagnose irritable bowel syndrome and classify it by predominant bowel habit subtype.
2. Explain the pathophysiologic mechanisms underlying irritable bowel syndrome, including visceral hypersensitivity, motility disturbance, and postinfectious onset.
3. Apply a structured diagnostic approach that excludes organic disease before assigning a functional diagnosis, and apply dietary and pharmacologic therapy by IBS subtype.
4. Classify chronic constipation by mechanism and apply a stepwise diagnostic and treatment approach, including recognition of dyssynergic defecation.
5. Apply a structured approach to chronic diarrhea that remains unexplained after initial evaluation.

**Chapter Outline**

This chapter develops irritable bowel syndrome as the prototypical disorder of gut-brain interaction affecting the lower gastrointestinal tract, covering its Rome IV diagnostic criteria and subtypes, pathophysiology, structured diagnostic approach, and dietary and pharmacologic management, before addressing chronic constipation and its mechanistic subtypes and closing with a structured approach to chronic diarrhea that remains unexplained after the disease-specific evaluations developed in earlier chapters. Each section connects a specific diagnostic threshold to a defined management pathway.

## Irritable Bowel Syndrome

### Rome IV Criteria and Subtypes

Irritable bowel syndrome is diagnosed by the Rome IV criteria, requiring recurrent abdominal pain, on average at least one day per week over the preceding three months, associated with two or more of the following: a relationship to defecation, a change in stool frequency, or a change in stool form, with symptom onset at least six months before diagnosis, and, as with functional dyspepsia discussed in an earlier chapter, this diagnosis requires positive symptom criteria rather than functioning as a default label applied whenever an organic workup is unrevealing. Subtyping by predominant stool pattern using the Bristol stool form scale, IBS with constipation, IBS with diarrhea, mixed IBS with alternating patterns, or unclassified IBS when stool pattern does not fit one of these categories clearly, carries direct treatment relevance, since the pharmacologic approaches developed later in this chapter differ substantially by subtype, mirroring the subtype-matched treatment principle already established for functional dyspepsia.

Symptom severity itself varies considerably even within a single subtype, and this variation, rather than the subtype label alone, should also inform how aggressively treatment is escalated at the outset.

### Pathophysiology: Visceral Hypersensitivity, Motility, and the Microbiome

Visceral hypersensitivity, an exaggerated perception of normal intestinal distension and motility, is a consistent finding across irritable bowel syndrome subtypes and reflects the same disordered gut-brain signaling mechanism discussed in earlier chapters for functional dyspepsia and functional esophageal disorders, reinforcing the unifying disorders-of-gut-brain-interaction framework introduced there. Altered gastrointestinal motility, distinct from but related to this sensory disturbance, contributes to the bowel habit pattern that defines each subtype, with accelerated transit contributing to diarrhea-predominant disease and delayed transit contributing to constipation-predominant disease, though the correlation between measured transit time and symptom severity is imperfect, similar to the dissociation between objective and subjective findings already noted for gastroparesis. Postinfectious irritable bowel syndrome, developing after an acute episode of infectious gastroenteritis in a meaningful proportion of affected individuals, provides a specific, well-documented mechanistic pathway in which the acute infection triggers persistent low-grade mucosal inflammation, altered gut microbiota composition, and increased mucosal permeability that outlasts the resolved infection itself, a pathway that offers a concrete explanation for how a discrete infectious trigger can produce a chronic, ongoing functional disorder, and one that patients often find clarifying when their symptom onset genuinely followed a documented gastrointestinal infection. Emerging research into low-grade mucosal immune activation and mast cell infiltration in a subset of IBS patients further supports the concept that measurable, if subtle, biological changes underlie a condition sometimes still mischaracterized as having no identifiable physical basis.

**Figure 10.1: Bristol Stool Form Scale**

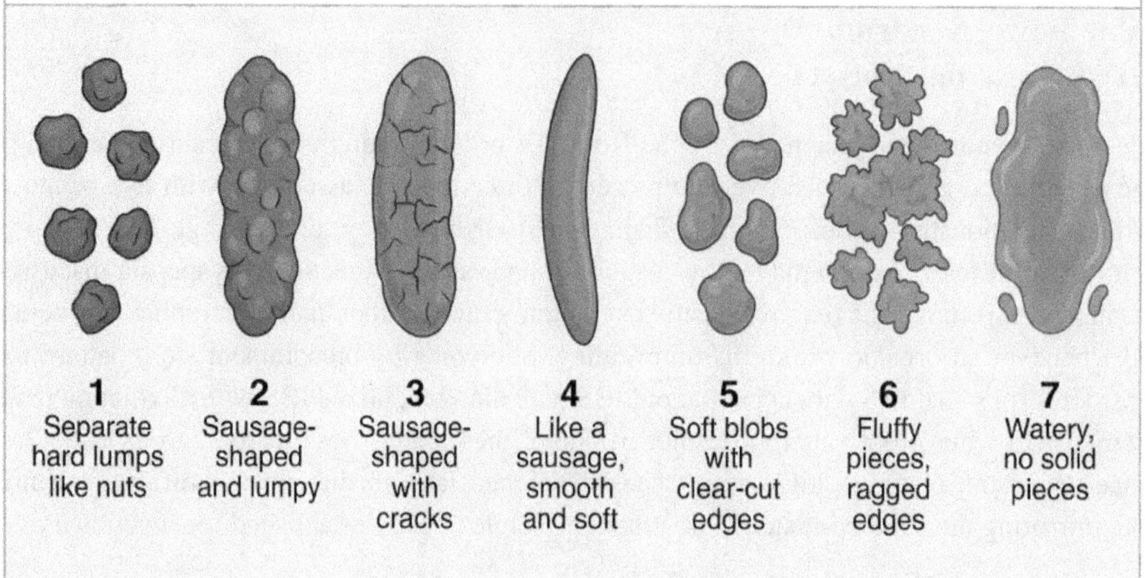

## Diagnostic Approach and Alarm Features

A structured, limited evaluation, rather than an open-ended organic workup, is appropriate for a patient meeting Rome IV criteria without alarm features: celiac serology given its relative prevalence and the low cost and yield of testing, established in the seventh chapter, fecal calprotectin or, in appropriate settings, a stool inflammatory marker to help distinguish IBS from inflammatory bowel disease when the clinical picture is ambiguous, and, in diarrhea-predominant disease specifically, consideration of the bile acid malabsorption evaluation developed in the seventh chapter given its substantial symptomatic overlap with and frequent misdiagnosis as IBS-D. Alarm features, applying the same threshold-based reasoning established in the first chapter, including gastrointestinal bleeding, unintentional weight loss, nocturnal symptoms, onset after age 50, and a family history of colorectal cancer or inflammatory bowel disease, lower the threshold for a more extensive evaluation, including colonoscopy, before a functional diagnosis is accepted, since these features raise the pretest probability of an organic explanation sufficiently to warrant more than the limited standard workup. Ordering these limited tests together at the initial visit, rather than sequentially across multiple follow-up appointments, respects the patient's time and reaches a working diagnosis more efficiently.

### THE GI THRESHOLD DECISION SYSTEM — Bowel Habit Thresholds — Distinguishing IBS-D from Its Organic Mimics

**Presentation Signature:** A patient meets Rome IV criteria for diarrhea-predominant IBS, and the clinician must decide how extensively to evaluate for an organic mimic before accepting the functional diagnosis.

**Threshold Point:** The absence of alarm features and a limited standard workup, celiac serology, inflammatory marker, and consideration of bile acid malabsorption testing or empiric sequestrant trial, define the threshold below which a functional diagnosis can be accepted with confidence; any alarm feature, or an inadequate response to appropriately sequenced first-line IBS-D therapy, crosses the threshold requiring colonoscopy and, where relevant, random biopsy to exclude microscopic colitis.

**The Call:** Patients without alarm features and a negative limited workup are managed as IBS-D with the dietary and pharmacologic strategies developed below; patients with alarm features, or those failing to respond to an adequately sequenced trial of first-line therapy, proceed to colonoscopy with biopsy, which can identify microscopic colitis, discussed in the previous chapter, or inflammatory bowel disease that the limited initial workup did not capture.

**Trap Logic:** Treating a diagnosis of IBS-D as permanent and unquestionable once assigned, rather than revisiting it when treatment response is inadequate, is a common source of diagnostic inertia that delays recognition of bile acid malabsorption, microscopic colitis, or another treatable mimic.

**Decision Anchor:** Apply the limited standard workup and alarm-feature screen before accepting an IBS-D diagnosis, and revisit the diagnosis, rather than simply escalating IBS-directed therapy, when an adequately sequenced treatment trial fails to produce the expected response.

## Dietary Management: The Low-FODMAP Diet

The low-fermentable oligosaccharide, disaccharide, monosaccharide, and polyol, or low-FODMAP, diet restricts a specific group of poorly absorbed, rapidly fermentable short-chain carbohydrates that, in a susceptible individual, draw water into the intestinal lumen osmotically and undergo rapid colonic fermentation producing gas, and this combination of luminal distension and gas production is thought to provoke symptoms specifically through the visceral hypersensitivity mechanism discussed above, explaining why an otherwise nutritionally unremarkable set of foods produces disproportionate symptoms in this population. The diet is implemented in three structured phases, an elimination phase restricting high-FODMAP foods for two to six weeks, a systematic reintroduction phase testing individual FODMAP subgroups sequentially to identify specific triggers, and a personalized long-term maintenance phase restricting only the identified trigger foods, and skipping the reintroduction phase, remaining on the restrictive elimination diet indefinitely, is a common and avoidable error that unnecessarily limits dietary variety and nutritional adequacy without additional symptomatic benefit beyond what the personalized maintenance phase would achieve; dietitian involvement, given the diet's complexity, meaningfully improves both adherence and the successful completion of the reintroduction phase. Common high-FODMAP foods include onions, garlic, wheat, certain fruits such as apples and pears, and legumes, and a practical, printed food list organized by FODMAP category helps patients navigate grocery shopping and meal planning during the elimination phase without needing to memorize an extensive and initially unfamiliar set of dietary rules.

## Pharmacologic Management by Subtype

Pharmacologic therapy is matched to predominant bowel habit subtype, paralleling the subtype-matched approach already established for functional dyspepsia. IBS-C management includes fiber supplementation, osmotic laxatives, and, for inadequate response, secretagogues such as linaclotide or plecanatide, which increase intestinal fluid secretion and accelerate transit through a mechanism distinct from osmotic laxation, or prokinetic-adjacent agents targeting specific receptor pathways. IBS-D management includes antidiarrheal agents, bile acid sequestrants when the bile acid malabsorption overlap discussed above is suspected or confirmed, and, for more refractory cases, rifaximin, the same antibiotic introduced in the eighth chapter for small intestinal bacterial overgrowth, reflecting accumulating evidence for a microbiome-modulating mechanism of benefit in a subset of IBS-D patients independent of confirmed bacterial overgrowth. Neuromodulator therapy, most commonly a low-dose tricyclic antidepressant for IBS-D given its additional antidiarrheal, transit-slowing effect, or a selective serotonin reuptake inhibitor for IBS-C given its comparatively transit-neutral to mildly accelerating profile, addresses the underlying visceral hypersensitivity directly and is reserved, as with functional dyspepsia, for patients with inadequate response to subtype-matched first-line therapy or with a prominent pain component disproportionate to bowel habit alone. Combining a dietary and a pharmacologic approach from the outset, rather than sequentially trialing one before introducing the other, is reasonable in patients with more severe symptoms at presentation, since the two approaches act through distinct, complementary mechanisms rather than competing for the same therapeutic effect.

**PATIENT EDUCATION:** Explain irritable bowel syndrome using the same disorder-of-gut-brain-interaction framing developed for functional dyspepsia: the gut is genuinely oversensitive and its movement genuinely altered, not merely perceived to be so, and this framing supports engagement with treatment without implying the symptoms are imagined or less legitimate than a structural diagnosis.

## Opioid-Induced Constipation and Broader Opioid-Induced Gastrointestinal Dysfunction

Opioid-induced constipation, resulting from direct activation of mu-opioid receptors within the enteric nervous system that slows motility and increases fluid absorption throughout the gastrointestinal tract, occurs in a substantial proportion of patients on chronic opioid therapy and, unlike many medication side effects, does not reliably improve with continued use, meaning that ongoing, proactive bowel regimen management, rather than a reactive response only after constipation becomes symptomatic, should accompany any chronic opioid prescription from the outset. Standard laxative therapy, particularly osmotic and stimulant laxatives, is first-line treatment, but a subset of patients have an inadequate response to standard laxative therapy despite adequate dosing, and peripherally acting mu-opioid receptor antagonists, a drug class specifically designed to block the peripheral gastrointestinal opioid effect without crossing the blood-brain barrier and reversing central analgesia, offer a targeted option in this specific, laxative-refractory population, addressing the underlying receptor-level mechanism directly rather than only its downstream consequence. A proactive, prophylactic bowel regimen prescribed alongside the opioid at the time it is first started, rather than added only after constipation has already become established and symptomatic, is generally more effective and prevents the added distress of an entirely avoidable complication.

### Broader Opioid Bowel Dysfunction

Beyond constipation specifically, chronic opioid use produces a broader pattern of gastrointestinal dysfunction, including the delayed gastric emptying discussed in the sixth chapter and the small intestinal bacterial overgrowth risk discussed in the eighth chapter, both mediated by the same enteric opioid receptor mechanism, reinforcing why a patient on chronic opioid therapy presenting with any new upper or lower gastrointestinal symptom should have opioid-related dysfunction specifically considered as a contributing factor, applying the same systematic medication-review discipline emphasized throughout this book, rather than each new symptom being evaluated as an entirely separate, unrelated clinical problem. A single, comprehensive opioid-effects discussion at the time therapy is started, covering all of these downstream gastrointestinal consequences together, is more efficient than addressing each one separately as it arises over subsequent visits.

## Food-Related Triggers Beyond FODMAPs

While the low-FODMAP diet addresses the most extensively studied dietary trigger category in irritable bowel syndrome, other food-related factors warrant consideration in patients whose response to FODMAP restriction is incomplete. Caffeine and alcohol can independently provoke symptoms through direct effects on intestinal motility and secretion distinct from any FODMAP content, and a brief, targeted trial of reducing these specific exposures is a reasonable, low-burden adjunct for patients who have not already tried this on their own. Gluten, distinct from the FODMAP fructan content also present in wheat, has been proposed as an independent trigger in some IBS patients even after celiac disease has been excluded, a phenomenon overlapping conceptually with the non-celiac gluten sensitivity discussed in the seventh chapter, though careful blinded challenge studies suggest that fructan content, a FODMAP component of wheat, rather than gluten itself, explains symptoms in many of these patients, reinforcing the value of the structured FODMAP reintroduction process described earlier in this chapter to identify the actual culprit component rather than assuming gluten is responsible by default. This finding is a useful teaching point in itself, illustrating how a widely popularized dietary belief can be partially, but not entirely, correct once examined through rigorous blinded testing. Nuance beats blanket avoidance.

### Meal Timing and Eating Behavior

Beyond the specific content of meals, eating behavior itself, including eating too quickly, which increases aerophagia and reduces satiety signaling, and eating irregularly, which disrupts the normal gastrocolic reflex pattern that helps regulate bowel habit, can independently contribute to symptom burden, and simple behavioral counseling addressing meal pace and regularity, while less extensively studied than the FODMAP diet specifically, is a reasonable, low-risk component of a comprehensive dietary approach that costs little to recommend and can meaningfully improve symptoms in some patients. These are inexpensive, low-risk interventions worth mentioning even briefly during a visit already focused on more intensive dietary or pharmacologic planning. Small changes, real value.

## Other Disorders of Gut-Brain Interaction

### Centrally Mediated Abdominal Pain Syndrome

Centrally mediated abdominal pain syndrome describes chronic or frequently recurring abdominal pain that is poorly related to eating, defecation, or menstrual cycle, distinguishing it from irritable bowel syndrome's defecation-related pain pattern, and reflects a more purely centrally driven pain amplification process with minimal peripheral gut sensory or motor contribution, meaning that the peripheral, gut-directed therapies effective in IBS, including the dietary and secretagogue approaches discussed above, are correspondingly less effective in this condition. Management centers on centrally acting neuromodulator therapy, often at doses closer to those used for primary psychiatric indications than the low, pain-modulating doses used in IBS, combined with psychological therapies including cognitive behavioral therapy specifically adapted for chronic pain, and setting accurate expectations, that treatment aims to reduce pain burden and improve function rather than eliminate pain entirely, supports more sustainable long-term engagement with what is typically a chronic condition. Distinguishing this condition from IBS accurately at the outset avoids a prolonged, frustrating trial of gut-directed dietary and pharmacologic therapies that were never well matched to its predominantly central mechanism in the first place.

### Narcotic Bowel Syndrome

Narcotic bowel syndrome describes a paradoxical worsening of abdominal pain with escalating opioid dosing in a patient using opioids chronically, typically for an unrelated or a previously diagnosed gastrointestinal pain condition, and its recognition requires actively considering opioids as a cause of worsening pain rather than only as a treatment for it, since the intuitive clinical response to worsening pain, increasing the opioid dose, is precisely the action that perpetuates this specific syndrome through opioid-induced changes in central pain processing. Management requires a structured, supervised opioid tapering program, ideally with concurrent management of the anticipated withdrawal-related symptom exacerbation that typically occurs before improvement, and this counterintuitive treatment, reducing rather than increasing pain medication in a patient reporting worsening pain, requires clear, sustained communication with the patient about the syndrome's mechanism to support adherence to a taper that will predictably feel worse before it feels better. Involving a multidisciplinary pain or addiction medicine team, where available, supports both the physical taper and the psychological adjustment this counterintuitive treatment approach requires, particularly in patients whose opioid use has continued for an extended period before the diagnosis is recognized.

## Structural and Special Population Considerations in Constipation

Rectal prolapse, rectocele, and rectal intussusception, structural abnormalities of pelvic floor anatomy, can coexist with or mimic dyssynergic defecation, and defecography, introduced in the second chapter, adds structural information beyond what manometry alone provides, visualizing these anatomic abnormalities directly and helping determine whether a surgical, rather than purely behavioral, intervention is needed once biofeedback therapy for a coexisting functional component has been optimized. A large rectocele that fails to empty adequately during defecation, sometimes requiring the patient to apply manual vaginal or perineal pressure to complete evacuation, a detail patients may not volunteer unless specifically asked given its sensitive nature, indicates a structural contribution that behavioral therapy alone is unlikely to fully resolve, and surgical referral for rectocele repair is a reasonable consideration in this specific, well-defined scenario once conservative measures have been adequately trialed. Asking specifically and directly about the need for manual assistance during defecation, rather than waiting for the patient to volunteer this detail, is necessary given how uncomfortable many patients feel raising it unprompted, even though the information changes management meaningfully once obtained. A joint clinic visit or close communication between gastroenterology and colorectal surgery, when structural findings are identified, ensures the surgical and behavioral treatment plans are coordinated rather than pursued independently.

## Constipation in Older Adults

Constipation in older adults warrants particular attention to medication review, given the substantial number of common medications, including anticholinergics, calcium channel blockers, and opioids, that slow colonic transit as a recognized effect, applying the same systematic medication-review principle emphasized throughout this book, and to the possibility that new constipation in an older adult represents an early symptom of colorectal malignancy rather than a purely functional process, which is why new-onset constipation after age 50, particularly when accompanied by any other alarm feature, should prompt colonoscopy rather than being managed as routine functional constipation from the outset, mirroring the age-based threshold already established for other gastrointestinal presentations throughout this book. Fecal impaction, a specific complication more common in older or institutionalized patients with reduced mobility, presents with paradoxical liquid stool leakage around an impacted, immobile fecal mass and should not be mistaken for diarrhea, since treating it with antidiarrheal therapy rather than disimpaction would worsen rather than resolve the underlying problem. A rectal examination specifically checking for a palpable fecal mass should be performed in any older or immobile patient presenting with unexplained diarrhea or overflow incontinence, since this bedside step alone can immediately clarify a presentation that might otherwise be pursued through an extensive and unnecessary diarrhea workup. A brief digital rectal exam takes only moments and can immediately redirect an evaluation that might otherwise proceed down an incorrect and time-consuming diagnostic path.

## Choosing Among Fiber and Laxative Formulations

Not all fiber supplements behave identically, and this distinction is worth explaining to patients who may have tried one type and concluded fiber generally does not help them: soluble, fermentable fiber, such as psyllium, softens stool and adds bulk effectively but can worsen bloating in a patient with coexisting visceral hypersensitivity or overlapping IBS, while less fermentable fiber sources produce less gas-related bloating but may be somewhat less effective at softening stool consistency, meaning that fiber selection, like the medication selection developed elsewhere in this book, benefits from being matched to the individual patient's specific symptom profile rather than treated as an interchangeable, one-size-fits-all category. Osmotic laxatives, primarily polyethylene glycol, draw water into the colonic lumen through an osmotic gradient and are generally well tolerated with a low risk of electrolyte disturbance at standard doses, while saline osmotic laxatives, including magnesium-based products, carry a meaningful risk of electrolyte disturbance in patients with renal impairment and should be used more cautiously or avoided in this population, a distinction that is easy to overlook when recommending an over-the-counter product without considering the patient's renal function specifically. Starting at a low dose and titrating gradually upward over one to two weeks, regardless of which fiber type is chosen, reduces the initial bloating and gas that can otherwise cause a patient to abandon fiber therapy prematurely before it has had adequate time to produce benefit. Match the fiber to the patient. Simple, effective.

### Addressing Outdated Concerns About Stimulant Laxatives

The historical concern that stimulant laxatives cause colonic dependence or damage with regular use, once widely taught and still commonly repeated by patients and even some clinicians, has not been supported by more recent, better-designed studies, and current evidence supports stimulant laxatives as a safe and effective option for both intermittent and sustained use when needed, a reassurance that should be communicated proactively to patients who may otherwise avoid an effective treatment option out of an outdated concern, and this specific myth-correction is a useful, concrete example of the value of directly addressing a patient's preexisting beliefs about a medication rather than assuming silence means acceptance of the recommended treatment. Framing this correction as an update to outdated information, rather than a dismissal of the patient's prior concern, tends to land better and preserves the collaborative tone of the visit. Old myths persist; correct them plainly.

## Chronic Constipation

### Classification: Normal Transit, Slow Transit, and Outlet Dysfunction

Chronic constipation is classified mechanistically into normal-transit constipation, in which colonic transit is objectively normal despite the patient's perception of constipation, often reflecting a primarily sensory or perceptual disturbance overlapping with IBS-C, slow-transit constipation, in which colonic motility itself is genuinely impaired, and outlet dysfunction, more completely termed dyssynergic defecation and introduced in the second chapter, in which paradoxical pelvic floor and anal sphincter contraction impairs evacuation despite normal or even accelerated proximal colonic transit. This mechanistic classification, rather than symptom severity alone, determines treatment selection, since a patient with dyssynergic defecation will not benefit from escalating laxative therapy, the correct response to slow-transit constipation, and instead requires the biofeedback therapy developed below, meaning that mechanistic misclassification produces predictable, avoidable treatment failure. Explaining this three-way classification to the patient in plain terms, rather than treating it as an internal diagnostic detail not worth sharing, helps them understand why the specific test being ordered next, rather than simply another medication trial, is the appropriate next step.

### Diagnostic Evaluation

Anorectal manometry with balloon expulsion testing, introduced in the second chapter, is the key test distinguishing dyssynergic defecation from the other constipation subtypes and should be considered in any patient with chronic constipation refractory to an adequate trial of fiber and osmotic laxative therapy, since dyssynergic defecation is common enough, and different enough in its correct treatment, that ruling it out specifically before escalating laxative therapy further prevents a predictable pattern of treatment failure. Colonic transit studies, using radiopaque markers, wireless motility capsule technology introduced in the second chapter, or scintigraphy, distinguish slow-transit from normal-transit constipation in patients whose manometry has excluded dyssynergic defecation, and this testing sequence, evaluating for outlet dysfunction before assessing transit time, reflects the practical reality that dyssynergic defecation is both common and correctable with a fundamentally different, nonpharmacologic therapy, making its exclusion or confirmation the higher-yield first diagnostic step. This sequencing, testing for the mechanism that has the most specific and most different treatment first, applies the same efficient diagnostic-sequencing logic developed in the seventh chapter for the broader malabsorption workup, prioritizing the test most likely to change the treatment pathway rather than proceeding in an arbitrary or purely historical order.

**Management: Fiber, Laxatives, Secretagogues, and Biofeedback**

Fiber supplementation and osmotic laxatives, most commonly polyethylene glycol, remain appropriate first-line therapy for normal-transit and mild slow-transit constipation, and stimulant laxatives, historically avoided due to unfounded concerns about colonic dependence with long-term use, are increasingly recognized as safe and effective for both intermittent and, when needed, longer-term use, a reassurance worth communicating explicitly to patients who may have heard the older, now largely discredited concern from another source. Secretagogues, the same class introduced above for IBS-C, and prokinetic agents targeting colonic motility specifically are reserved for inadequate response to fiber and osmotic laxative therapy, applying the same stepwise escalation principle used throughout this book. Dyssynergic defecation, once confirmed by manometry and balloon expulsion testing, is treated with biofeedback therapy, a structured behavioral retraining program teaching the patient to coordinate pelvic floor relaxation with defecation effort, and this therapy, rather than escalating laxative dosing, is the evidence-based first-line treatment for this specific mechanistic subtype, with response rates substantially exceeding those achieved by laxative therapy alone in confirmed dyssynergic defecation. Adequate fluid intake alongside fiber supplementation is essential, since fiber without sufficient accompanying fluid can paradoxically worsen constipation by creating a bulkier but still poorly hydrated stool mass, a practical point that is easy to omit when recommending fiber but that meaningfully affects whether the recommendation actually helps.

**Figure 10.2: Anorectal Manometry Pressure Tracings in Dyssynergic Defecation**

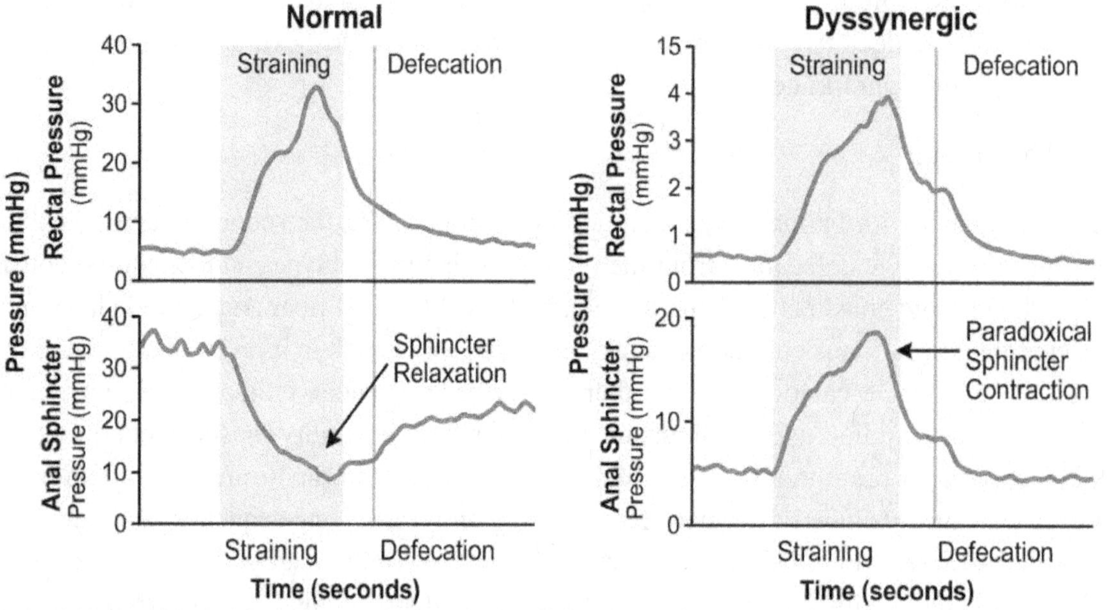

**THE GI THRESHOLD DECISION SYSTEM — Constipation Thresholds — When to Test for Dyssynergic Defecation**

---

**Presentation Signature:** A patient with chronic constipation has not responded adequately to an initial trial of fiber and osmotic laxative therapy, and the clinician must decide whether to escalate pharmacotherapy further or pursue anorectal function testing.

**Threshold Point:** Inadequate response to an adequate trial of first-line fiber and osmotic laxative therapy defines the threshold for anorectal manometry with balloon expulsion testing, performed before, not after, a trial of escalating secretagogue or prokinetic therapy, given the different and specific treatment dyssynergic defecation requires.

**The Call:** Confirmed dyssynergic defecation is treated with biofeedback therapy as first-line treatment; confirmed normal-transit or slow-transit constipation without dyssynergia proceeds to secretagogue or prokinetic escalation as the next pharmacologic step.

**Trap Logic:** Escalating through multiple pharmacologic agents sequentially before ever testing for dyssynergic defecation delays effective treatment in a patient whose actual mechanism, an evacuation disorder rather than a transit or secretory disorder, no escalating medication will adequately address.

**Decision Anchor:** Test for dyssynergic defecation before, not after, escalating pharmacotherapy in constipation refractory to first-line fiber and osmotic laxative treatment, since its correct treatment, biofeedback, is fundamentally different from every pharmacologic option that would otherwise be tried next.

## Psychosocial Factors and the Gut-Brain Axis in IBS Management

Anxiety, depression, and a history of adverse life experiences are more prevalent among patients with irritable bowel syndrome than in the general population, and this association, mirroring the pattern already discussed for functional dyspepsia, reflects the bidirectional gut-brain relationship underlying the disorder's core pathophysiology rather than implying that the bowel symptoms are secondary to or less legitimate than a psychiatric condition, a distinction worth restating explicitly to patients given how easily this framing can be misheard as dismissive. Gut-directed hypnotherapy and cognitive behavioral therapy specifically adapted for IBS have a substantial evidence base supporting their use, comparable in some studies to pharmacologic therapy, and referral to practitioners with specific training in these gut-directed techniques, rather than general psychotherapy without this specific focus, improves the likelihood of a meaningful symptomatic response, since the therapeutic techniques used differ meaningfully from general anxiety- or depression-focused psychotherapy in their specific content and targets. Screening every IBS patient with a brief, validated instrument as a routine part of the initial evaluation, rather than reserving this screening for patients who appear visibly distressed, identifies patients who would benefit from this referral even when they have not raised the topic themselves. This matters more than it seems.

### The Brain-Gut Behavior Therapy Referral Conversation

Introducing a referral for psychological therapy in the context of a gastrointestinal complaint requires deliberate framing, since patients may otherwise interpret the referral as a sign their symptoms are being dismissed as psychological rather than physical, and explaining the referral explicitly in terms of the shared gut-brain signaling pathway, using concrete, accessible language about how the brain and gut communicate bidirectionally through the same nervous system, helps patients understand the referral as an additional, complementary treatment avenue targeting a real physiologic mechanism rather than a redirection away from their gastrointestinal care. Offering to remain closely involved in ongoing gastroenterology follow-up alongside the behavioral referral, rather than presenting it as a full transfer of care, also reduces the perception that the patient is being handed off elsewhere. Frame it as addition.

## Epidemiology and Overlap With Other Disorders of Gut-Brain Interaction

Irritable bowel syndrome affects a substantial proportion of the general population, making it, alongside functional dyspepsia introduced in an earlier chapter, one of the most common conditions encountered across primary care and gastroenterology practice, and its economic and quality-of-life burden, including reduced work productivity and healthcare utilization comparable to more structurally visible chronic diseases, is frequently underappreciated for the same reasons already discussed regarding functional dyspepsia's underappreciated burden. Overlap between IBS and functional dyspepsia is substantial, with a meaningful proportion of patients meeting criteria for both conditions simultaneously, and this overlap, rather than representing two independent coincidental diagnoses, likely reflects the shared underlying gut-brain dysregulation mechanism discussed throughout this chapter and the previous one, extending across multiple regions of the gastrointestinal tract in the same susceptible individual. Recognizing and explicitly documenting this overlap, rather than treating each region's symptoms in isolation, supports the same unified, whole-patient management philosophy introduced in the sixth chapter, including the possibility that a single neuromodulator agent may address symptoms across both the upper and lower gastrointestinal tract simultaneously. This economic and quality-of-life burden should be communicated within healthcare systems and to payers advocating for adequate coverage of the dietary counseling and behavioral therapies developed throughout this chapter, which are sometimes reimbursed less consistently than pharmacologic therapy despite comparable or superior evidence in appropriately selected patients.

### IBS Subtype Fluidity Over Time

A patient's IBS subtype is not necessarily fixed over the long term, and a meaningful proportion of patients transition between subtypes, most commonly between mixed and either constipation- or diarrhea-predominant patterns, over months to years, which has practical implications for long-term management: a treatment plan matched to a patient's subtype at diagnosis should be reassessed periodically rather than assumed to remain appropriate indefinitely, and a patient reporting a new, sustained change in bowel habit pattern should have their subtype reclassified and their treatment adjusted accordingly rather than having their prior subtype-matched therapy simply continued unchanged despite a clear shift in the underlying symptom pattern. Documenting subtype explicitly at each visit, rather than relying on the label recorded years earlier at initial diagnosis, keeps this reassessment from being inadvertently skipped during routine follow-up. Truly.

## Considerations Across the Lifespan and Special Populations in Functional Bowel Disease

Functional gastrointestinal disorders in adolescents and young adults transitioning from pediatric to adult care benefit from the same structured transition principles already developed in earlier chapters for celiac disease and inflammatory bowel disease, and adult clinicians receiving a young adult patient with a pediatric-onset diagnosis of IBS or functional abdominal pain should specifically review the treatments already trialed and their response, since the diagnostic label alone, without this history, provides insufficient information to plan the next treatment step efficiently. Pregnancy commonly provokes new or worsening constipation, related to progesterone-mediated smooth muscle relaxation and mechanical compression from the enlarging uterus, and management follows a stepped approach favoring the safest available options first, fiber and osmotic laxatives, before considering stimulant laxatives or other agents, applying the same pregnancy-specific stepwise safety consideration already established in earlier chapters for reflux and inflammatory bowel disease management during pregnancy. Family dynamics around a child's chronic symptoms, including well-intentioned but potentially counterproductive parental accommodation of avoidance behaviors, are worth exploring specifically during this transition, since patterns established during childhood can persist into adult presentation if not addressed directly. This takes patience.

### Functional Bowel Disorders in Older Adults

Diagnosing a new functional bowel disorder for the first time in a patient over 50 requires particular caution, since Rome IV criteria were developed and validated predominantly in younger populations and the pretest probability of an organic explanation, particularly colorectal neoplasia, rises substantially with age, reinforcing why the alarm-feature and age-based thresholds developed throughout this chapter and this book should be applied especially rigorously before a functional diagnosis is accepted for the first time in an older patient, even when the symptom pattern otherwise fits Rome IV criteria closely. This heightened caution should not, however, translate into an assumption that older adults cannot have a genuine functional disorder at all; the goal is a rigorous, not a reflexively dismissive, evaluation. Balance is the goal, not suspicion.

## Emerging Therapies and Multidisciplinary Care in Functional Bowel Disease

The gut microbiome's role in disorders of gut-brain interaction continues to be an area of active investigation, and while probiotic therapy has shown benefit for specific symptoms in some studies, the marked heterogeneity across probiotic strains, doses, and study populations means that no single, universally recommended probiotic regimen currently has strong enough evidence to be considered standard first-line therapy, and patients interested in trying a probiotic should be counseled honestly about this evidence limitation rather than given either an overly enthusiastic or a dismissive response. Fecal microbiota transplantation, with an established, well-defined role in recurrent Clostridioides difficile infection outside the scope of this chapter, has been investigated for irritable bowel syndrome specifically with mixed and generally underwhelming results to date, and it should not currently be offered or sought outside of a formal research protocol for this indication given the absence of a clear, established benefit demonstrated in adequately designed trials. Patients following microbiome-related health information from nonclinical sources should be gently redirected toward this evidence-based, cautious framing rather than either dismissed outright or given false confidence in an unproven intervention. Patients should be told plainly that this option is not currently recommended outside of research settings for their condition, even if they have heard about its use for a different indication.

### The Role of the Multidisciplinary Gut-Brain Clinic

Comprehensive management of complex or refractory disorders of gut-brain interaction increasingly occurs within dedicated multidisciplinary clinics combining gastroenterology, dietetics, and gut-directed behavioral health expertise under one coordinated program, and referral to such a program, where available, is a reasonable option for patients whose symptoms remain refractory despite an adequately sequenced trial of the dietary, pharmacologic, and single-modality behavioral therapies developed throughout this chapter, since the combined, simultaneous application of these modalities within a coordinated program has evidence suggesting superior outcomes to the same modalities applied sequentially and independently by separate, uncoordinated providers. Where such a coordinated program is not locally available, gastroenterologists can approximate its benefits by proactively coordinating directly with the dietitian and behavioral health provider involved in a given patient's care, rather than making each referral in isolation and hoping the pieces come together on their own. This coordination effort is worth the extra time.

## Communicating Functional Diagnoses and Setting Long-Term Expectations

How a functional gastrointestinal diagnosis is communicated at the time it is delivered shapes a patient's subsequent engagement with treatment substantially, and applying the same concrete, mechanism-based framing already established in the sixth chapter for functional dyspepsia, explaining that the gut's sensation and movement are genuinely, physiologically altered rather than the symptoms being imagined, dismissed, or attributed vaguely to stress alone, supports a more productive therapeutic relationship than a diagnosis delivered as an exclusionary afterthought once other, more serious possibilities have been ruled out. Patients who have undergone extensive prior testing, often across multiple providers, before reaching a functional diagnosis may arrive skeptical or frustrated, and acknowledging this history explicitly, along with a clear explanation of why the current diagnosis is being made now with confidence rather than by default, helps rebuild the diagnostic trust that a long, inconclusive workup can erode. Involving the patient explicitly in the reasoning behind the diagnosis, rather than delivering it as an unexplained conclusion, similarly reinforces engagement and reduces the likelihood of the patient seeking a second opinion out of a sense that something was overlooked. Empathy paired with clarity, not empathy alone, is what ultimately rebuilds this trust.

### Setting Realistic, Durable Expectations

Disorders of gut-brain interaction are chronic, relapsing-remitting conditions for most affected patients, mirroring the long-term course already discussed for functional dyspepsia and gastroparesis in earlier chapters, and setting this expectation explicitly at diagnosis, along with a specific, written plan for periodic reassessment and treatment adjustment over time, supports more sustainable long-term engagement than allowing a patient to expect a single successful treatment course to produce permanent, complete resolution. Providing patients with a written summary of their working diagnosis, current treatment plan, and the specific triggers that would prompt reassessment or escalation, applying the same plan-anchored communication principle emphasized throughout this book, gives them a concrete reference point for navigating symptom fluctuations without needing to seek reassurance through repeat, often unnecessary testing each time symptoms flare. Reviewing and updating this written plan at each follow-up visit, rather than drafting it once at diagnosis and never revisiting it, keeps it accurate as treatment evolves over the years. A brief version given physically to the patient is more useful in practice than one buried only within a portal message they may not revisit.

## Chronic Diarrhea Beyond IBS

### A Structured Approach to Unexplained Chronic Diarrhea

Chronic diarrhea that remains unexplained after the disease-specific evaluations developed throughout this book, celiac serology, inflammatory markers, bile acid malabsorption testing, and structural evaluation with colonoscopy and biopsy to exclude microscopic colitis and inflammatory bowel disease, warrants a final, systematic reconsideration rather than a default IBS-D label applied simply because the more common causes have been excluded. Factitious diarrhea from surreptitious laxative use, uncommon but underrecognized, can be screened for with a stool osmotic gap calculation and, where specifically suspected, laxative screening, and this possibility, while sensitive to raise directly with a patient, should not be omitted from the differential simply because it is an uncomfortable conversation to initiate. Carbohydrate malabsorption, including lactose and, less commonly, fructose intolerance, produces osmotic diarrhea through a mechanism analogous to the FODMAP mechanism discussed earlier in this chapter, and hydrogen breath testing using the specific suspected carbohydrate as substrate, distinct from the SIBO breath testing introduced in the eighth chapter though using similar technology, can confirm a specific carbohydrate intolerance when clinically suspected. Endocrine causes, including hyperthyroidism and, rarely, a hormone-secreting neuroendocrine tumor, round out the differential for genuinely refractory, unexplained chronic diarrhea and should be considered specifically when the clinical picture includes systemic features, such as flushing or wheezing suggesting carcinoid syndrome, that point beyond a purely gastrointestinal process. Revisiting the full differential systematically at this stage, rather than continuing to escalate empiric antidiarrheal therapy indefinitely, reflects the same diagnostic discipline emphasized throughout this book whenever an initial working diagnosis fails to explain a persistent clinical picture. A brief, direct conversation acknowledging that this possibility is part of a thorough evaluation, rather than an accusation, generally preserves rapport even when the topic is sensitive. A targeted review of systems covering these features specifically, rather than a generic open-ended question, is more likely to surface the clue that redirects the workup appropriately. A dietary elimination trial of the specific suspected carbohydrate, alongside or instead of formal breath testing, is a reasonable, low-cost pragmatic alternative when testing access is limited.

Case Presentation: A 38-year-old woman presents with three years of urgent, watery diarrhea occurring six to eight times daily, previously diagnosed as IBS-D and treated sequentially with an antispasmodic, a bile acid sequestrant trial that produced no improvement, and dietary modification with limited benefit. She reports the diarrhea is not clearly related to meals and occasionally wakes her at night. Applying the reasoning developed in this chapter, nocturnal symptoms are an alarm feature that should not simply be absorbed into an existing IBS-D label without reconsideration, particularly given her inadequate response to an appropriately sequenced treatment trial including a bile acid sequestrant, which should have helped if bile acid malabsorption were the primary mechanism. Colonoscopy with random biopsy, prompted by this alarm feature and treatment-refractory course, identifies a thickened subepithelial collagen band on histology despite a grossly normal-appearing colon, confirming collagenous colitis. She is started on budesonide with substantial improvement in stool frequency and resolution of nocturnal symptoms within weeks. This case illustrates the chapter's central principle for chronic diarrhea: an alarm feature or inadequate response to appropriately sequenced therapy should prompt genuine diagnostic reconsideration, including colonoscopy with biopsy, rather than continued escalation within an increasingly doubtful functional diagnosis.

Case Presentation: A 52-year-old man presents with two years of infrequent bowel movements, occurring every four to five days, straining, and a sensation of incomplete evacuation despite regular use of an osmotic laxative at an adequate dose, which he reports provides minimal benefit. He denies alarm features. Applying the reasoning developed in this chapter, inadequate response to an adequate trial of osmotic laxative therapy defines the threshold for anorectal manometry testing before further pharmacologic escalation is pursued, since his sensation of incomplete evacuation despite regular bowel movement attempts is a specific clue suggesting a possible outlet dysfunction component rather than a purely transit-related problem. Anorectal manometry with balloon expulsion testing demonstrates paradoxical anal sphincter contraction during simulated defecation and an inability to expel the rectal balloon within the expected time, confirming dyssynergic defecation. Rather than escalating to a secretagogue or prokinetic agent, which would not address this specific mechanism, he is referred for biofeedback therapy, a structured program teaching him to coordinate pelvic floor relaxation with defecation effort. Over eight sessions, he achieves substantial improvement in both stool frequency and the sensation of complete evacuation. This case illustrates the chapter's core constipation-management principle: testing for dyssynergic defecation before escalating pharmacotherapy identified the correct, fundamentally different treatment that laxative escalation alone would never have achieved.

| Condition | Key Distinguishing Feature | First-Line Treatment |
|---|---|---|
| IBS-D | Defecation-related pain, no alarm features | Low-FODMAP diet, antidiarrheals, rifaximin |
| IBS-C | Defecation-related pain, constipation-predominant | Fiber, osmotic laxative, secretagogue |
| Centrally mediated abdominal pain syndrome | Pain poorly related to defecation or meals | Central neuromodulator, CBT |
| Dyssynergic defecation | Paradoxical sphincter contraction on manometry | Biofeedback therapy |
| Slow-transit constipation | Delayed transit without dyssynergia | Osmotic laxative, secretagogue, prokinetic |

**THE GI THRESHOLD DECISION SYSTEM — Functional Bowel and Constipation Thresholds**

**Presentation Signature:** This chapter's threshold instances addressed distinguishing IBS-D from its organic mimics and determining when to test for dyssynergic defecation in refractory constipation.

**Threshold Point:** Alarm features and inadequate response to sequenced first-line therapy gate reconsideration of an IBS-D diagnosis; inadequate response to first-line fiber and laxative therapy gates anorectal manometry testing in constipation.

**The Call:** Both thresholds prevent a functional diagnosis from becoming a permanent, unquestioned label, ensuring that treatment failure prompts diagnostic reconsideration rather than simple escalation within the existing diagnostic framework.

**Trap Logic:** Treating a functional bowel diagnosis as fixed once assigned, and escalating constipation pharmacotherapy repeatedly without ever testing for dyssynergic defecation, are this chapter's most consequential threshold misapplications.

**Decision Anchor:** Revisit an IBS-D diagnosis when alarm features emerge or first-line therapy fails, and test for dyssynergic defecation before escalating pharmacotherapy in refractory constipation, since its correct treatment is fundamentally different from any medication that would otherwise be tried next.

## Summary and Key Concepts

Irritable bowel syndrome is diagnosed by Rome IV symptom criteria and subtyped by predominant bowel habit, which directly determines the appropriate dietary and pharmacologic treatment approach.

A limited, structured workup, not an open-ended search, is appropriate before accepting an IBS diagnosis, and alarm features or treatment failure should prompt reconsideration rather than continued escalation.

The low-FODMAP diet follows a three-phase structure, elimination, reintroduction, and personalized maintenance, and skipping reintroduction unnecessarily restricts long-term dietary variety.

Centrally mediated abdominal pain syndrome and narcotic bowel syndrome are distinct disorders of gut-brain interaction requiring centrally directed therapy and, in narcotic bowel syndrome, counterintuitive opioid tapering rather than escalation.

Chronic constipation is classified as normal-transit, slow-transit, or outlet dysfunction (dyssynergic defecation), and this mechanistic classification, not symptom severity, determines whether biofeedback or pharmacotherapy is the appropriate treatment.

Chronic diarrhea unexplained after standard evaluation warrants systematic reconsideration, including screening for factitious diarrhea, carbohydrate malabsorption, and endocrine causes, before a default functional label is accepted.

# CHAPTER 11: COLORECTAL NEOPLASIA, POLYPOSIS SYNDROMES, AND COLORECTAL CANCER SCREENING

**Learning Objectives**

1. Apply current average-risk and increased-risk colorectal cancer screening guidelines, including modality selection and interval determination.
2. Classify colorectal polyps by histology and apply appropriate polypectomy technique and surveillance intervals.
3. Recognize clinical features suggesting a hereditary colorectal cancer syndrome and apply an appropriate genetic evaluation and management pathway.
4. Distinguish Lynch syndrome, familial adenomatous polyposis, and other polyposis syndromes by their clinical and genetic features.
5. Describe the staging, treatment overview, and surveillance approach for colorectal cancer after curative-intent treatment.

**Chapter Outline**

This chapter develops colorectal cancer prevention as a threshold-driven, risk-stratified process, covering average-risk and increased-risk screening, polyp classification and surveillance, the major hereditary colorectal cancer syndromes and the clinical features that should prompt genetic evaluation, and an overview of colorectal cancer staging, treatment, and post-treatment surveillance. Each section connects a specific risk or histologic threshold to a defined screening, surveillance, or referral pathway.

## Colorectal Cancer Screening

### Average-Risk Screening Modalities and Intervals

Colorectal cancer screening in average-risk individuals begins at age 45, reflecting a lowered starting age adopted in response to rising incidence in younger adults, and continues through age 75 in most guidance, with the decision to continue screening between ages 76 and 85 individualized based on overall health status, prior screening history, and patient preference rather than applied uniformly. Colonoscopy, examining the entire colon directly with the ability to perform biopsy or polypectomy within the same procedure, remains the reference standard, while stool-based tests, including fecal immunochemical testing performed annually and multi-target stool DNA testing performed at a longer interval, offer noninvasive alternatives with lower single-test sensitivity for advanced neoplasia that is partially offset by more frequent testing in the case of annual fecal immunochemical testing; any positive stool-based test result must be followed by colonoscopy to complete the evaluation, meaning that a stool-based screening strategy is not equivalent to declining colonoscopy altogether but rather defers it unless and until a positive result occurs. Flexible sigmoidoscopy and CT colonography represent additional, less commonly used options in current practice, and the specific choice among all available modalities should reflect a genuine discussion of the trade-offs between invasiveness, sensitivity, and required follow-up, since patient adherence to whichever modality is chosen matters more for actual cancer prevention than the theoretical superiority of one modality over another if the higher-performing test is one the patient will not actually complete. Documenting the specific modality choice and the shared decision-making conversation that led to it protects continuity of care if the patient is later seen by a different clinician who might otherwise default to a different modality without knowing this history.

**Risk Stratification and Family History-Based Screening**

A first-degree relative with colorectal cancer or an advanced adenoma diagnosed before age 60, or two or more first-degree relatives diagnosed at any age, shifts screening initiation earlier, generally to age 40 or ten years before the youngest affected relative's diagnosis age, whichever is earlier, and this family-history-based threshold, applying the same risk-stratified screening principle already established in this book for Barrett esophagus and hepatocellular carcinoma surveillance, should be assessed and documented explicitly at every relevant primary care or gastroenterology visit rather than assumed unchanged from a prior encounter, since family history can evolve as relatives receive new diagnoses over time. Inflammatory bowel disease-related surveillance, developed in detail in the ninth chapter, and the hereditary syndromes developed later in this chapter represent further, more intensive risk categories with their own specific screening protocols that supersede average-risk or family-history-based guidance entirely once identified. A dedicated family history questionnaire completed by the patient before the visit, rather than relying entirely on a verbal recollection during a time-limited appointment, can improve the completeness and accuracy of this information.

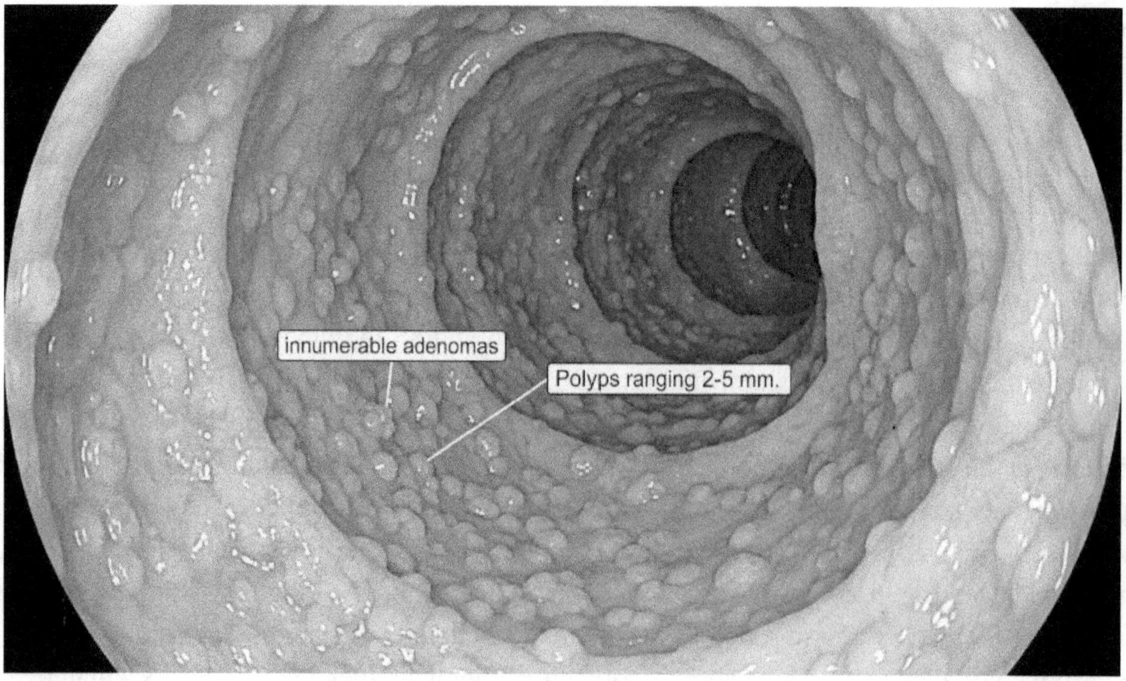

**THE GI THRESHOLD DECISION SYSTEM — Colorectal Thresholds — Selecting Screening Modality and Initiation Age by Risk Category**

**Presentation Signature:** A patient presents for a routine health maintenance visit, and the clinician must determine the appropriate colorectal cancer screening initiation age and modality based on personal and family history.

**Threshold Point:** Average risk, with no qualifying family history, personal history, or hereditary syndrome, defines screening initiation at age 45 with any guideline-endorsed modality; a qualifying family history defines earlier initiation, generally age 40 or ten years before the youngest affected relative's age, whichever is earlier, with colonoscopy specifically as the preferred modality given its superior detection and the shorter recommended intervals in this population.

**The Call:** Average-risk patients select among colonoscopy, annual fecal immunochemical testing, or multi-target stool DNA testing based on informed patient preference; increased-risk patients due to family history are directed to colonoscopy specifically, generally at a shortened interval relative to average-risk colonoscopy screening.

**Trap Logic:** Applying average-risk screening intervals and starting ages to a patient with a qualifying family history, because the family history was not specifically asked about or was not updated since a prior visit, is a common and consequential gap in preventive care.

**Decision Anchor:** Reassess family history explicitly at relevant visits, and shift both starting age and modality preference toward colonoscopy whenever a qualifying family history, personal history, or hereditary syndrome is identified, rather than defaulting to average-risk guidance by omission.

## Colorectal Polyps

### Polyp Classification and Malignant Potential

Conventional adenomas, the most common colorectal polyp type with recognized malignant potential, are classified by architecture, tubular, tubulovillous, or villous, and by the presence and grade of dysplasia, and villous architecture and high-grade dysplasia both independently increase the risk of an adenoma harboring or progressing to invasive carcinoma, information that should be reflected explicitly in the surveillance interval assigned rather than treated as incidental pathologic detail. Serrated lesions, encompassing hyperplastic polyps, which carry minimal malignant potential when small and located in the rectosigmoid colon, and sessile serrated lesions, which follow a distinct molecular pathway to carcinoma involving epigenetic gene silencing rather than the chromosomal instability pathway characteristic of conventional adenomas, require this histologic distinction to be made accurately, since sessile serrated lesions, unlike small distal hyperplastic polyps, carry meaningful malignant potential and require the same surveillance attention as a conventional adenoma of comparable size. Traditional serrated adenomas, an uncommon but distinct third serrated category with mixed morphologic features, similarly carry malignant potential requiring surveillance attention comparable to conventional adenomas. Piecemeal resection of a large polyp, in which the lesion is removed in multiple fragments rather than as a single intact specimen, complicates definitive histologic assessment of margins and increases local recurrence risk, which is why endoscopists should clearly document when a resection was piecemeal versus en bloc and why a shortened surveillance interval, following a repeat examination of the resection site specifically, is generally warranted after piecemeal resection of a large lesion. Pathologists should be encouraged to specify sessile serrated lesion versus hyperplastic polyp explicitly in every report rather than using ambiguous or inconsistent terminology, since this specific distinction, more than almost any other single pathology report detail in this chapter, directly determines the surveillance interval that follows.

**Figure 11.1: Adenoma-to-Carcinoma Progression Pathway**

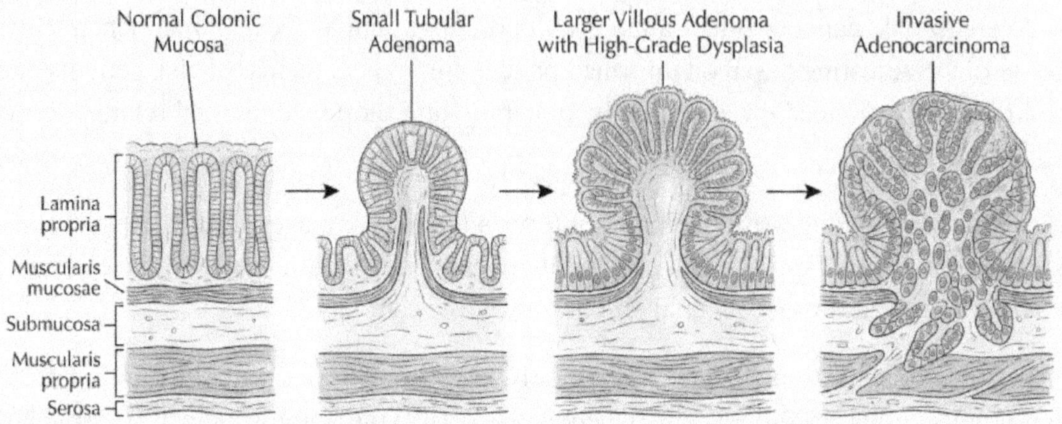


### Polypectomy Technique and Surveillance Intervals

Polypectomy technique is selected based on polyp size and morphology: cold snare polypectomy, removing the polyp without cautery, is preferred for small polyps given its favorable safety profile and adequate complete resection rates, while larger or more complex lesions may require endoscopic mucosal resection, injecting fluid beneath the lesion to create a safety cushion before snare resection, or, for the most complex lesions, endoscopic submucosal dissection, introduced in the third chapter for Barrett esophagus-related neoplasia, allowing en bloc removal of larger lesions than conventional techniques can reliably achieve in a single piece. Surveillance intervals following polypectomy are determined by the number, size, and histology of resected polyps considered together rather than by any single polyp in isolation, with more numerous, larger, or higher-risk-histology polyps warranting shorter surveillance intervals, and communicating the specific interval and its rationale clearly to the patient at the time of the procedure, rather than leaving this information solely within a pathology report the patient may never see, applies the same plan-anchored communication principle emphasized throughout this book. Documenting whether a resection was complete, and if margins were assessed, adds important information for the pathologist and for any future clinician reviewing this record, particularly if the lesion recurs at the same site during subsequent surveillance.

## The Genetic Counseling and Testing Process

Pretest genetic counseling, ideally performed by a certified genetic counselor rather than delivered informally by the referring gastroenterologist alone, establishes informed consent covering the implications of a positive, negative, and variant-of-uncertain-significance result before testing proceeds, and this structured counseling process, rather than testing performed reflexively once a red-flag feature is identified, ensures the patient understands what each possible result would mean for their own management and for their relatives before that information is obtained. A variant of uncertain significance, a genetic finding that cannot currently be classified as clearly pathogenic or clearly benign, should not be used to guide clinical management as though it were a confirmed pathogenic finding, and patients receiving this result should be counseled that classification may change as scientific understanding evolves, with periodic reclassification review a reasonable long-term practice for any patient carrying an unresolved variant result. Adequate time allocated for this counseling conversation, rather than compressing it into the final minutes of an already time-constrained visit, reflects the genuine complexity and emotional weight of the decision the patient is being asked to make. Written materials summarizing this counseling discussion give the patient something to refer back to after the visit. Contacting patients when a variant reclassification occurs, rather than only at the time of the original result, requires a systematic tracking process most centers are still developing. Clarity supports consent.

### Cascade Testing and Family Communication

Once a pathogenic variant is confirmed in an index patient, cascade testing, offering targeted testing for the identified specific variant to at-risk first-degree relatives, is far more efficient and less costly than repeating comprehensive panel testing in each relative, and facilitating this cascade process, including providing the index patient with clear, written information to share with relatives about the specific variant identified and the recommended next step of contacting a genetic counselor, supports family-wide risk identification that the index patient alone often cannot coordinate effectively without this structured support. Family communication about a hereditary cancer diagnosis can be complicated by estrangement, geographic distance, or the emotional difficulty of raising the topic, and acknowledging these barriers explicitly, rather than assuming family communication will happen automatically once the index patient is informed, allows the care team to provide additional support, such as a letter the patient can share directly, where this communication proves difficult. Some centers now offer direct outreach programs contacting at-risk relatives, with the index patient's consent, to further reduce the burden of family communication falling entirely on the newly diagnosed patient during an already difficult time. Recognizing that not every relative will choose to pursue testing, and that this choice is theirs to make once informed, respects patient and family autonomy even when more complete family-wide testing uptake might otherwise be hoped for. This letter approach reduces the burden of a difficult conversation falling entirely on the patient. Every relative matters.

## Hereditary Colorectal Cancer Syndromes

### Lynch Syndrome

Lynch syndrome, caused by a germline pathogenic variant in one of the DNA mismatch repair genes, produces microsatellite instability and a substantially elevated lifetime risk of colorectal cancer along with an elevated risk of endometrial, ovarian, gastric, and several other cancers, and its recognition depends on a combination of family history meeting defined clinical criteria and, increasingly, universal tumor testing, screening every newly diagnosed colorectal or endometrial cancer for mismatch repair deficiency or microsatellite instability regardless of family history, since a meaningful proportion of confirmed Lynch syndrome cases would be missed by family history criteria alone given incomplete or unknown family cancer history in many patients. A tumor identified as mismatch repair deficient or microsatellite unstable should prompt germline genetic testing to distinguish true Lynch syndrome from sporadic mismatch repair deficiency, most commonly from acquired hypermethylation of the MLH1 promoter, a distinction with substantial implications since sporadic cases do not carry the same hereditary cancer risk to the patient's relatives that confirmed Lynch syndrome does. Confirmed Lynch syndrome carriers require colonoscopy beginning at a substantially younger age than average-risk screening and repeated at a shortened interval given the syndrome's accelerated adenoma-to-carcinoma progression, alongside gynecologic cancer risk-reduction counseling and, in appropriately selected patients, consideration of risk-reducing gynecologic surgery once childbearing is complete. The specific mismatch repair gene involved carries prognostic and management nuance of its own, since MSH2 and MSH6 pathogenic variants are associated with a higher lifetime endometrial cancer risk than MLH1 or PMS2 variants, information that should specifically inform the intensity of gynecologic surveillance and the timing discussion around risk-reducing surgery for an individual carrier. BRAF mutation testing on the tumor further supports this distinction, since a BRAF-mutated tumor with MLH1 loss strongly favors a sporadic mechanism, whereas the absence of a BRAF mutation in this setting increases the likelihood that germline testing will confirm true Lynch syndrome.

### Familial Adenomatous Polyposis

Familial adenomatous polyposis, caused by a germline pathogenic variant in the APC gene, produces hundreds to thousands of colorectal adenomas beginning in adolescence, with colorectal cancer developing with near-certainty by mid-adulthood if colectomy is not performed prophylactically, and its recognition, whether through family history or the identification of innumerable polyps on an index colonoscopy performed for another indication, should prompt genetic counseling and testing along with early, intensive endoscopic surveillance beginning in the early teenage years in at-risk family members. Extracolonic manifestations, including duodenal and periampullary adenomas carrying their own independent malignant potential requiring dedicated upper endoscopic surveillance, desmoid tumors, and osteomas, mean that familial adenomatous polyposis management extends well beyond colorectal surveillance alone, and attenuated familial adenomatous polyposis, a milder phenotype with fewer polyps and later onset, should be considered in a patient with a suggestive but less dramatic polyp burden than classic disease, since it is caused by the same gene and carries substantial though somewhat delayed colorectal cancer risk requiring its own structured surveillance program. Prophylactic colectomy timing is individualized based on polyp burden and size trajectory on surveillance, but is generally recommended once polyps become too numerous to manage endoscopically or once high-grade dysplasia is identified, and this decision benefits from being made collaboratively between the patient, gastroenterology, and colorectal surgery well before an emergency or a missed cancer forces the decision under less favorable circumstances. Spigelman staging classifies the severity of duodenal polyposis and directly informs the interval for upper endoscopic surveillance, with more advanced staging warranting more frequent examination and, in severe cases, consideration of intervention directed at the duodenum itself.

**Other Polyposis Syndromes**

MUTYH-associated polyposis, an autosomal recessive condition requiring pathogenic variants in both MUTYH alleles to produce the full polyposis phenotype, presents similarly to attenuated familial adenomatous polyposis and should be considered when APC testing is negative in a patient with a compatible adenomatous polyposis phenotype, given the different inheritance pattern this distinction implies for family counseling. Peutz-Jeghers syndrome, caused by a pathogenic variant in the STK11 gene, produces characteristic hamartomatous polyps throughout the gastrointestinal tract alongside distinctive mucocutaneous pigmentation, most visibly around the lips and buccal mucosa, and carries an elevated risk not only of colorectal cancer but of several extraintestinal malignancies, requiring a broader, multi-organ surveillance program beyond the colon alone. Juvenile polyposis syndrome and serrated polyposis syndrome, the latter defined by a specific quantitative threshold of serrated polyps rather than by a currently identified single causative gene in most cases, each carry meaningfully elevated colorectal cancer risk and require intensive colonoscopic surveillance, with serrated polyposis syndrome specifically illustrating that a hereditary or familial colorectal cancer risk pattern can be recognized and managed even before, or without ever identifying, the specific underlying genetic cause. Genetic counseling for MUTYH-associated polyposis should explicitly address its recessive inheritance pattern with parents and siblings of an affected patient, since this pattern implies a different risk calculation for these relatives than the autosomal dominant inheritance seen in Lynch syndrome and familial adenomatous polyposis, a distinction that is easy to blur if the counseling conversation does not address inheritance pattern explicitly for each specific syndrome. Recurrent small bowel intussusception from Peutz-Jeghers hamartomatous polyps is a specific, well-recognized acute complication that can present as an emergency in a young patient and should be considered in the differential when a known carrier presents with acute abdominal pain. Juvenile polyposis syndrome should also prompt evaluation for a coexisting hereditary hemorrhagic telangiectasia phenotype in a subset of patients carrying an overlapping SMAD4 pathogenic variant, since this genetic overlap carries additional vascular malformation risks requiring their own dedicated screening beyond gastrointestinal surveillance alone.

**THE GI THRESHOLD DECISION SYSTEM — Colorectal Thresholds — Red Flags Warranting Genetic Evaluation**

**Presentation Signature:** A patient presents with colorectal cancer, a personal history of multiple colorectal polyps, or a family history pattern that may reflect an underlying hereditary syndrome, and the clinician must decide whether genetic counseling and testing are warranted.

**Threshold Point:** Colorectal or endometrial cancer diagnosed at any age now warrants universal tumor testing for mismatch repair deficiency regardless of family history; cancer diagnosed before age 50, ten or more cumulative adenomas, any hamartomatous polyp, or a family history meeting defined hereditary cancer criteria each independently cross the threshold for genetic counseling referral.

**The Call:** Any patient meeting one or more of these threshold criteria is referred for formal genetic counseling and, where indicated, germline testing, rather than being managed with standard-risk or even generically increased-risk screening alone, since a confirmed hereditary syndrome changes both the patient's own surveillance intensity and the screening recommendations that must be communicated to at-risk relatives.

**Trap Logic:** Relying on family history alone without universal tumor testing misses a meaningful proportion of true Lynch syndrome cases, since family cancer history is often incomplete, unknown, or simply not obtained in sufficient detail during a routine clinical encounter.

**Decision Anchor:** Apply universal tumor testing to every new colorectal and endometrial cancer diagnosis regardless of family history, and refer for genetic counseling whenever any of the specific red-flag criteria above is met, since identifying a hereditary syndrome changes management for the patient and their relatives alike.

## Special Considerations in Colorectal Cancer Screening

Colorectal cancer screening participation remains suboptimal across many populations, and disparities in screening completion by race, ethnicity, insurance status, and geographic access to endoscopic services contribute to disparities in colorectal cancer mortality that mirror, rather than reflect any biological difference in disease behavior, differences in screening access and completion, meaning that improving screening participation specifically in underserved populations is a meaningful, evidence-based intervention for reducing these outcome disparities. Patient navigation programs, providing dedicated support to help patients complete the scheduling, preparation, and follow-up steps of colorectal cancer screening, have demonstrated measurable improvements in screening completion rates in underserved populations and represent a practical, systems-level intervention that individual clinicians can advocate for within their own practice settings even when they cannot single-handedly address the broader structural barriers to screening access. Culturally tailored educational materials addressing specific, documented barriers within a given community, rather than a generic, one-size-fits-all screening reminder, further improve the effectiveness of these navigation efforts. Health systems evaluating the cost-effectiveness of navigation programs should account for the downstream cost savings of earlier-stage cancer detection and prevention, not only the upfront program cost, when assessing this investment. Small investments, real returns.

### Screening in Patients With Limited Life Expectancy

Colorectal cancer screening in patients with substantially limited life expectancy from advanced age, frailty, or serious comorbid illness requires individualized judgment rather than mechanical application of the age-based intervals developed earlier in this chapter, since the multi-year lag time between polyp detection and the clinical benefit of its removal means that screening a patient unlikely to survive long enough to benefit exposes them to procedural risk without the corresponding benefit that justifies that risk in a patient with a longer life expectancy. This individualized approach requires an honest, direct conversation about life expectancy and goals of care, which some clinicians find uncomfortable to initiate, but which is a necessary component of avoiding both under-screening a patient with genuine remaining life expectancy and over-screening a patient for whom the procedure's risk clearly outweighs its potential benefit. Documenting this individualized decision explicitly, including the reasoning discussed with the patient, protects against a later clinician reflexively resuming screening simply because a prior deferral was not clearly explained in the record. Framing this conversation around what matters most to the patient given their remaining time and priorities, rather than around abstract statistics alone, tends to be better received and more useful for the shared decision that follows. Every conversation counts.

## Colonoscopy Quality and Interval Colorectal Cancer

Interval colorectal cancer, a cancer diagnosed after a colonoscopy that did not identify it, most commonly results from a missed lesion, an incompletely resected lesion, or a rapidly progressing biologically aggressive tumor arising after an adequate examination, and understanding this distinction matters both for individual patient counseling and for the quality improvement efforts already introduced in the second chapter's discussion of adenoma detection rate as a key endoscopist-level quality benchmark. A patient developing colorectal cancer within a shorter interval than would be expected based on the adenoma-to-carcinoma progression timeline discussed earlier in this chapter should prompt review of the prior colonoscopy, including bowel preparation adequacy, withdrawal time, and cecal intubation confirmation, since this review can identify a systemic quality issue relevant to that endoscopist's broader practice rather than being dismissed as an isolated, unexplainable occurrence. Communicating with the patient about this review process, when it is undertaken, in a transparent, non-defensive manner, rather than avoiding the conversation out of discomfort, supports both the immediate therapeutic relationship and the broader trust in the screening program that this specific patient's case has, understandably, called into question for them. Sharing this quality review, in appropriate detail, with the endoscopy unit's broader quality committee, rather than treating it as strictly a private matter for the individual endoscopist, supports the kind of systemic learning that benefits future patients beyond the one directly affected.

### The Right-Sided Colon and Detection Challenges

Right-sided colonic lesions, particularly flat or subtly elevated sessile serrated lesions discussed earlier in this chapter, are disproportionately represented among interval cancers, reflecting both their inherently more difficult endoscopic detection given their flat morphology and blending with surrounding mucosa, and, in some studies, a more rapid progression pathway than the classic adenoma-carcinoma sequence, reinforcing why meticulous, unhurried inspection technique specifically in the right colon during colonoscope withdrawal, applying the withdrawal-time and technique principles introduced in the second chapter, deserves particular attention beyond a generic, uniform inspection pace applied to the entire colon. Adjunctive imaging techniques and dye-based or virtual chromoendoscopy, introduced in the second chapter, may further improve detection of these subtle right-sided lesions in appropriately selected higher-risk patients, though their routine use across all average-risk screening colonoscopies has not been established as a universal standard of care. Endoscopists should specifically document withdrawal time and technique in the right colon distinctly, when feasible, rather than reporting only a single, undifferentiated total withdrawal time for the entire examination.

## Molecular Testing and Targeted Therapy in Colorectal Cancer

Beyond mismatch repair and microsatellite instability testing, already introduced in this chapter for Lynch syndrome identification, molecular profiling of colorectal tumors, particularly in metastatic disease, has become standard practice for guiding targeted therapy selection. KRAS, NRAS, and BRAF mutation status determine eligibility for anti-epidermal growth factor receptor therapy, since tumors harboring these mutations do not respond to this drug class and, in the case of certain mutations, may even experience worse outcomes with its use, making this testing essential before this specific therapy is considered rather than an optional refinement. High microsatellite instability or mismatch repair deficiency, beyond its hereditary-syndrome implications discussed earlier in this chapter, also predicts a favorable response to immune checkpoint inhibitor therapy in metastatic disease, reflecting the increased tumor mutational burden and resulting immunogenicity characteristic of mismatch-repair-deficient tumors, meaning that this single test result now carries both hereditary-risk and therapeutic-selection implications that should each be acted upon. Repeat molecular testing on a metastatic biopsy at the time of disease progression, rather than relying solely on the original primary tumor's molecular profile, is increasingly recommended given the possibility of clonal evolution and acquired resistance mutations emerging over the course of treatment. Communicating a complex molecular result and its treatment implications to a patient without extensive scientific background requires the same plain-language framing already emphasized throughout this book for other technical findings. Clarity always helps.

### The Expanding Role of Circulating Tumor DNA

Circulating tumor DNA testing, detecting tumor-derived genetic material in a peripheral blood sample, is an emerging tool with investigational and, increasingly, clinical applications in colorectal cancer, including detection of minimal residual disease after curative-intent surgery that may identify patients at higher recurrence risk who could benefit from adjuvant therapy intensification, and monitoring for recurrence during surveillance with potentially greater sensitivity than conventional carcinoembryonic antigen monitoring, though its precise role in routine clinical decision-making continues to evolve and its use should be guided by current, actively updated professional society guidance rather than adopted uniformly ahead of that evolving evidence base. Patients should be counseled that this remains an evolving area, and a negative circulating tumor DNA result does not currently provide the same level of reassurance against recurrence that a truly mature, long-term surveillance dataset would eventually support once this technology's role is more fully established. Insurance coverage for this testing also varies considerably by region and payer, a practical consideration alongside the evolving evidence base itself.

## Early-Onset Colorectal Cancer

Colorectal cancer diagnosed before age 50, termed early-onset colorectal cancer, has risen in incidence over recent decades even as overall age-adjusted colorectal cancer incidence has declined, a divergent trend that prompted the lowered average-risk screening age discussed earlier in this chapter, and this rising incidence occurs predominantly in patients without an identifiable hereditary syndrome despite the younger age at diagnosis, meaning that most early-onset cases reflect a genuinely sporadic process whose underlying drivers, possibly related to dietary, microbiome, or other environmental factors accumulating across a birth cohort, remain incompletely understood. Because a younger patient's symptoms are more likely to be attributed to a benign or functional cause given the lower baseline pretest probability of malignancy at younger ages, discussed as a general principle in earlier chapters, diagnostic delay is a recognized and significant problem in early-onset colorectal cancer specifically, and clinicians should maintain a genuinely low threshold for colonoscopy in a younger patient presenting with rectal bleeding, iron deficiency anemia, or a persistent, unexplained change in bowel habits, resisting the instinct to attribute these findings reflexively to hemorrhoids or a functional disorder without at least considering, and often pursuing, endoscopic evaluation. Ongoing research into diet, the gut microbiome, antibiotic exposure history, and other early-life environmental factors continues to investigate potential contributors to this trend, though no single factor has yet been conclusively established as the primary driver. Explicitly documenting the reasoning for pursuing or deferring colonoscopy in a younger patient with these symptoms protects against this reasoning being lost or unclear if the patient re-presents later with persistent or progressive symptoms. This trend deserves continued study. Vigilance matters most here.

### Universal Germline Testing Considerations in Early-Onset Disease

Given the disproportionate, though still minority, representation of hereditary syndromes among early-onset colorectal cancer cases relative to average-onset disease, many centers now apply a broader, multi-gene hereditary cancer panel rather than mismatch repair testing alone in patients diagnosed before age 50, capturing not only Lynch syndrome but also the polyposis syndromes and other hereditary cancer predisposition genes discussed throughout this chapter, reflecting an evolution in practice toward more comprehensive genetic evaluation specifically triggered by young age at diagnosis regardless of the specific tumor's mismatch repair status. This broader panel approach also captures rarer hereditary conditions not otherwise discussed in detail in this chapter, reflecting the evolving, increasingly comprehensive nature of hereditary cancer risk assessment as genetic testing technology and its cost-effectiveness continue to improve. Insurance coverage and cost considerations similarly apply to broader panel testing, and discussing these practical factors alongside the clinical rationale supports a fully informed decision. This trend continues to evolve.

## Chemoprevention and Lifestyle Factors in Colorectal Cancer Risk

Aspirin has demonstrated colorectal cancer risk reduction in several large studies, and current guidance supports its consideration specifically in average-risk adults within a defined age range who also have an independent cardiovascular indication for aspirin therapy, weighing the colorectal cancer risk-reduction benefit alongside the bleeding risk that must be considered for any aspirin therapy decision, applying the same multi-factor risk-benefit framework already established in earlier chapters for gastroprotective strategy selection in patients on antiplatelet or anticoagulant therapy. Aspirin is not currently recommended as a dedicated chemoprevention strategy in patients without an independent cardiovascular indication, given that the bleeding risk of aspirin therapy is not clearly outweighed by colorectal cancer risk reduction alone in this population, a nuance worth communicating clearly to patients who may have heard about aspirin's colorectal cancer benefit without the accompanying risk-benefit context. Ongoing periodic reassessment of this risk-benefit balance, rather than a one-time decision made at a single visit and never revisited, is appropriate as a patient ages and their bleeding risk profile potentially changes over time. Shared decision-making documentation for this specific choice, noting the factors discussed and the patient's preference, protects continuity if the aspirin decision is later revisited by a different clinician.

### Dietary and Lifestyle Modification

Red and processed meat consumption, sedentary lifestyle, obesity, and heavy alcohol use are each independently associated with increased colorectal cancer risk, while adequate physical activity, maintenance of a healthy body weight, and adequate dietary fiber intake are associated with reduced risk, and while none of these lifestyle factors substitutes for appropriate screening, counseling patients on these modifiable risk factors as a complementary, not alternative, component of colorectal cancer risk reduction is a reasonable and evidence-supported part of a comprehensive preventive care conversation, particularly given that many of these same modifications carry independent cardiovascular and metabolic health benefits beyond colorectal cancer risk reduction alone. Framing these lifestyle recommendations as broadly beneficial for overall health, not solely as a colorectal cancer prevention strategy, may improve their reception and adoption relative to a narrower, single-disease framing that can feel less personally relevant to some patients. Referral to a dietitian for structured dietary counseling is reasonable for motivated patients seeking more detailed, individualized guidance beyond general recommendations.

## Anal Neoplasia and Its Distinction From Colorectal Cancer

Anal squamous cell carcinoma, distinct histologically and etiologically from colorectal adenocarcinoma, is predominantly caused by human papillomavirus infection and shares risk factors and a screening rationale with cervical cancer, including elevated risk in patients with HIV infection, a history of receptive anal intercourse, and other HPV-related anogenital dysplasia, and anal cytology screening, analogous to cervical Papanicolaou testing, is recommended in specific high-risk populations, most notably people living with HIV, at intervals determined by CD4 count and other risk factors. High-resolution anoscopy, performed by clinicians with specific training in this technique, evaluates abnormal cytology results further and allows targeted biopsy of visible dysplastic lesions, and this evaluation pathway, distinct from the colonoscopic surveillance developed throughout this chapter for colorectal neoplasia, should not be conflated with or substituted by routine colorectal cancer screening, since the two conditions, despite their anatomic proximity, require entirely separate risk assessment and screening protocols. Coordinating this screening with an infectious disease or HIV primary care provider, when the patient has one, ensures the anal cytology recommendation is integrated into the patient's overall preventive care plan rather than existing as an isolated, easily forgotten recommendation from a single gastroenterology encounter. Patients should understand that a diagnosis of anal HPV-related dysplasia is separate from and does not increase their colorectal cancer risk specifically, since these are anatomically adjacent but biologically distinct entities.

### Anal Intraepithelial Neoplasia Management

Anal intraepithelial neoplasia, the precursor lesion to anal squamous cell carcinoma identified on high-resolution anoscopy-directed biopsy, is managed with ablative or excisional therapy for high-grade lesions in appropriately selected patients, paralleling the dysplasia-grade-driven management threshold already established in this book for Barrett esophagus and colorectal adenomas, though the evidence base for anal intraepithelial neoplasia treatment reducing progression to invasive cancer is less mature than the corresponding evidence for colorectal polypectomy, and this evolving evidence landscape should be communicated honestly to patients making decisions about treatment versus continued surveillance alone. Referral to a high-resolution anoscopy specialist, where this evolving field's expertise is concentrated at present, is reasonable for patients requiring this evaluation given the specialized equipment and training the procedure requires.

## Psychosocial Impact and Survivorship Care in Colorectal Cancer

A colorectal cancer diagnosis and its treatment, including surgery, chemotherapy, and, for many rectal cancer patients, a temporary or permanent ostomy, carry substantial psychosocial burden, and structured survivorship care, extending beyond the surveillance protocol developed earlier in this chapter, should address ostomy adjustment support, sexual and bowel function concerns following pelvic surgery or radiation, and screening for anxiety and depression, applying the same routine mental health screening standard already established throughout this book for other chronic gastrointestinal conditions, rather than treating survivorship as purely a matter of recurrence surveillance. Cascade genetic counseling for family members, when a hereditary syndrome has been identified as developed earlier in this chapter, is itself a component of comprehensive survivorship care, since the psychological impact of a new hereditary cancer risk diagnosis extends to the patient's relatives and requires its own dedicated support and counseling resources distinct from the patient's own cancer treatment and recovery. Peer support programs connecting newly diagnosed patients with survivors who have navigated similar treatment, including ostomy adjustment specifically, provide a form of practical, lived-experience support that clinical staff, however well-intentioned, cannot fully replicate. Sexual health concerns specifically are often underaddressed unless a clinician raises the topic directly, since patients frequently do not volunteer this concern unprompted. Ask directly.

### Coordinating Survivorship Care Across Specialties

Long-term colorectal cancer survivorship care benefits from explicit coordination between oncology, gastroenterology, and primary care, with a clearly documented survivorship care plan specifying which surveillance test is performed by which service and at what interval, applying the same plan-anchored, explicit coordination principle emphasized throughout this book for other complex, multidisciplinary conditions, since ambiguity about which specialty is responsible for ordering a given surveillance test is a recognized and avoidable cause of surveillance gaps in long-term cancer survivors. Electronic health record tools flagging upcoming surveillance due dates, where available, provide an additional systems-level safeguard against these gaps beyond individual clinician vigilance alone. This plan should be revisited at each visit, not only created once at the transition from active treatment. Revisit often.

## Colorectal Cancer Staging and Management Overview

### Staging and Initial Workup

Colorectal cancer staging follows the tumor-node-metastasis system, incorporating depth of tumor invasion through the bowel wall, regional lymph node involvement, and distant metastasis, and the initial workup after tissue diagnosis includes cross-sectional imaging of the chest, abdomen, and pelvis to assess for metastatic disease, carcinoembryonic antigen as a baseline marker for later surveillance rather than as a diagnostic test given its limited sensitivity and specificity as discussed in an earlier chapter, and, for rectal cancer specifically, pelvic MRI to assess local tumor extent and mesorectal lymph node involvement with a precision that guides the specific choice between upfront surgery and neoadjuvant chemoradiation in this anatomic location. Multidisciplinary tumor board review, incorporating input from surgery, medical oncology, radiation oncology where relevant, radiology, and pathology together, is standard practice for treatment planning in colorectal cancer, particularly for rectal cancer where the sequencing of surgery, chemotherapy, and radiation requires careful, individualized coordination rather than a single specialty determining the plan independently. Stage-specific five-year survival estimates, while useful for general prognostic counseling, should be communicated with appropriate individualization, since a given patient's specific tumor biology, comorbidities, and response to treatment can meaningfully shift their actual prognosis away from a population-level statistic.

### Surgical and Adjuvant Treatment Overview

Surgical resection with adequate lymph node harvest remains the primary curative treatment for localized colorectal cancer, and adjuvant chemotherapy is added for node-positive disease and select high-risk node-negative disease to reduce recurrence risk, reflecting the tumor biology risk stratification that pathologic staging after resection provides. Rectal cancer management specifically often incorporates neoadjuvant chemoradiation before surgery for locally advanced disease, and a small but growing subset of rectal cancer patients achieving a complete clinical response to neoadjuvant therapy are candidates for a watch-and-wait, organ-preserving surveillance strategy rather than immediate radical surgery, an evolving area of practice that requires close, structured surveillance and should be pursued only within an experienced multidisciplinary program given the consequences of a missed local recurrence in a patient who deferred definitive surgical resection. Minimally invasive laparoscopic or robotic surgical approaches, when performed by an experienced surgeon with appropriate oncologic technique, achieve comparable oncologic outcomes to open surgery with the benefit of faster recovery, and the choice between approaches should reflect surgeon experience and tumor-specific technical factors rather than a uniform preference for one approach regardless of individual case complexity. Adjuvant chemotherapy regimen selection and duration are further individualized based on specific pathologic risk features and, increasingly, the circulating tumor DNA findings discussed later in this chapter, reflecting a gradual shift toward biomarker-informed rather than purely stage-based adjuvant treatment decisions. Total neoadjuvant therapy, delivering both chemotherapy and radiation before surgery rather than sequencing chemotherapy afterward, has shown improved rates of complete clinical response supporting the watch-and-wait approach and is increasingly adopted at centers with the multidisciplinary expertise to manage this more intensive upfront treatment sequence.

## Post-Treatment Surveillance

Surveillance after curative-intent colorectal cancer treatment follows a structured protocol combining periodic carcinoembryonic antigen measurement, cross-sectional imaging, and colonoscopy at defined intervals, generally more intensive in the initial years after treatment when recurrence risk is highest and de-escalating over time as the cumulative recurrence-free interval lengthens, mirroring the same risk-proportionate surveillance intensity principle already established throughout this book for other conditions. A rising carcinoembryonic antigen during surveillance, even in the absence of a localized recurrence identified on imaging, warrants further evaluation rather than reassurance, since a rising trend can precede radiographically detectable recurrence, and this pattern should prompt closer monitoring or additional imaging rather than being dismissed as an isolated laboratory fluctuation. Communicating the full surveillance schedule to the patient in writing at the time treatment concludes, rather than relying on the treating oncologist alone to remember and initiate each subsequent test at the correct interval, supports continuity as the patient transitions from active treatment to a longer-term survivorship phase, potentially under the care of a different set of clinicians. A single, isolated modest elevation without a clear rising trend across successive measurements is less concerning than a consistent upward trajectory, and interpreting the trend over several data points, rather than reacting to any single value, is the more clinically meaningful approach.

Case Presentation: A 44-year-old woman is diagnosed with colon cancer, and universal tumor testing performed per standard protocol demonstrates loss of MSH2 and MSH6 expression on immunohistochemistry, consistent with mismatch repair deficiency. Applying the reasoning developed in this chapter, this finding, obtained regardless of her family history, warrants germline genetic testing to distinguish true Lynch syndrome from a sporadic cause, and because MSH2 and MSH6 loss, unlike MLH1 loss, is rarely explained by sporadic promoter hypermethylation, Lynch syndrome is strongly suspected even before germline results return. Germline testing confirms a pathogenic MSH2 variant, establishing a diagnosis of Lynch syndrome. She undergoes cascade genetic counseling discussions for testing her siblings and children, and her own subsequent surveillance plan incorporates earlier and more frequent colonoscopy following her cancer treatment, along with gynecologic cancer risk counseling given her elevated endometrial and ovarian cancer risk. This case illustrates the chapter's central hereditary-syndrome principle: universal tumor testing, applied regardless of family history, identified a hereditary syndrome that specifically changes both her own long-term surveillance and the screening recommendations for her at-risk relatives.

Case Presentation: A 51-year-old man undergoes screening colonoscopy and is found to have twelve sessile serrated lesions distributed throughout the colon, several exceeding one centimeter, meeting quantitative criteria for serrated polyposis syndrome. He has no known family history of colorectal cancer, and germline genetic testing for known polyposis genes is negative. Applying the reasoning developed in this chapter, a negative genetic test does not exclude serrated polyposis syndrome, since this diagnosis is defined by a specific quantitative polyp burden rather than by a currently identified single causative gene in most affected individuals, and he is managed with intensive surveillance colonoscopy at a substantially shortened interval regardless of the negative genetic result. His first-degree relatives are also counseled regarding their own increased colorectal cancer risk and offered earlier screening initiation, applying the same family-based risk stratification developed earlier in this chapter even though no specific causative gene was identified to test them for directly. This case illustrates that a hereditary or familial colorectal cancer risk pattern can be recognized and managed effectively through phenotypic criteria alone, without requiring a positive genetic test to justify intensive surveillance.

Figure 11.2

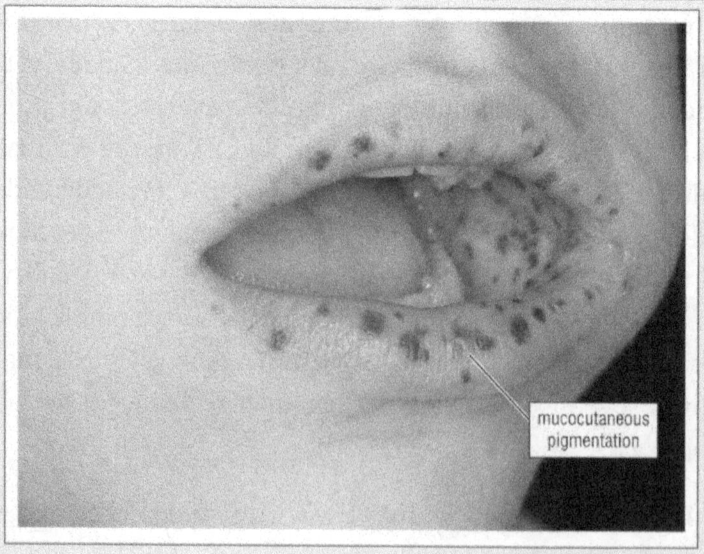


| Syndrome | Gene(s) | Key Extracolonic Feature |
|---|---|---|
| Lynch syndrome | MLH1, MSH2, MSH6, PMS2, EPCAM | Endometrial, ovarian, gastric cancer risk |
| Familial adenomatous polyposis | APC | Duodenal adenomas, desmoid tumors, osteomas |
| MUTYH-associated polyposis | MUTYH (biallelic) | Attenuated polyposis phenotype |

| | | |
|---|---|---|
| Peutz-Jeghers syndrome | STK11 | Mucocutaneous pigmentation, multi-organ cancer risk |
| Serrated polyposis syndrome | Largely unknown | Defined by quantitative serrated polyp burden |

**THE GI THRESHOLD DECISION SYSTEM — Colorectal Neoplasia Thresholds**

**Presentation Signature:** This chapter's threshold instances addressed matching screening modality and initiation age to personal and family risk, and recognizing when a colorectal cancer or polyp presentation warrants genetic evaluation.

**Threshold Point:** Family history and personal history define the screening initiation age and preferred modality; universal tumor testing criteria and specific red-flag features define the threshold for genetic counseling referral.

**The Call:** Both thresholds ensure that risk stratification, not a uniform default protocol, determines the intensity of screening and evaluation applied to each individual patient.

**Trap Logic:** Relying on family history alone without universal tumor testing, and failing to reassess family history at follow-up visits as it evolves over time, are this chapter's most consequential threshold misapplications.

**Decision Anchor:** Apply universal tumor testing to every new colorectal and endometrial cancer, reassess family history at relevant visits, and shift screening intensity upward whenever a qualifying risk factor or red-flag feature is identified rather than defaulting to average-risk protocols by omission.

## Summary and Key Concepts

Average-risk colorectal cancer screening begins at age 45 with colonoscopy or a stool-based alternative, while qualifying family history shifts both starting age and preferred modality toward earlier, colonoscopy-based screening.

Sessile serrated lesions carry malignant potential comparable to conventional adenomas and require accurate histologic distinction from low-risk hyperplastic polyps to assign appropriate surveillance intervals.

Universal tumor testing for mismatch repair deficiency, applied to every new colorectal and endometrial cancer regardless of family history, identifies Lynch syndrome cases that family history criteria alone would miss.

Familial adenomatous polyposis, MUTYH-associated polyposis, Peutz-Jeghers syndrome, and serrated polyposis syndrome each have distinguishing clinical and genetic features that determine surveillance intensity and extracolonic screening needs.

A hereditary or familial colorectal cancer risk pattern can be managed through phenotypic criteria alone even when genetic testing is negative or no causative gene has been identified, as with serrated polyposis syndrome.

Post-treatment colorectal cancer surveillance intensity is highest in the early years after treatment and de-escalates over time, and a rising CEA trend warrants further evaluation even without an imaging-confirmed recurrence.

# CHAPTER 12: ACUTE AND CHRONIC PANCREATITIS

## Learning Objectives

1. Apply diagnostic criteria for acute pancreatitis and identify its major etiologies.
2. Apply severity stratification tools to acute pancreatitis and select an appropriate initial fluid resuscitation, nutrition, and monitoring strategy.
3. Recognize and manage the local complications of acute pancreatitis, including necrosis, pseudocyst, and walled-off necrosis.
4. Evaluate and manage chronic pancreatitis, including pain, exocrine insufficiency, and endocrine insufficiency.
5. Distinguish autoimmune pancreatitis from other causes of pancreatic disease and apply an appropriate diagnostic and treatment approach.

## Chapter Outline

This chapter develops acute pancreatitis from diagnostic criteria through severity-stratified initial management and local complications, then addresses chronic pancreatitis, its pathophysiology, diagnostic evaluation, and the pain, exocrine, and endocrine management this progressive disease requires, and closes with autoimmune pancreatitis as a distinct, steroid-responsive entity requiring its own recognition pathway. Each section connects a specific severity or diagnostic threshold to a defined management pathway.

## Acute Pancreatitis

### Etiology and Diagnostic Criteria

Acute pancreatitis is diagnosed when at least two of three criteria are met: characteristic abdominal pain, typically epigastric with radiation to the back, lipase or amylase elevated at least three times the upper limit of normal, with lipase preferred given its longer diagnostic window and greater specificity for pancreatic injury, and characteristic findings on cross-sectional imaging, and this two-of-three framework matters clinically because it permits the diagnosis to be made confidently even when imaging has not yet been obtained, provided the clinical and biochemical criteria are both satisfied. Gallstones and alcohol together account for the substantial majority of cases, and the remaining etiologies, including hypertriglyceridemia, generally provoking pancreatitis only once triglyceride levels exceed a very high threshold, medications, a growing and often overlooked category given the wide range of implicated drug classes, post-endoscopic retrograde cholangiopancreatography pancreatitis discussed in the second chapter, and, in a meaningful minority of cases, no identifiable cause despite thorough evaluation, should each be systematically considered rather than assuming a gallstone or alcohol etiology by default in every patient. Amylase, while historically the more familiar test, rises and falls more rapidly than lipase and can be normal by the time a patient presents several days into a pancreatitis episode, which is why lipase alone is now generally sufficient and preferred, and ordering both tests together rarely adds diagnostic value beyond lipase alone. A thorough, structured search for an identifiable cause should always precede an idiopathic label, since true idiopathic disease should be a diagnosis of exclusion reached only after this systematic evaluation, not a default conclusion adopted whenever the initial history and basic testing do not immediately suggest an obvious etiology.

**Severity Assessment and Risk Stratification**

Severity stratification, performed within the first 24 to 48 hours of presentation, distinguishes mild pancreatitis, without organ failure or local complications, from moderately severe disease, with transient organ failure or local complications resolving within 48 hours, and severe disease, with persistent organ failure beyond 48 hours, and this classification carries direct implications for monitoring intensity, admission location, and the aggressiveness of the interventions discussed throughout this chapter. The bedside index for severity in acute pancreatitis, incorporating blood urea nitrogen, impaired mental status, systemic inflammatory response syndrome criteria, age, and pleural effusion, provides an early, simple risk stratification tool calculable at admission before the full 48-hour severity picture has developed, and a score of three or more identifies patients at substantially increased risk of mortality who warrant closer monitoring, ideally in a higher level of care setting, from the time of admission rather than only after clinical deterioration has already occurred. Reassessing severity classification at multiple points during the admission, rather than assigning a single classification at presentation and never revisiting it, captures patients who evolve from mild to moderately severe or severe disease over the following days, a trajectory that a single, static initial assessment would miss entirely. Calculating this score should become a routine, automatic part of admission order entry rather than an optional additional step performed inconsistently depending on clinician habit or time pressure at the point of admission.

**Initial Management: Fluid Resuscitation, Nutrition, and Pain Control**

Goal-directed intravenous fluid resuscitation, using a balanced crystalloid solution rather than normal saline given evidence of reduced hyperchloremic acidosis and, in some studies, reduced systemic inflammatory response with balanced solutions, is the cornerstone of early management, and resuscitation adequacy should be assessed against specific, objective targets, including urine output, heart rate, and hematocrit trend, rather than a fixed volume prescribed uniformly regardless of the individual patient's response, since both inadequate resuscitation, worsening pancreatic microcirculatory injury, and excessive resuscitation, contributing to abdominal compartment syndrome and pulmonary complications, carry meaningful risk. Early oral or enteral nutrition, initiated within 24 to 72 hours in patients able to tolerate it rather than the traditional practice of prolonged bowel rest, is now standard practice given evidence that early feeding reduces infectious complications and length of stay by maintaining gut mucosal integrity and limiting bacterial translocation, and this represents a significant evolution from older management paradigms that patients or family members who have witnessed a prior pancreatitis admission may not be aware has changed, making explicit communication about this updated approach a useful part of admission counseling. Serial hematocrit and blood urea nitrogen trends, checked at defined intervals during the first

24 to 48 hours, provide objective feedback on resuscitation adequacy that should guide ongoing fluid rate adjustment rather than continuing a fixed initial rate unchanged throughout the resuscitation period regardless of the patient's actual physiologic response.

**THE GI THRESHOLD DECISION SYSTEM — Pancreatic Thresholds — Severity-Stratified Monitoring and Resuscitation Intensity**

---

**Presentation Signature:** A patient is admitted with acute pancreatitis, and the clinician must determine the appropriate monitoring level and resuscitation intensity at admission before the full 48-hour severity picture has developed.

**Threshold Point:** A bedside index for severity in acute pancreatitis score of three or more, or the presence of any organ dysfunction at presentation, defines the threshold for higher-acuity monitoring, ideally in an intensive or step-down care setting, and for more frequent reassessment of fluid resuscitation adequacy than standard ward-level monitoring would provide.

**The Call:** Patients below this threshold are managed with standard ward-level monitoring and goal-directed resuscitation; patients meeting or exceeding this threshold are triaged to higher-acuity monitoring with more frequent vital sign and laboratory reassessment, recognizing that early identification of evolving organ dysfunction changes outcomes more than intervention initiated only after overt organ failure has developed.

**Trap Logic:** Waiting for the full 48-hour severity classification to determine monitoring level delays the higher-acuity triage that an early risk score can already suggest is warranted, since early, simple risk tools exist specifically to identify high-risk patients before the more complete severity picture has fully developed.

**Decision Anchor:** Calculate an early severity risk score at admission, before the 48-hour window has elapsed, and triage monitoring intensity accordingly rather than waiting for organ failure to become clinically apparent before escalating the level of care.

### Local Complications: Necrosis, Pseudocyst, and Walled-Off Necrosis

Pancreatic necrosis, identified on contrast-enhanced cross-sectional imaging as non-enhancing pancreatic or peripancreatic tissue, is classified as sterile or infected, and this distinction carries substantial management implications, since infected necrosis, suspected when a patient with necrosis develops new or persistent fever, leukocytosis, or clinical deterioration beyond the expected recovery trajectory, generally requires intervention, while sterile necrosis, even when extensive, can often be managed conservatively with continued supportive care, deferring intervention unless a specific indication develops. Fine-needle aspiration for culture, once used routinely to confirm infected necrosis, has been largely supplanted by clinical judgment and the presence of gas within the necrotic collection on imaging, a finding essentially diagnostic of infection given that gas-forming organisms rarely arise from any process other than infection in this specific anatomic context, reducing the need for an invasive diagnostic procedure that itself carries infection-introduction risk. Pancreatic pseudocyst, a fluid collection with a defined wall developing after four or more weeks, and walled-off necrosis, a similarly matured collection but containing solid necrotic debris rather than purely fluid contents, are distinguished by their contents on imaging, and this distinction directly determines drainage technique, since walled-off necrosis requires an approach capable of removing solid debris, most commonly endoscopic transmural drainage with direct endoscopic necrosectomy performed through the same access route, while a purely fluid pseudocyst can be adequately managed with simple drainage alone. Timing of imaging matters as well, since contrast-enhanced CT obtained too early in the disease course, generally within the first 48 to 72 hours, can understate the eventual extent of necrosis before it has fully demarcated, meaning that a repeat study later in the clinical course, rather than relying solely on an early scan, provides a more accurate assessment when necrosis is genuinely suspected clinically despite an initially reassuring early study. When aspiration is still performed in genuinely ambiguous cases, obtaining the sample under image guidance with appropriate antibiotic coverage minimizes the risk of introducing infection into a previously sterile collection during the procedure itself. Asymptomatic pseudocysts and walled-off necrosis collections, even when large, do not automatically require intervention, and the decision to drain should be driven by symptoms, infection, or growth on serial imaging rather than size alone, echoing the symptom-driven intervention threshold already applied throughout this book to other incidentally discovered findings. Safety first, always. Patience prevents unneeded risk.

**Figure 12.2:** Endoscopic Transmural Drainage of Walled-Off Necrosis

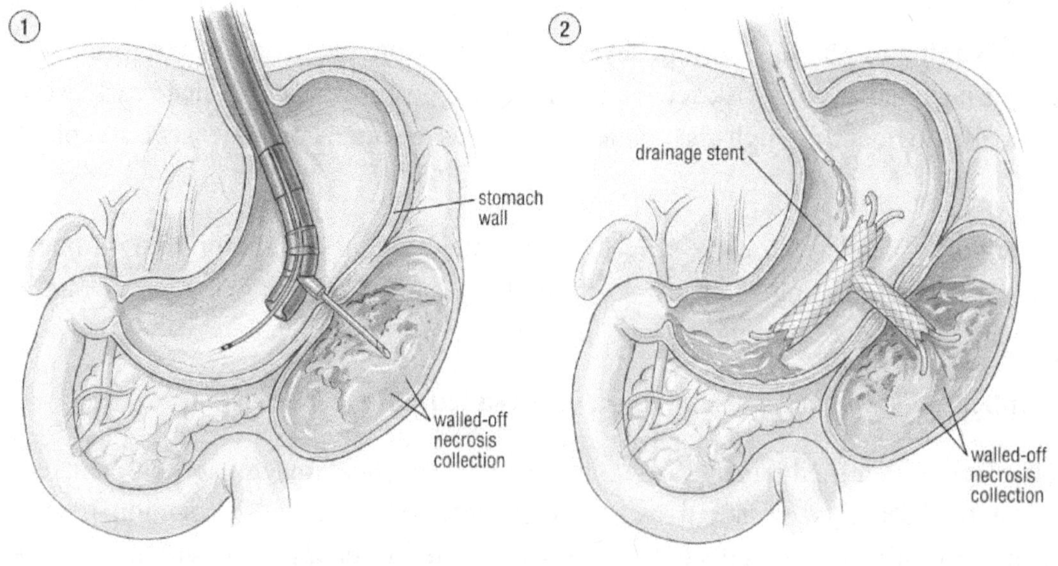


## Gallstone Pancreatitis: Timing of Cholecystectomy

Cholecystectomy during the index admission for mild gallstone pancreatitis, rather than the traditional practice of delaying surgery for several weeks after the pancreatitis has resolved, reduces the risk of recurrent biliary events, including recurrent pancreatitis, cholecystitis, and biliary colic, that occur during a delayed interval, and current guidance supports same-admission cholecystectomy once the patient has clinically recovered from the acute pancreatitis episode, reserving delayed cholecystectomy specifically for patients with more severe disease or significant local complications where the surgical risk of proceeding during the same admission outweighs the benefit of avoiding a delayed-interval recurrent event. Endoscopic retrograde cholangiopancreatography with sphincterotomy is reserved for gallstone pancreatitis complicated by concurrent cholangitis or persistent biliary obstruction, applying the same ERCP indication reasoning developed in the second chapter, rather than performed routinely in every gallstone pancreatitis admission regardless of whether obstruction persists, since the procedure carries its own complication risk that is not justified once the inciting stone has passed spontaneously, as occurs in a substantial proportion of gallstone pancreatitis cases. Coordinating this same-admission surgical timing explicitly with the surgical team at the point of pancreatitis diagnosis, rather than waiting until clinical resolution to initiate this conversation, prevents an avoidable delay in surgical scheduling that could otherwise result in a missed same-admission opportunity and an unnecessary readmission for a recurrent biliary event. In practice, distinguishing a passed stone from one still lodged in the distal duct can be genuinely difficult without direct imaging, and MRCP or endoscopic ultrasound, rather than clinical improvement alone, provides more reliable confirmation before deciding that ERCP is unnecessary in a borderline case.

## Chronic Pancreatitis

### Etiology and Pathophysiology

Chronic pancreatitis results from recurrent or sustained pancreatic injury producing irreversible fibrosis, glandular atrophy, and progressive exocrine and endocrine insufficiency, and alcohol use, generally requiring heavy, sustained consumption over years, remains the most commonly identified etiology, though a substantial proportion of cases involve genetic susceptibility, including pathogenic variants in genes such as PRSS1, SPINK1, and CFTR, that lower the threshold for pancreatic injury from a given degree of alcohol exposure or, in some patients, produce chronic pancreatitis in the absence of significant alcohol use altogether. Recurrent acute pancreatitis, whether from gallstones, alcohol, or another cause, can itself progress to chronic pancreatitis through cumulative, repeated injury, meaning that recurrent acute pancreatitis episodes should prompt evaluation for an underlying, correctable predisposing factor and genuine counseling about the risk of eventual progression to irreversible chronic disease, rather than each episode being managed in isolation without addressing this cumulative risk explicitly with the patient. Smoking, independent of alcohol use, is an established, additive risk factor for chronic pancreatitis progression, and this specific point is worth communicating clearly to patients, since smoking cessation counseling is sometimes deprioritized in this population relative to alcohol cessation despite carrying its own substantial, independent benefit for slowing disease progression. Family history of pancreatitis, unexplained recurrent episodes at a young age, or a personal history suggestive of cystic fibrosis-related disease should each independently prompt consideration of an underlying genetic evaluation even in a patient who also has a plausible acquired risk factor such as modest alcohol use, since more than one contributing factor can coexist. Framing each recurrent episode as a data point contributing to a cumulative injury narrative, rather than a fully independent event unrelated to prior episodes, helps both clinician and patient appreciate the stakes of ongoing risk factor modification over time.

Figure 12.3: Chronic Pancreatitis: Ductal Changes on MRCP

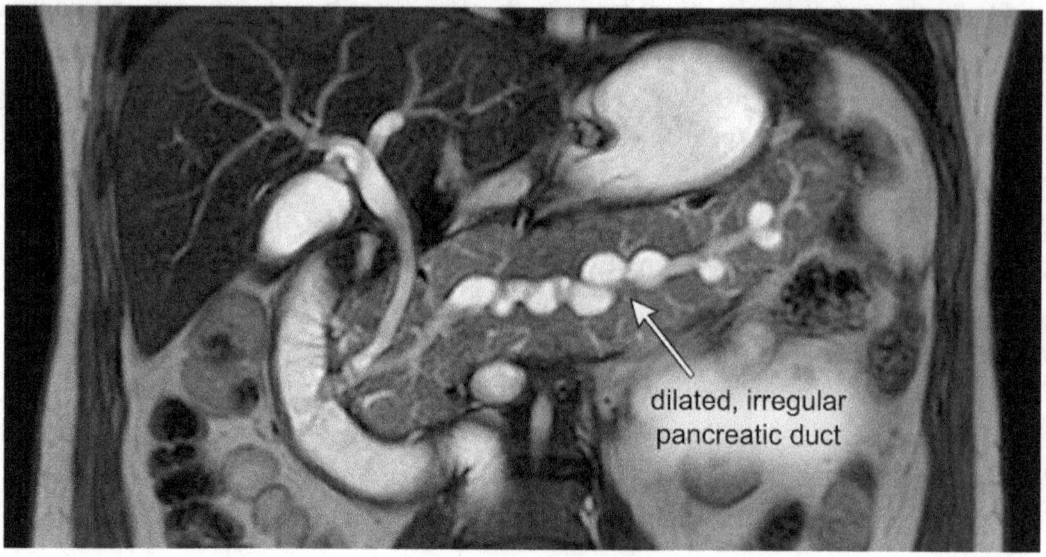


**Diagnostic Evaluation**

Cross-sectional imaging, most commonly CT or MRI with MRCP, identifies the characteristic findings of established chronic pancreatitis, including pancreatic ductal dilation and irregularity, parenchymal calcification, and glandular atrophy, and these findings are generally sufficient to confirm the diagnosis in a patient with a compatible clinical history without requiring more invasive testing. Endoscopic ultrasound, introduced in the second chapter, provides superior detection of the early, subtle parenchymal and ductal changes that precede the more advanced findings visible on standard cross-sectional imaging, and it is particularly valuable in a patient with a compatible clinical presentation and risk factors but nondiagnostic standard imaging, where its higher sensitivity for early disease can confirm a diagnosis that would otherwise remain uncertain. Fecal elastase, introduced in the seventh chapter as a screen for pancreatic exocrine insufficiency, should be checked in any patient with confirmed or suspected chronic pancreatitis given the high prevalence of exocrine insufficiency in this population, and a low value confirms the need for pancreatic enzyme replacement therapy discussed later in this section. Secretin-enhanced MRCP, administering secretin to stimulate pancreatic fluid secretion during the MRI examination, improves visualization of ductal architecture and can also provide a functional estimate of exocrine reserve, offering additional diagnostic information beyond standard MRCP alone in select equivocal cases. Interobserver variability in interpreting these subtle early endoscopic ultrasound findings has been a recognized limitation, and standardized criteria, developed and refined over recent years, have improved diagnostic consistency across different examiners and centers. Reassessment over time is reasonable as exocrine function can decline further as the disease progresses. This consistency benefits patients across sites.

## Pain Management

Chronic pancreatitis pain management follows a stepwise approach, beginning with lifestyle modification, most importantly alcohol and tobacco cessation given both substances' independent contributions to ongoing pancreatic injury and pain, and non-opioid analgesics, before escalating to neuromodulator therapy targeting the same central pain sensitization mechanism discussed in earlier chapters for other chronic visceral pain conditions, reflecting the recognition that chronic pancreatitis pain, like the functional pain syndromes discussed in the tenth chapter, often involves a central sensitization component that persists even when peripheral pancreatic inflammation has stabilized. Endoscopic or surgical intervention, including pancreatic duct stenting or drainage procedures for a dominant, obstructing stricture or stone, and, in appropriately selected patients with diffuse, small-duct disease not amenable to duct-directed intervention, total pancreatectomy with islet autotransplantation, preserving endocrine function by reimplanting the patient's own islet cells while removing the diseased, painful gland, are reserved for patients with severe, refractory pain despite optimized medical management, and this treatment escalation should be pursued at a center with specific expertise in these complex interventions given their technical demands and the careful patient selection they require. Referral to a chronic pain specialist or multidisciplinary pain program is a reasonable adjunct at any point in this stepwise sequence, not only after every other option has been exhausted, given the substantial overlap between chronic pancreatitis pain and the central sensitization mechanisms that specialized pain management expertise is specifically trained to address. Preoperative counseling for total pancreatectomy with islet autotransplantation should explicitly address the certainty of resulting exocrine insufficiency requiring lifelong enzyme replacement, and the variable degree of residual endocrine function achieved, since autotransplantation reduces but does not always eliminate subsequent diabetes risk. Careful counseling prevents later regret.

## Exocrine and Endocrine Insufficiency Management

Pancreatic enzyme replacement therapy, dosed with meals and confirmed against current dosing guidance based on meal fat content and patient response, is the primary treatment for exocrine insufficiency, and inadequate response to an apparently appropriate dose should prompt evaluation for concurrent small intestinal bacterial overgrowth, applying the reasoning developed in the eighth chapter, since impaired pancreatic secretion itself, including reduced bicarbonate output that would otherwise help maintain a duodenal pH unfavorable to bacterial overgrowth, is a recognized risk factor for this specific complicating condition. Endocrine insufficiency, producing a distinct form of diabetes termed pancreatogenic or type 3c diabetes, differs from typical type 1 or type 2 diabetes in its combined loss of both insulin and glucagon secretion, producing a pattern of glycemic lability and a higher hypoglycemia risk than typical type 2 diabetes management would predict, and this distinction should be communicated explicitly to any endocrinology or primary care colleague co-managing the patient's diabetes, since a standard type 2 diabetes management approach applied without this specific pancreatogenic context can produce more hypoglycemic events than expected. Concurrent acid suppression is sometimes added when enzyme response remains suboptimal despite adequate dosing and confirmed exclusion of bacterial overgrowth, since an excessively acidic duodenal environment can inactivate pancreatic enzymes before they have adequate opportunity to act on ingested food, representing a third mechanistic explanation for inadequate response beyond simple underdosing or coexisting bacterial overgrowth. Referral to an endocrinologist with specific familiarity with pancreatogenic diabetes, rather than management under a standard type 2 diabetes protocol alone, is reasonable once this diagnosis is confirmed, given the meaningfully different glycemic management approach this population often requires. This coordination reduces avoidable hypoglycemic episodes. Every detail counts here.

**THE GI THRESHOLD DECISION SYSTEM — Pancreatic Thresholds — Escalating Chronic Pancreatitis Pain Management**

**Presentation Signature:** A patient with confirmed chronic pancreatitis has ongoing pain despite lifestyle modification and initial non-opioid analgesic therapy, and the clinician must determine whether further medical management, endoscopic intervention, or surgical referral is appropriate.

**Threshold Point:** Persistent, functionally limiting pain despite optimized medical therapy, particularly in the presence of a dominant, imageable ductal stricture or stone, defines the threshold for endoscopic or surgical intervention rather than continued escalation of medical pain management alone.

**The Call:** Patients with a dominant, correctable ductal obstruction are referred for endoscopic or surgical duct-directed intervention; patients with diffuse, small-duct disease without a correctable target lesion are considered for total pancreatectomy with islet autotransplantation at an experienced center once medical management has been genuinely optimized and exhausted.

**Trap Logic:** Escalating opioid therapy indefinitely in a patient with a correctable ductal obstruction, rather than pursuing duct-directed intervention, both fails to address the underlying mechanical cause and risks the same narcotic bowel syndrome pattern discussed in the tenth chapter.

**Decision Anchor:** Image the pancreatic duct specifically to identify a correctable, dominant lesion before escalating medical pain management indefinitely, and refer to an experienced center for islet autotransplantation consideration once medical therapy is genuinely exhausted in diffuse, small-duct disease.

## Hypertriglyceridemia-Induced and Other Metabolic Pancreatitis

Hypertriglyceridemia-induced pancreatitis, generally occurring only once triglyceride levels substantially exceed a very high threshold, requires acute management targeting rapid triglyceride reduction, including insulin infusion, which activates lipoprotein lipase and accelerates triglyceride clearance independent of any coexisting hyperglycemia, and, in the most severe cases, apheresis to physically remove triglyceride-rich lipoproteins from the circulation when insulin-based management alone is insufficient or when the severity of presentation warrants more rapid intervention. Long-term management of the underlying hypertriglyceridemia, including dietary fat restriction, weight management, glycemic control in patients with underlying diabetes, and pharmacologic triglyceride-lowering therapy, is essential to prevent recurrence, and genetic testing for a primary lipid disorder is reasonable in a patient with recurrent severe hypertriglyceridemia-induced pancreatitis or triglyceride levels disproportionate to identifiable secondary causes such as poorly controlled diabetes or alcohol use. A rapid downward trend in triglyceride levels over the first 24 to 48 hours, rather than a single threshold value that must be reached before treatment can be considered successful, is the practical target guiding when insulin infusion or apheresis can be discontinued in favor of the longer-term management strategies discussed below. Coordinating this apheresis decision with a lipid specialist or intensivist experienced in the technique ensures it is deployed appropriately given its resource intensity and the more selective indication it carries relative to insulin infusion alone. Referral to a lipid clinic, where available, provides more specialized, sustained long-term management than a general primary care approach alone can typically offer for this often complex, multifactorial condition. Small margins matter clinically.

### Hypercalcemia and Other Metabolic Causes

Hypercalcemia, most commonly from primary hyperparathyroidism, is a less common but recognized cause of acute pancreatitis, thought to act through calcium-mediated premature activation of pancreatic proteolytic enzymes within the gland itself, and identifying and treating the underlying cause of hypercalcemia, in addition to managing the acute pancreatitis episode itself, prevents recurrence in a way that symptomatic pancreatitis management alone would not achieve; a calcium level should be included in the standard initial laboratory evaluation of any patient with new acute pancreatitis specifically to screen for this treatable, recurrence-preventable etiology. Once the acute hypercalcemia has been corrected and the acute pancreatitis episode has resolved, referral for definitive management of the underlying hyperparathyroidism, typically parathyroidectomy in appropriately selected patients, should be pursued rather than treating the hypercalcemia as an isolated acute finding without addressing its underlying cause. A calcium level, checked routinely alongside triglycerides in the standard initial pancreatitis panel, catches this treatable cause even when it is not the clinician's leading initial suspicion based on the presenting history alone. Simple tests, real value.

## Nutritional Support Strategy in Severe Acute Pancreatitis

While early oral or enteral feeding is preferred whenever tolerated, as established earlier in this chapter, a subset of patients with severe pancreatitis, significant ileus, or intolerance of oral or gastric feeding require a more structured nutritional support approach, and nasojejunal feeding, bypassing the stomach and reducing pancreatic stimulation relative to gastric or oral feeding, was historically favored in this population, though more recent evidence suggests nasogastric feeding is often equally well tolerated and avoids the additional procedural step of jejunal tube placement, making nasogastric feeding a reasonable first attempt in most patients requiring enteral access, with nasojejunal feeding reserved for patients who do not tolerate the gastric route. Parenteral nutrition is reserved for patients who cannot tolerate any enteral feeding despite appropriate attempts, since enteral feeding, even in small amounts, provides the gut mucosal integrity and bacterial translocation benefits discussed earlier in this chapter that parenteral nutrition alone cannot replicate, and this hierarchy, enteral preferred over parenteral whenever feasible, mirrors the same general nutritional support principle already established in earlier chapters for short bowel syndrome and inflammatory bowel disease. The specific choice between nasogastric and nasojejunal access should also account for local institutional expertise and the availability of fluoroscopic or endoscopic placement resources, since a delay in obtaining jejunal access purely for a theoretical benefit can itself delay the initiation of nutrition that early feeding is specifically intended to achieve promptly. Even a small volume of trophic enteral feeding administered alongside parenteral nutrition, when full enteral tolerance is not yet achievable, provides some of this gut-protective benefit and should be attempted whenever any degree of enteral tolerance exists.

### Reintroducing Oral Diet After an Acute Episode

Diet advancement after an acute pancreatitis episode, once the patient is clinically improving and pain is adequately controlled, can generally proceed directly to a low-fat solid diet rather than the traditional stepwise progression through clear liquids and gradually advancing consistency, since evidence supports that this traditional cautious approach does not improve outcomes and unnecessarily prolongs hospitalization, reflecting the same evidence-based departure from historical practice already discussed for early feeding initiation more broadly in this chapter. Educating both patients and other clinical staff about this updated, evidence-based diet advancement pathway helps overcome the institutional inertia that older, more cautious practices can otherwise perpetuate simply through habit and unfamiliarity with the more recent evidence. Discharge instructions summarizing this diet plan in writing, alongside the general recovery expectations, prevent confusion when a patient tries to reconcile current advice with outdated information they may have encountered elsewhere.

## Recurrent Acute Pancreatitis and Idiopathic Disease Evaluation

Recurrent acute pancreatitis, defined as two or more discrete episodes with symptom resolution between episodes, warrants a more thorough etiologic evaluation than a single, isolated episode, particularly when the initial standard workup, including triglycerides, calcium, and a careful medication and alcohol history, has not identified a clear cause, and this evaluation should include endoscopic ultrasound to assess for occult microlithiasis or biliary sludge not visible on transabdominal ultrasound, subtle chronic pancreatitis changes as discussed later in this chapter, or a small pancreatic mass or intraductal papillary mucinous neoplasm, discussed in the following chapter, that might not otherwise be apparent. Genetic testing for the hereditary pancreatitis-associated genes mentioned earlier in this chapter is reasonable in a patient with recurrent idiopathic pancreatitis, particularly with a younger age of onset or a family history of pancreatitis or pancreatic cancer, since confirmed hereditary pancreatitis carries both management implications for the patient's own care and family counseling and screening implications given the substantially elevated pancreatic cancer risk associated with certain hereditary pancreatitis genes over a patient's lifetime. A dedicated, structured re-evaluation visit specifically for this purpose, rather than addressing the recurrent-pancreatitis workup piecemeal across multiple unrelated appointments, ensures the full etiologic evaluation is completed systematically rather than left incomplete. Thoroughness here pays dividends later.

### Sphincter of Oddi Dysfunction as a Consideration

Sphincter of Oddi dysfunction, a functional disorder of the biliary and pancreatic sphincter complex, is a controversial and diminishingly invoked explanation for recurrent idiopathic pancreatitis or biliary-type pain after cholecystectomy, and current evidence has substantially narrowed the population in whom empiric sphincterotomy is considered beneficial, given data showing that empiric intervention in patients without objective biliary or pancreatic ductal abnormality does not reliably improve outcomes and carries meaningful procedural risk; this diagnosis should therefore be considered cautiously and only after more common and better-established causes of recurrent pancreatitis have been genuinely excluded, rather than invoked as a default explanation once other causes are not readily identified. Referral to a center with specific expertise in this controversial area, rather than proceeding directly to empiric sphincterotomy in a general practice setting, supports the more cautious, evidence-based evaluation this diagnosis now warrants. Patients who have heard of this diagnosis from other sources should be counseled honestly about the evolving and now more cautious evidence base, rather than either dismissed or offered intervention without this context. Context matters most.

## Psychosocial Burden and Alcohol Use Disorder Management in Pancreatitis

Chronic pancreatitis, and recurrent acute pancreatitis, carry substantial psychosocial burden, including chronic pain-related disability, dietary restriction, and, particularly in alcohol-related disease, the layered burden of managing both a chronic physical illness and an underlying substance use disorder simultaneously, and screening for anxiety, depression, and alcohol use disorder using validated instruments, applying the routine mental health and substance use screening standard already established throughout this book, should be integrated into ongoing pancreatitis care rather than addressed only reactively when a crisis prompts the conversation. A nonjudgmental, direct approach to alcohol use discussion, applying the same communication principle developed in the first chapter, is particularly important in this population, since the stigma surrounding alcohol-related pancreatitis can itself become a barrier to patients seeking care or disclosing ongoing use, and framing the conversation around shared goals, reducing pain and preventing further pancreatic injury, rather than around judgment, supports more productive engagement with both alcohol treatment resources and ongoing pancreatitis management. Integrating this screening into a routine template used at every follow-up visit, rather than relying on memory to raise it periodically, makes consistent screening more achievable across a busy practice managing many other clinical priorities simultaneously. Training clinical staff broadly in this communication approach, rather than assuming it comes naturally without deliberate practice, improves consistency across an entire care team managing this vulnerable patient population. People, not just diseases.

### Integrated Care for Alcohol-Related Pancreatitis

Referral to addiction medicine or a structured alcohol treatment program should be offered proactively to every patient with alcohol-related pancreatitis, rather than only to patients who explicitly request this support, given that alcohol cessation is the single most impactful intervention available for preventing further episodes and slowing progression to chronic disease in this population, and coordinating this referral at the time of an acute admission, when motivation for change may be highest, rather than deferring the conversation to a later outpatient visit, takes advantage of this window of opportunity that may not remain open indefinitely. Following up on whether the patient actually attended a referred program, rather than considering the referral itself as thc completed task, closes the loop on this intervention and allows for adjustment if barriers to attendance are identified. Small, consistent efforts add up over a long-term relationship.

## Pancreatitis in Pregnancy and Pediatric Patients

Acute pancreatitis in pregnancy, most commonly gallstone-related given the increased biliary sludge and stone formation that pregnancy's hormonal and mechanical changes promote, requires the same diagnostic and severity-stratification approach developed throughout this chapter, adapted with the imaging and medication safety considerations already established in earlier chapters for other conditions in pregnancy; endoscopic ultrasound and MRI without gadolinium are preferred over CT when advanced imaging is needed, and endoscopic retrograde cholangiopancreatography, when a clear indication such as choledocholithiasis or cholangitis exists, is performed with the same fluoroscopy-minimization and shielding precautions discussed in the second chapter, since the risks of untreated biliary obstruction or infection generally outweigh the radiation exposure risk when the procedure is genuinely indicated. Delivery timing and mode are generally not altered by an episode of pancreatitis alone in the absence of other obstetric indications, and close coordination between gastroenterology and maternal-fetal medicine throughout the pregnancy, applying the same coordinated care principle emphasized in earlier chapters, supports management decisions that account for both maternal and fetal considerations simultaneously. Anesthesia consultation, when a procedure requiring sedation is planned during pregnancy, should specifically address the physiologic changes of pregnancy relevant to sedation safety, applying the same collaborative, condition-specific planning already emphasized for other procedures performed during pregnancy in earlier chapters of this book. Patient anxiety about fetal safety during any needed procedure is common and understandable, and directly addressing this concern with clear, specific information about the precautions taken supports informed, less anxious decision-making. Reassurance helps outcomes.

### Pediatric Pancreatitis Considerations

Pediatric acute pancreatitis, while less common than adult disease, has risen in reported incidence in recent years, and its etiology differs somewhat from the adult pattern, with biliary disease, systemic illness, trauma, and medications representing more prominent causes relative to the alcohol-predominant pattern seen in many adult populations, and genetic and structural causes, including pancreas divisum and the hereditary pancreatitis genes discussed earlier in this chapter, are considered more readily in a child or adolescent with recurrent pancreatitis given the lower baseline prevalence of the acquired risk factors, alcohol and typical adult-onset gallstone disease, that dominate the adult differential. Coordination with pediatric gastroenterology, where the pediatric patient's care is not already being managed by a specialist in that field, ensures age-appropriate diagnostic and treatment approaches are applied rather than a direct, unmodified extrapolation of adult management protocols to a substantially different patient population. Family-centered communication, engaging both the pediatric patient at an age-appropriate level and their caregivers, differs meaningfully from the adult-patient communication approach used throughout the rest of this chapter. Age-appropriate care matters most.

## Pancreas Divisum and Other Congenital Ductal Anomalies

Pancreas divisum, the most common congenital pancreatic ductal anomaly, results from incomplete fusion of the dorsal and ventral pancreatic duct systems during embryologic development, and the resulting predominant drainage of the pancreatic gland through the smaller minor papilla, rather than the main ampulla, is thought to predispose to recurrent pancreatitis in a subset of affected individuals through relative outflow obstruction at this narrower drainage route, though the majority of individuals with this common anatomic variant, present in a meaningful proportion of the general population, remain entirely asymptomatic throughout their lives. Endoscopic minor papilla sphincterotomy, facilitating drainage through the smaller papilla, is considered in patients with recurrent pancreatitis and confirmed pancreas divisum once other causes have been excluded, though patient selection for this intervention should be careful and individualized, given that the anatomic variant's high prevalence in asymptomatic individuals means the finding alone, without a compelling clinical correlation, does not necessarily explain a given patient's pancreatitis and does not automatically warrant intervention. Discussing this uncertain causal relationship candidly with patients, rather than presenting the anatomic finding as a definitive explanation for their symptoms, supports realistic expectations about the likelihood that intervention directed at the finding will actually resolve their recurrent pancreatitis episodes. Population-level prevalence data for this variant should be shared with anxious patients who discover the finding incidentally, to contextualize how common and usually benign it is.

### Annular Pancreas and Other Rare Anomalies

Annular pancreas, in which pancreatic tissue encircles the duodenum, can present with duodenal obstruction in infancy or, less commonly, with recurrent pancreatitis or obstructive symptoms first recognized in adulthood, and its recognition on cross-sectional imaging should prompt consideration as a contributing factor in a patient with otherwise unexplained recurrent pancreatitis or duodenal obstruction, though, similar to pancreas divisum, its presence alone does not always indicate causation and clinical correlation remains essential before attributing a patient's symptoms definitively to this anatomic finding. Surgical bypass is generally reserved for cases with clear, symptomatic duodenal obstruction rather than pursued for an incidentally identified anomaly without a corresponding clinical picture that the anomaly plausibly explains. This same caution against overattribution applies broadly whenever an incidental anatomic variant is discovered in the course of an unrelated evaluation.

## Autoimmune Pancreatitis

### Type 1 and Type 2 Distinction and Diagnosis

Autoimmune pancreatitis, an uncommon but important and highly treatable cause of pancreatic disease, presents in two histologically and clinically distinct subtypes: type 1, associated with elevated serum IgG4 and frequently accompanied by other IgG4-related disease manifestations affecting the bile duct, salivary glands, kidneys, or retroperitoneum, and type 2, which lacks the IgG4 association but is more strongly linked to coexisting inflammatory bowel disease, and this distinction matters because type 1 disease has a higher relapse rate after treatment and warrants closer long-term follow-up than type 2 disease. Autoimmune pancreatitis characteristically presents with painless obstructive jaundice and a pancreatic mass on imaging that closely mimics pancreatic adenocarcinoma, making this distinction one of the most consequential in pancreatic disease, since a missed diagnosis of autoimmune pancreatitis can lead to unnecessary pancreatic resection for presumed malignancy, while a missed diagnosis of actual malignancy misattributed to autoimmune pancreatitis delays essential cancer treatment; diagnosis integrates imaging characteristics, serum IgG4 level, other organ involvement, and, where the diagnosis remains uncertain, tissue biopsy demonstrating the characteristic histologic pattern, and a dramatic, rapid response to a corticosteroid trial, while sometimes used as a supportive diagnostic clue, should never substitute for adequate diagnostic certainty before excluding malignancy definitively, given the serious consequences of missing a genuine cancer diagnosis. Both subtypes respond well to corticosteroid induction therapy, generally achieving rapid clinical, biochemical, and radiographic improvement within weeks, a response pattern distinct enough from typical pancreatic malignancy behavior that it can itself, though cautiously, support the diagnosis retrospectively once malignancy has already been reasonably excluded through the diagnostic evaluation described above. Multidisciplinary review, involving gastroenterology, radiology, and pathology together when the diagnosis is genuinely uncertain, applies the same tumor-board-style collaborative decision-making already established in the previous chapter for colorectal cancer, and this approach is particularly valuable given the serious consequences of an incorrect diagnosis in either direction. Long-term follow-up after successful treatment should specifically monitor for relapse, particularly in type 1 disease and its associated IgG4-related organ involvement, since relapse, when it occurs, may involve a different organ system than the initial presentation. Vigilance protects patients long-term.

Case Presentation: A 52-year-old man with known gallstones presents with severe epigastric pain radiating to the back, and lipase returns at eight times the upper limit of normal, confirming acute pancreatitis. His bedside index for severity in acute pancreatitis score is 4, and he is admitted to a step-down monitoring unit per the threshold developed in this chapter. Over the following 72 hours he develops persistent fever and clinical deterioration despite adequate fluid resuscitation, and contrast-enhanced CT demonstrates extensive pancreatic necrosis with gas locules within the collection. Applying the reasoning developed in this chapter, the presence of gas within the necrotic collection is essentially diagnostic of infected necrosis without requiring fine-needle aspiration for confirmation, and broad-spectrum antibiotics are initiated with interventional radiology and advanced endoscopy consulted for eventual drainage once the collection has matured sufficiently for a minimally invasive approach, following a step-up strategy that defers the most invasive intervention until less invasive options have been attempted. He undergoes endoscopic transmural drainage with direct endoscopic necrosectomy several weeks later once the collection has walled off adequately, with clinical improvement following the procedure. Once recovered, he undergoes cholecystectomy during the same overall hospitalization course rather than a delayed interval, per the gallstone pancreatitis timing principle developed in this chapter. This case illustrates the integrated application of this chapter's thresholds: early severity risk stratification determined his monitoring level, imaging findings determined the infected-necrosis diagnosis without invasive testing, and same-admission cholecystectomy addressed his underlying gallstone etiology definitively.

Case Presentation: A 58-year-old woman with a 20-year history of heavy alcohol use presents with recurrent epigastric pain, unintentional 15-pound weight loss, and greasy, foul-smelling stools. CT demonstrates pancreatic calcifications and ductal dilation consistent with chronic pancreatitis. Fecal elastase returns markedly low, confirming exocrine insufficiency. Applying the reasoning developed in this chapter, pancreatic enzyme replacement therapy is initiated at an appropriate weight-based starting dose with meals, alongside counseling on alcohol cessation given its role in both ongoing pancreatic injury and pain. At follow-up eight weeks later, her steatorrhea has improved only partially despite confirmed medication adherence and appropriate dosing technique. Rather than simply escalating the enzyme replacement dose further, small intestinal bacterial overgrowth is considered given the reasoning developed in this chapter connecting impaired pancreatic bicarbonate secretion to bacterial overgrowth risk, and glucose breath testing confirms this diagnosis. She is treated with rifaximin, and her steatorrhea improves substantially on the existing enzyme replacement dose once the coexisting bacterial overgrowth is addressed. This case illustrates why inadequate response to appropriately dosed pancreatic enzyme replacement therapy should prompt evaluation for this specific, mechanistically linked coexisting condition rather than escalating enzyme dosing indefinitely.

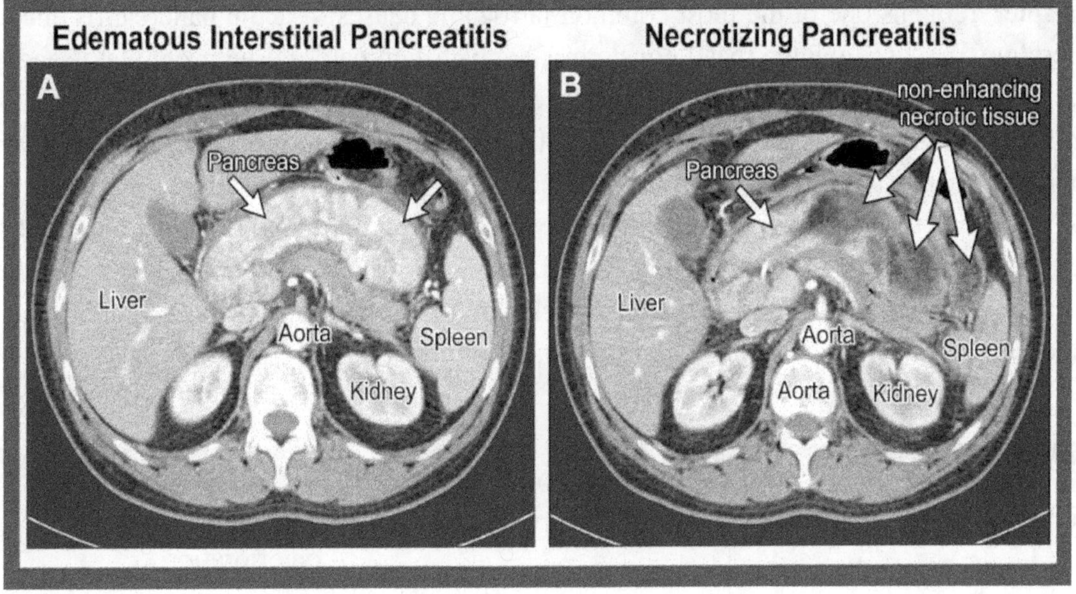

Figure 12.1: CT Findings in Acute Pancreatitis: Edematous vs Necrotizing

## Drug-Induced Pancreatitis and Post-ERCP Prophylaxis

Drug-induced pancreatitis is likely underrecognized given the wide range of implicated medications, including certain diuretics, antiretroviral agents, immunosuppressants used in inflammatory bowel disease treatment discussed in the ninth chapter, and several diabetes medications, and establishing this diagnosis requires a temporal relationship between medication initiation and symptom onset, exclusion of the more common gallstone and alcohol etiologies, and, ideally, resolution with medication discontinuation and, where rechallenge would be clinically informative and safe, recurrence with reintroduction, though rechallenge is rarely pursued deliberately given the unnecessary risk it would impose. A structured medication timeline, reviewed specifically for any drug started within the preceding weeks to months before the pancreatitis episode, applying the same systematic medication-history discipline emphasized throughout this book, is a more reliable approach to identifying a drug-induced cause than relying on spontaneous patient recall of recent medication changes. Reporting a suspected drug-induced pancreatitis case to the relevant pharmacovigilance system, where such systems exist, contributes to the broader evidence base that individual case reports, accumulated over time, have historically provided for establishing many of the drug associations now recognized in this category. Recognition benefits future patients too.

### Post-ERCP Pancreatitis Prophylaxis Revisited

Post-endoscopic retrograde cholangiopancreatography pancreatitis, introduced mechanistically in the second chapter, remains one of the most common iatrogenic causes of acute pancreatitis encountered in gastroenterology practice, and the rectal nonsteroidal anti-inflammatory drug prophylaxis and, in higher-risk cases, prophylactic pancreatic duct stenting discussed in that earlier chapter should be applied consistently and proactively in appropriately identified higher-risk patients rather than reserved only for cases where risk factors are recognized in retrospect after a complication has already occurred, reinforcing the proactive-rather-than-reactive complication-prevention principle emphasized throughout this book. Building this prophylaxis protocol into a standardized, checklist-based pre-procedure workflow, rather than relying on individual endoscopist recall for each case, improves consistency of application across an entire endoscopy unit and reduces the variability that individual practice patterns alone would otherwise produce.

| Feature | Sterile Necrosis | Infected Necrosis |
|---|---|---|
| Clinical course | Stable or improving | New/persistent fever, deterioration |
| Imaging clue | No gas within collection | Gas locules within collection |
| Confirmatory test | Not routinely needed | Clinical + imaging; FNA rarely needed |
| Management | Conservative, defer intervention | Antibiotics; drainage once walled off |

## THE GI THRESHOLD DECISION SYSTEM — Pancreatic Disease Thresholds

**Presentation Signature:** This chapter's threshold instances addressed early severity-based monitoring triage in acute pancreatitis and escalation to duct-directed or surgical intervention in refractory chronic pancreatitis pain.

**Threshold Point:** An early bedside severity score of three or more triages monitoring intensity in acute pancreatitis; a dominant, correctable ductal lesion or exhausted medical therapy triages escalation to intervention in chronic pancreatitis.

**The Call:** Both thresholds convert an evolving or refractory clinical picture into a proactive escalation decision rather than a reactive one triggered only after further deterioration or prolonged, ineffective therapy has already occurred.

**Trap Logic:** Waiting for the full 48-hour severity picture before triaging monitoring level, and escalating opioid therapy indefinitely in chronic pancreatitis without imaging the duct for a correctable lesion, are this chapter's most consequential threshold misapplications.

**Decision Anchor:** Calculate an early severity score at acute pancreatitis admission to guide monitoring intensity, and image the pancreatic duct specifically before escalating chronic pancreatitis pain management indefinitely without addressing a potentially correctable structural cause.

## Summary and Key Concepts

Acute pancreatitis is diagnosed by two of three criteria: characteristic pain, lipase at least three times normal, and characteristic imaging, with gallstones and alcohol as the dominant etiologies.

Early severity risk stratification, using tools like the bedside index for severity in acute pancreatitis, should guide monitoring intensity from admission rather than waiting for the full 48-hour severity classification.

Goal-directed balanced crystalloid resuscitation and early oral or enteral nutrition, rather than prolonged bowel rest, are now standard, evidence-based initial management for acute pancreatitis.

Gas within a necrotic collection is essentially diagnostic of infection without requiring fine-needle aspiration, and same-admission cholecystectomy is preferred for mild gallstone pancreatitis to prevent recurrent biliary events.

Chronic pancreatitis pain management follows a stepwise approach from lifestyle modification and medical therapy through duct-directed endoscopic or surgical intervention, and exocrine insufficiency unresponsive to adequate enzyme dosing should prompt evaluation for coexisting small intestinal bacterial overgrowth.

Autoimmune pancreatitis mimics pancreatic malignancy on imaging, and distinguishing type 1 from type 2 disease, along with adequate diagnostic certainty before excluding cancer, prevents both unnecessary surgery and missed malignancy.

# CHAPTER 13: BILIARY TRACT DISEASE AND GALLSTONE-RELATED DISORDERS

**Learning Objectives**

1. Distinguish asymptomatic cholelithiasis, biliary colic, and acute cholecystitis, and apply appropriate diagnostic and management strategies for each.
2. Apply risk stratification for choledocholithiasis and select an appropriate diagnostic and therapeutic pathway.
3. Recognize and manage acute cholangitis, including severity-based urgency of biliary decompression.
4. Evaluate and manage acalculous cholecystitis, gallbladder polyps, porcelain gallbladder, and biliary dyskinesia.
5. Recognize post-cholecystectomy syndrome and bile duct injury, and apply an appropriate evaluation and management approach.

**Chapter Outline**

This chapter develops gallstone disease along its natural clinical spectrum, from asymptomatic cholelithiasis through biliary colic and acute cholecystitis, then addresses choledocholithiasis and the risk-stratified pathway to its diagnosis and treatment, acute cholangitis and its severity-based urgency, several important gallbladder disease variants, and the recognition and management of postcholecystectomy complications. Each section connects a specific clinical or risk threshold to a defined management pathway.

## Cholelithiasis and Its Complications

### Epidemiology and Risk Factors

Gallstones affect a substantial proportion of adults, with cholesterol stones predominating in most populations and pigment stones, black pigment stones associated with hemolytic conditions and cirrhosis, and brown pigment stones associated with biliary infection and stasis, representing a distinct minority with their own specific associated conditions. The classic risk factor mnemonic, female, forty, fertile, and family history, while imperfect and incomplete, captures genuine epidemiologic associations including female sex hormone effects on cholesterol saturation, increasing age, and genetic predisposition, and additional recognized risk factors include obesity, rapid weight loss, particularly after bariatric surgery, pregnancy, and total parenteral nutrition, each of which alters bile composition or gallbladder motility in ways that favor stone formation. Ethnic and geographic variation in gallstone prevalence is substantial, with certain populations, including some Native American and Hispanic communities, demonstrating markedly higher cholesterol gallstone prevalence than other populations, likely reflecting a combination of genetic and dietary factors that remain incompletely characterized despite decades of epidemiologic study. Counseling should be realistic about the modest magnitude of this benefit rather than overpromising a dramatic reduction from gradual weight loss alone.

### Asymptomatic Gallstones and Biliary Colic

Asymptomatic gallstones, discovered incidentally on imaging obtained for another indication, generally do not require prophylactic cholecystectomy given their low annual rate of progression to symptomatic disease, and this conservative approach, rather than proceeding directly to surgery for an incidental finding, applies the same restraint already emphasized throughout this book for other incidentally discovered, low-risk findings. Biliary colic, the first symptomatic manifestation in patients who do progress, produces episodic, postprandial right upper quadrant or epigastric pain, typically lasting thirty minutes to several hours and resolving spontaneously between episodes, and this self-limited, episodic pattern distinguishes biliary colic from the persistent, progressively worsening pain of acute cholecystitis discussed next; once biliary colic has developed, elective cholecystectomy is generally recommended given the substantial risk of recurrent symptoms and progression to a complication if the gallbladder is left in place. Exceptions to this conservative approach exist in specific higher-risk populations, including patients with sickle cell disease, in whom distinguishing a vaso-occlusive pain crisis from biliary colic can be genuinely difficult, and select patients undergoing bariatric surgery, where concurrent prophylactic cholecystectomy is sometimes considered given the elevated stone-formation risk from rapid postoperative weight loss discussed earlier in this chapter. Distinguishing biliary colic from other causes of upper abdominal pain, including peptic ulcer disease and functional dyspepsia discussed in earlier chapters, relies on the specific postprandial, self-limited timing pattern and right upper quadrant location, and a presentation that does not fit this pattern cleanly should prompt reconsideration of the diagnosis rather than automatic attribution to known gallstones simply because they are present on imaging. Careful history-taking pays off here.

### Acute Cholecystitis: Diagnosis and Management

Acute cholecystitis, resulting from sustained cystic duct obstruction by a stone producing gallbladder wall inflammation, presents with persistent right upper quadrant pain, often with a positive Murphy sign, fever, and leukocytosis, and diagnosis integrates this clinical picture with ultrasound findings, including gallbladder wall thickening, pericholecystic fluid, and a sonographic Murphy sign, or, when ultrasound is equivocal, hepatobiliary scintigraphy demonstrating nonvisualization of the gallbladder, confirming cystic duct obstruction functionally when structural imaging alone has not clarified the diagnosis. Early laparoscopic cholecystectomy, generally within 72 hours of symptom onset, is preferred over delayed surgery or a trial of antibiotics alone in appropriately fit surgical candidates, given evidence that early surgery reduces overall hospital length of stay and complication rates compared with delayed intervention, representing a similar evidence-based departure from older, more conservative practice patterns already discussed in the previous chapter for pancreatitis management. The Tokyo Guidelines, a widely adopted international consensus framework, provide standardized diagnostic and severity grading criteria for acute cholecystitis that parallel the severity-based approach already established in this chapter for cholangitis, and applying this same standardized framework consistently supports more reproducible communication between clinicians managing a shared patient across different points in their care. Communicating this evidence-based timing preference to referring emergency medicine and hospitalist colleagues, who may still default to consulting surgery only after a trial of conservative management, supports timely referral that allows the early-window opportunity to actually be realized in practice. Timely recognition saves both time and morbidity.

**THE GI THRESHOLD DECISION SYSTEM — Biliary Thresholds — Surgical Timing and Candidacy in Acute Cholecystitis**

**Presentation Signature:** A patient presents with acute cholecystitis, and the clinician must determine whether early cholecystectomy, delayed cholecystectomy, or a nonoperative bridging strategy is appropriate.

**Threshold Point:** Presentation within 72 hours of symptom onset in a fit surgical candidate defines the threshold favoring early laparoscopic cholecystectomy; presentation beyond this window, significant surgical risk from comorbidity, or severe, complicated cholecystitis defines the threshold favoring either delayed surgery after a trial of antibiotics or a nonoperative bridging strategy.

**The Call:** Patients within the early window and reasonable surgical candidates proceed to early laparoscopic cholecystectomy; patients beyond the window or at elevated surgical risk are managed with antibiotics and, in select high-risk patients unable to tolerate any surgery, percutaneous cholecystostomy tube drainage as a bridging or, in some cases, definitive strategy.

**Trap Logic:** Reflexively delaying surgery in every patient with acute cholecystitis out of a now-outdated preference for interval cholecystectomy denies appropriately fit patients the shorter hospital stay and lower complication rate that early surgery, within the appropriate window, has been shown to provide.

**Decision Anchor:** Assess symptom duration and surgical fitness promptly at presentation, and pursue early laparoscopic cholecystectomy in appropriate candidates within the 72-hour window rather than defaulting to delayed surgery as a matter of routine practice.

## Choledocholithiasis and Cholangitis

### Risk Stratification for Choledocholithiasis

Suspected choledocholithiasis, a common bile duct stone, is risk-stratified using a combination of clinical, laboratory, and imaging findings, including a visualized duct stone on transabdominal ultrasound, a dilated common bile duct, and elevated liver biochemistries, particularly a rising or persistently elevated bilirubin, and this risk stratification determines the diagnostic pathway pursued, avoiding both under-evaluation of a patient with a genuine stone and over-utilization of invasive endoscopic retrograde cholangiopancreatography in a patient whose probability of choledocholithiasis is actually low. High-probability patients, generally those with a visualized duct stone or classic cholangitis, discussed below, proceed directly to therapeutic ERCP, while intermediate-probability patients are further evaluated with magnetic resonance cholangiopancreatography or endoscopic ultrasound, both introduced in the second chapter, to confirm or exclude the presence of a stone before committing to the more invasive ERCP procedure, and low-probability patients proceed to cholecystectomy alone with intraoperative cholangiography available to evaluate the duct at the time of surgery if intraoperative findings raise concern. Liver biochemistry trends over time, rather than a single isolated value, provide additional diagnostic information, since a rising bilirubin trend is more suggestive of ongoing obstruction than a stable, mildly elevated value that may instead reflect a resolved or intermittent process, an important nuance when interpreting laboratory results obtained at different points during a patient's evaluation. This tiered approach avoids the two failure modes at either extreme: subjecting a low-probability patient to unnecessary ERCP with its associated pancreatitis risk discussed in the previous chapter, and delaying necessary intervention in a high-probability patient through excessive additional imaging that adds little diagnostic value once the probability of a stone is already high. Balance matters most.

**Acute Cholangitis: Diagnosis and Management**

Acute cholangitis, resulting from biliary obstruction combined with infection within the obstructed system, classically presents with Charcot's triad of fever, jaundice, and right upper quadrant pain, though this complete triad is present in only a minority of cases, and the addition of altered mental status and hypotension, forming Reynolds' pentad, identifies the more severe, suppurative form of the disease carrying substantially higher mortality if decompression is delayed. Diagnosis integrates clinical suspicion with laboratory evidence of cholestasis and inflammation and imaging confirmation of biliary obstruction, and unlike many of the conditions in this book where diagnostic certainty is pursued deliberately before treatment, cholangitis management follows a more urgent logic: broad-spectrum antibiotics should be initiated immediately upon clinical suspicion, without waiting for imaging confirmation, given the risk of rapid deterioration to septic shock in this specific infectious process.

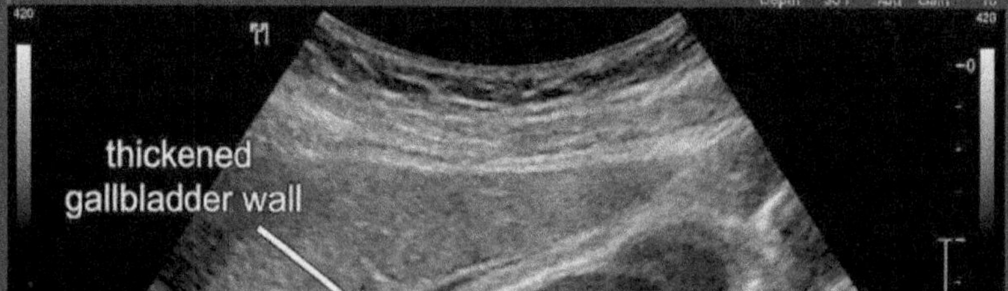


Figure 13.1: Ultrasound Findings in Acute Cholecystitis

Recognizing that atypical or incomplete presentations, particularly in older or immunocompromised patients whose inflammatory response may be blunted, are common, rather than requiring the complete Charcot triad before considering the diagnosis, prevents a dangerous delay in a patient whose presentation does not fit the classic textbook description precisely. This urgency-first approach, treating before full diagnostic certainty is established, mirrors reasoning applied elsewhere in medicine to other rapidly progressive infectious or hemorrhagic emergencies, where the cost of delay meaningfully exceeds the marginal diagnostic value of additional confirmatory testing before treatment begins. Act first, confirm alongside.

**THE GI THRESHOLD DECISION SYSTEM — Biliary Thresholds — Severity-Based Urgency of Decompression in Acute Cholangitis**

---

**Presentation Signature:** A patient is diagnosed with acute cholangitis, and the clinician must determine the appropriate timing for biliary decompression, most commonly via ERCP, relative to initial antibiotic therapy and resuscitation.

**Threshold Point:** Severe cholangitis, meeting criteria including septic shock, altered mental status, or organ dysfunction, defines the threshold for emergent biliary decompression, generally within 24 hours regardless of hour of presentation; moderate cholangitis without these features allows decompression within a somewhat longer, though still urgent, window, generally within 24 to 48 hours, once initial resuscitation and antibiotics have been established.

**The Call:** Severe cholangitis triggers immediate mobilization of an emergent ERCP team, including after-hours activation when necessary, rather than waiting for the next routine procedural slot; moderate cholangitis is decompressed urgently within the broader window once the patient has been appropriately resuscitated and stabilized.

**Trap Logic:** Treating cholangitis as a condition that can wait for routine next-day endoscopy scheduling, regardless of severity, ignores the mortality difference between emergent and delayed decompression in the severe subgroup specifically, where delay meaningfully worsens outcomes.

**Decision Anchor:** Classify cholangitis severity explicitly at diagnosis, and mobilize emergent, after-hours ERCP for severe disease rather than allowing routine scheduling logistics to dictate the timing of decompression in a patient who meets severe criteria.

## Gallbladder Disease Variants

### Acalculous Cholecystitis

Acalculous cholecystitis, gallbladder inflammation without an obstructing stone, occurs predominantly in critically ill patients, including those with prolonged fasting, mechanical ventilation, or severe trauma or burns, and results from gallbladder stasis and ischemia rather than mechanical obstruction, meaning that a critically ill patient with unexplained sepsis or clinical deterioration should have acalculous cholecystitis specifically considered even in the absence of gallstones on imaging, since this diagnosis is easily overlooked when the more familiar, stone-associated pattern of cholecystitis is used as the primary mental model. Percutaneous cholecystostomy tube drainage, rather than immediate cholecystectomy, is generally preferred initial management in this critically ill population given their frequently prohibitive surgical risk, with interval cholecystectomy or tube removal considered once the patient's overall clinical status has stabilized sufficiently to tolerate either intervention or a trial of tube removal. Maintaining acalculous cholecystitis explicitly on the differential for any critically ill patient with unexplained sepsis, alongside the more commonly considered sources such as central line infection, pneumonia, and urinary tract infection, ensures this diagnosis is not overlooked simply because it is less familiar than these more routinely considered sources of sepsis in the intensive care setting. A trial of tube clamping before formal removal, confirming the patient tolerates this without recurrent symptoms, is a reasonable practice before definitive removal, applying the same cautious, stepwise de-escalation principle already emphasized throughout this book for other temporary interventions being withdrawn. Patience pays off clinically.

## Gallbladder Polyps and Porcelain Gallbladder

Gallbladder polyps, most commonly benign cholesterol polyps discovered incidentally on ultrasound, are risk-stratified primarily by size, with polyps exceeding one centimeter carrying meaningfully increased malignant potential warranting cholecystectomy, while smaller polyps are generally managed with surveillance ultrasound at defined intervals, and additional risk factors independent of size, including patient age over fifty, concurrent gallstones, and rapid polyp growth on serial imaging, should also lower the threshold for cholecystectomy even in a polyp below the one-centimeter size threshold. Porcelain gallbladder, extensive calcification of the gallbladder wall visible on imaging, was historically associated with a substantially elevated gallbladder cancer risk prompting routine prophylactic cholecystectomy, though more recent evidence suggests this risk was previously overestimated, and current management is more individualized, generally still favoring cholecystectomy in fit surgical candidates given the residual, if lower than historically believed, cancer association, while reserving more conservative management for patients with prohibitive surgical risk. Distinguishing a true polyp from adherent sludge or a small, mobile stone artifact on ultrasound can occasionally be difficult, and repeat imaging or a different imaging modality is reasonable when this distinction remains genuinely unclear, since misclassifying sludge as a persistent polyp could otherwise lead to unnecessary surveillance imaging over an extended period. Multiple polyps, rather than a single dominant lesion, should each be individually measured and tracked, since the largest polyp typically drives the malignancy risk assessment and surveillance interval decision even when smaller polyps are also present. Patients found to have porcelain gallbladder incidentally should have the evolving nature of this risk estimate explained clearly, since older counseling that emphasized a very high cancer risk may have been based on outdated data and could cause disproportionate anxiety relative to the current, more moderate risk estimate. Track every lesion separately.

### Biliary Dyskinesia

Biliary dyskinesia, functional gallbladder disease producing biliary-type pain without gallstones, is diagnosed using hepatobiliary scintigraphy with cholecystokinin stimulation, calculating a gallbladder ejection fraction, and a low ejection fraction in a patient with a compatible clinical presentation supports the diagnosis and predicts symptomatic response to cholecystectomy, though patient selection should remain careful given that this functional diagnosis, similar to the functional disorders discussed in the tenth chapter, requires genuine clinical correlation rather than reflexive intervention based on a borderline ejection fraction value alone in a patient whose presentation does not otherwise fit the classic biliary-type pain pattern. Discussing the possibility of persistent symptoms even after cholecystectomy, given the imperfect predictive value of the ejection fraction threshold used for this diagnosis, sets realistic expectations before surgery is pursued for what remains, ultimately, a functional rather than structural diagnosis.

## Gallbladder and Biliary Malignancy

Gallbladder cancer, while uncommon, is frequently diagnosed at an advanced, incurable stage, since early disease produces few specific symptoms and is often discovered incidentally on pathology after cholecystectomy performed for presumed benign disease, and this diagnostic pattern reinforces why the risk factors discussed throughout this chapter, large or growing polyps, porcelain gallbladder, and chronic gallstone disease with recurrent inflammation, deserve careful attention rather than routine dismissal as low-risk findings, since they represent the field's best available early-warning signals for a cancer that otherwise presents late. Cholangiocarcinoma, arising from the bile duct epithelium itself rather than the gallbladder, is associated with primary sclerosing cholangitis, discussed further in a later chapter on cholestatic liver disease, choledochal cysts, and chronic biliary parasitic infection in endemic regions, and its presentation with painless jaundice from biliary obstruction can closely mimic pancreatic head adenocarcinoma, making cross-sectional imaging and, where the diagnosis remains unclear, tissue sampling via ERCP-directed brushing or biopsy essential before a management plan is finalized. Incidental gallbladder cancer discovered on pathology after a routine cholecystectomy performed for presumed benign disease requires prompt oncologic staging and, depending on the depth of invasion identified, may warrant reoperation for more extensive resection, a scenario that underscores the importance of routine pathologic examination of every cholecystectomy specimen rather than treating this step as a formality that can occasionally be skipped. Serum tumor markers, including CA 19-9, can provide supportive information but lack the sensitivity and specificity to serve as a standalone diagnostic test, and their primary utility lies in monitoring treatment response and surveillance for recurrence once a tissue diagnosis has already been established. Prognostic counseling for advanced gallbladder cancer should be honest about the generally limited treatment options and outcomes at this stage, while still ensuring the patient understands and can access appropriate palliative and supportive care resources alongside any remaining disease-directed treatment options that may be available. Compassion matters most.

### Approach to the Patient With Painless Jaundice

Painless jaundice, in contrast to the painful presentations of choledocholithiasis and cholangitis developed earlier in this chapter, should raise specific concern for a malignant biliary obstruction, whether from cholangiocarcinoma, pancreatic head adenocarcinoma discussed in the following chapter, or, less commonly, ampullary carcinoma, and this presentation warrants prompt, dedicated cross-sectional imaging and multidisciplinary evaluation rather than being managed with the same reflexive urgency-driven pathway developed for painful biliary obstruction in this chapter, since the diagnostic priority in painless jaundice centers on cancer staging and multidisciplinary planning rather than emergent decompression alone. Multidisciplinary tumor board discussion, involving hepatobiliary surgery, medical oncology, and radiation oncology as appropriate, should be pursued once malignant biliary obstruction is confirmed or strongly suspected, applying the same collaborative decision-making model already established in earlier chapters for other gastrointestinal malignancies.

## Advances in Cholecystectomy Technique and Difficult Gallbladder Management

The critical view of safety, a specific set of anatomic landmarks that must be confirmed before dividing the cystic duct and artery during laparoscopic cholecystectomy, is the standard safety technique aimed at preventing the bile duct injury discussed later in this chapter, and its consistent application, documented explicitly in the operative note, represents a systems-level safeguard against injury analogous to the timeout and checklist practices used elsewhere in surgery and endoscopy. When the critical view cannot be safely achieved due to severe inflammation or distorted anatomy, a subtotal cholecystectomy, leaving a portion of the gallbladder in place to avoid dissecting through dangerous, unclear anatomy, is an accepted and increasingly recognized alternative to pressing forward with a complete cholecystectomy under unsafe visualization conditions, reflecting a shift in surgical culture toward accepting a less complete operation in favor of avoiding a bile duct injury that carries far greater long-term morbidity than a retained gallbladder remnant. Formal training programs and simulation-based education specifically focused on achieving and documenting the critical view of safety have been proposed and, in some centers, implemented as part of surgical trainee education, reflecting growing recognition that consistent technique adoption benefits from structured teaching rather than relying solely on individual surgeon judgment developed through experience alone. Photodocumentation of the achieved critical view within the operative record provides an objective, reviewable record beyond a narrative description alone, supporting both individual case review and broader quality improvement efforts across an institution over time. Good records help everyone.

### Intraoperative Cholangiography and Conversion to Open Surgery

Intraoperative cholangiography, injecting contrast directly into the biliary tree during surgery to delineate anatomy and identify unsuspected common bile duct stones, is used selectively rather than routinely in most current practice, reserved for cases where anatomy is unclear or where the preoperative choledocholithiasis risk stratification developed earlier in this chapter has left genuine diagnostic uncertainty, and its selective rather than routine use reflects an evidence-based balance between diagnostic value and the added procedural time and resource utilization routine use would require. Conversion from laparoscopic to open cholecystectomy, once viewed by some as a marker of surgical failure, is increasingly recognized and taught as an appropriate, safety-oriented decision when laparoscopic visualization is inadequate to proceed safely, and this reframing, converting a stigmatized outcome into a recognized safety behavior, parallels the broader theme throughout this book that proactive escalation, whether surgical conversion, medical rescue therapy, or specialist referral, should be viewed as sound clinical judgment rather than a failure to manage a case independently. Surgeon and institutional experience with intraoperative cholangiography interpretation also varies, and this variability is worth acknowledging when deciding whether to rely on this technique versus a preoperative imaging-based risk stratification approach in a given clinical setting. Preoperative counseling that mentions the possibility of conversion, framed as a safety-oriented contingency rather than an unlikely worst-case scenario, prepares patients for this outcome without unnecessary alarm and supports informed consent that genuinely reflects the range of possible intraoperative findings. Framing conversion positively in surgical training and departmental culture, rather than treating it as a marker of individual surgeon shortcoming, reinforces the safety-first behavior this chapter emphasizes.

## Endoscopic Alternatives to Cholecystectomy and Gallbladder Preservation

Endoscopic ultrasound-guided gallbladder drainage, creating a transmural drainage tract between the gallbladder and the gastrointestinal lumen using a specialized stent, has emerged as an alternative to percutaneous cholecystostomy tube drainage in appropriately selected high-surgical-risk patients with acute cholecystitis, offering the advantage of internal, rather than external, drainage that avoids the ongoing catheter care burden and dislodgement risk associated with a percutaneous tube, though appropriate patient selection and referral to a center with specific expertise in this technique remain essential given its relative novelty and specialized skill requirements relative to the more widely available percutaneous approach. For patients who ultimately require long-term nonoperative gallbladder management, whether from prohibitive surgical risk or personal preference against surgery after appropriate informed discussion, structured follow-up addressing both the drainage device itself and ongoing symptom monitoring should be established explicitly rather than allowing this population to be lost to follow-up once the acute episode has resolved. Comparative outcome data between endoscopic and percutaneous drainage approaches continues to accumulate, and current practice at most centers still favors percutaneous drainage as the more widely available, familiar first-line approach, with endoscopic drainage reserved for centers with specific expertise or for patients in whom percutaneous access is technically difficult or anatomically unfavorable. As this technique matures and more comparative outcome data accumulates, its role relative to percutaneous drainage may continue to evolve, and clinicians should stay current with updated society guidance rather than relying on an initial impression formed when the technique was still novel. A clearly assigned point of contact for this ongoing management, whether gastroenterology, surgery, or interventional radiology depending on local practice patterns, prevents the ambiguity that can otherwise lead to this population falling through the cracks between specialties.

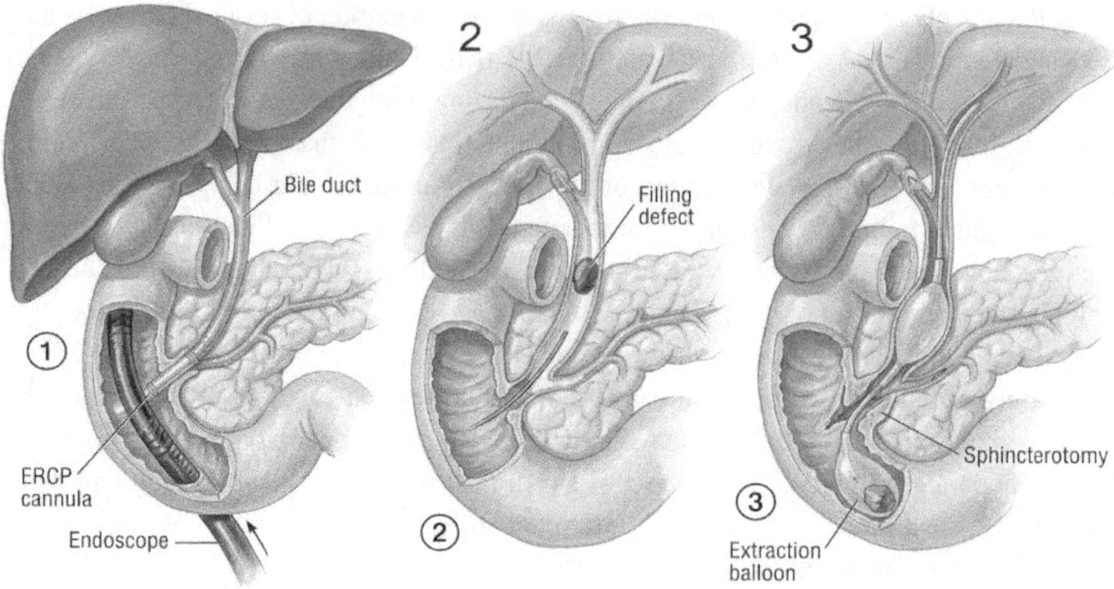


### Oral Dissolution Therapy and Extracorporeal Shock Wave Lithotripsy

Oral bile acid dissolution therapy and extracorporeal shock wave lithotripsy, both historically used as nonsurgical alternatives for symptomatic gallstone disease, have fallen out of favor in current practice given their limited efficacy, restricted to small, purely cholesterol stones in a functioning gallbladder, high recurrence rates after treatment discontinuation, and the widespread availability and superior efficacy of laparoscopic cholecystectomy, and clinicians should be aware that patients occasionally ask about these older approaches, sometimes having encountered outdated information, and can be counseled honestly that current evidence and practice guidelines favor surgical management in essentially all patients who are reasonable surgical candidates. Occasional narrow exceptions exist, such as a patient with prohibitive surgical risk and a small, purely cholesterol stone who has already declined percutaneous or surgical alternatives, but these represent rare, individualized scenarios rather than a return to routine use of these older modalities. These narrow exceptions require explicit multidisciplinary discussion and documentation before pursuing an approach that falls outside standard current practice.

## Antimicrobial Selection and Source Control in Biliary Infection

Antibiotic selection for acute cholangitis and cholecystitis should account for the typical biliary pathogen spectrum, predominantly gram-negative enteric organisms and enterococcus, and local antimicrobial resistance patterns, with severity of illness guiding the breadth of empiric coverage, broader, more aggressive coverage for severe or healthcare-associated infection and narrower coverage for mild, community-acquired disease in a patient without recent healthcare exposure, mirroring the same severity-matched, rather than uniformly maximal, antimicrobial selection principle used across other infectious presentations in medicine. Antibiotics alone, without source control, meaning biliary decompression in cholangitis or cholecystectomy or drainage in cholecystitis, are inadequate definitive therapy for either condition, and this point deserves explicit emphasis since a patient who initially improves on antibiotics alone can experience a false sense of resolution that delays the source-control intervention actually required to prevent relapse or progression. Blood cultures should be obtained before initiating empiric antibiotics whenever feasible without meaningfully delaying treatment, since culture data, when positive, allows the de-escalation to narrower, pathogen-directed therapy discussed below and provides valuable information about local resistance patterns that benefits future patients treated at the same institution. Communicating this explicitly to the patient, that clinical improvement on antibiotics is a bridge to definitive drainage rather than a substitute for it, prevents a scenario where a patient who feels better declines the recommended procedure believing antibiotics alone have resolved the underlying problem. Institutional antibiograms, reviewed periodically and reflected in local empiric therapy guidelines, ensure that empiric antibiotic choices remain aligned with actual local resistance patterns rather than a national or textbook default that may not reflect the specific microbial ecology of a given institution.

### De-escalation and Duration of Therapy

Antibiotic duration following adequate source control is generally short, often just several days once the biliary system has been adequately decompressed and the patient has clinically improved, reflecting current antimicrobial stewardship principles that favor the shortest effective duration over historically longer, less evidence-based courses, and de-escalating from broad empiric coverage to a narrower, culture-directed regimen once blood or bile culture results return, applying the same antimicrobial stewardship principle emphasized in other infectious contexts throughout medicine, should be a routine part of ongoing management rather than continuing broad-spectrum therapy by default throughout the treatment course. Institutional order sets built around these shortened, evidence-based durations, rather than defaulting to a longer standard course out of habit, help translate this evidence into consistent bedside practice across a busy hospital service. Consistency counts.

## Recurrent Choledocholithiasis and Difficult Bile Duct Stones

Recurrent common bile duct stones after apparently successful clearance, whether newly formed or representing incompletely cleared fragments from the index procedure, should prompt evaluation for a predisposing anatomic or physiologic factor, including biliary strictures, periampullary diverticula that can alter sphincter function and predispose to stone formation, or, in a patient without cholecystectomy yet performed, an ongoing source from the gallbladder itself, reinforcing why cholecystectomy is generally recommended after ERCP-based duct clearance in a patient with an intact gallbladder rather than leaving the gallbladder in place as an ongoing potential stone source. Large or difficult common bile duct stones, resistant to standard extraction techniques, may require adjunctive methods including mechanical lithotripsy, crushing the stone within a specialized basket device, or, for the most difficult stones, cholangioscopy-directed electrohydraulic or laser lithotripsy, performed under direct visualization of the stone using a dedicated cholangioscope introduced through the working channel of a standard duodenoscope, and referral to a center with this specific advanced expertise is reasonable when standard extraction techniques have proven inadequate rather than repeating standard technique attempts indefinitely. Periampullary diverticula specifically deserve careful documentation when identified, since their presence can also complicate future ERCP attempts and should be communicated to any endoscopist performing subsequent procedures on this patient. Preprocedural discussion with the patient about the possibility of a staged approach, before the index procedure rather than only if it becomes necessary mid-procedure, sets appropriate expectations and reduces anxiety if a second procedure ultimately proves necessary. Cholecystectomy timing relative to duct clearance is also worth explicit discussion with the patient, since a staged approach, clearing the duct first and performing cholecystectomy at a subsequent, closely timed procedure, is common and does not indicate incomplete treatment.

### Temporary Biliary Stenting as a Bridging Strategy

Temporary biliary stent placement, providing adequate drainage without complete stone clearance, is a reasonable bridging strategy in a patient with a difficult stone not amenable to complete extraction at the index procedure, particularly when the patient's overall clinical status does not permit a prolonged initial procedure, with definitive clearance planned at a subsequent, staged procedure once the patient has recovered or once specialized equipment or expertise can be arranged; communicating this staged plan explicitly to the patient, rather than allowing them to believe the problem has been fully resolved after the first procedure, prevents confusion and supports adherence to the necessary follow-up procedure.

## Patient Communication and Shared Decision-Making in Gallstone Disease

Patients newly diagnosed with symptomatic gallstone disease often have specific questions and misconceptions about life without a gallbladder, including concerns about long-term dietary restriction, and providing clear, accurate counseling, that most patients tolerate a normal diet well after recovery with only a minority experiencing persistent fat intolerance or altered bowel habits, supports informed decision-making and reduces unnecessary anxiety about the surgery's long-term lifestyle impact. Discussing the specific risks of continued nonoperative management, recurrent biliary colic, and the possibility of progression to the more serious complications developed throughout this chapter, alongside the risks of surgery itself, supports genuine shared decision-making for the subset of patients who are hesitant about proceeding with a recommended cholecystectomy, applying the same informed, balanced risk-benefit discussion principle emphasized throughout this book for other elective interventions. Written educational materials summarizing this information, provided at the time of surgical referral, give patients a reliable reference to revisit rather than relying entirely on their recall of a single verbal counseling conversation delivered during a busy clinic visit. Addressing common cultural or family-transmitted beliefs about diet after gallbladder removal directly, rather than assuming the patient has no preexisting views on the topic, allows any inaccurate information to be corrected proactively rather than discovered only after it has already influenced the patient's postoperative eating pattern unnecessarily.

### Addressing Surgical Hesitancy

A patient declining recommended cholecystectomy after being fully informed of the risks and benefits should have that decision respected, with clear documentation of the discussion and a specific plan for what symptoms or findings would prompt reconsideration of surgery, rather than either pressuring the patient toward a procedure they have declined or abandoning the topic without providing this specific, actionable guidance for future decision-making should their clinical picture change. Revisiting this decision periodically at subsequent visits, rather than treating a single documented conversation as permanently closing the topic, respects both patient autonomy and the possibility that circumstances or preferences may change over time. Culturally sensitive counseling, aware that attitudes toward surgery and bodily autonomy vary across patient populations, supports genuinely respectful shared decision-making rather than a uniform counseling script applied without regard to individual patient context.

## Mirizzi Syndrome and Complex Gallstone Presentations

Mirizzi syndrome, an uncommon complication in which a stone impacted in the gallbladder neck or cystic duct produces external compression and, in more advanced cases, erosion into the adjacent common hepatic duct, produces obstructive jaundice that can mimic malignant biliary obstruction both clinically and on imaging, and its recognition preoperatively, generally through MRCP demonstrating the characteristic anatomic relationship between the impacted stone and the compressed or eroded bile duct, is critical since standard laparoscopic cholecystectomy carries substantially elevated bile duct injury risk in this specific anatomic scenario and often requires a modified surgical approach or conversion to open surgery. Distinguishing Mirizzi syndrome from a malignant process preoperatively, while not always possible with complete certainty, meaningfully changes the surgical plan and the preoperative counseling provided to the patient, and a multidisciplinary discussion involving radiology and hepatobiliary surgery is reasonable whenever this diagnosis is genuinely being considered, given the technical complexity and injury risk this specific anatomic variant presents. Preoperative recognition, even when incomplete, allows the surgical and anesthesia teams to plan for a longer, potentially more complex procedure and to have the necessary specialized equipment and expertise available from the outset rather than discovering the anatomic complexity unexpectedly during an operation planned as routine. Prevention beats cure.

### Gallstone Ileus

Gallstone ileus, a rare mechanical small bowel obstruction caused by a large gallstone that has eroded through a cholecystoenteric fistula and migrated into the intestinal lumen, should be considered in an older patient presenting with small bowel obstruction, particularly when a history of prior gallstone disease is present, even though many affected patients have not had a prior cholecystectomy and may not recall significant prior biliary symptoms, since the fistula formation itself can develop silently over an extended period. The characteristic finding of pneumobilia, air within the biliary tree from the abnormal enteric communication, visible on cross-sectional imaging obtained for the obstruction workup, is a specific diagnostic clue that should prompt consideration of this unusual cause of obstruction rather than assuming a more common obstruction etiology, such as adhesions or a mass lesion, without reviewing the imaging specifically for this finding. Management typically requires surgical removal of the obstructing stone, with the decision to address the underlying fistula at the same operation versus a staged approach individualized based on the patient's overall clinical stability, given that these patients are often elderly with significant comorbidity that may favor the less physiologically demanding staged approach. Vigilance saves lives.

## Postcholecystectomy Considerations

### Post-Cholecystectomy Syndrome

Post-cholecystectomy syndrome, persistent or recurrent abdominal symptoms following cholecystectomy, encompasses a heterogeneous group of underlying causes rather than representing a single diagnosis, and systematic evaluation should distinguish biliary causes, including retained or recurrent common bile duct stones, bile duct injury discussed below, or sphincter of Oddi dysfunction, introduced in the previous chapter, from nonbiliary causes, including the functional gastrointestinal disorders discussed in the tenth chapter, peptic ulcer disease, or pancreatitis, that may have been coincidentally present or unmasked once the more obvious gallbladder pathology was removed and could no longer serve as a convenient explanation for ongoing symptoms. This differential should be approached with the same systematic, threshold-based diagnostic reasoning emphasized throughout this book rather than assuming persistent symptoms after cholecystectomy necessarily reflect an incomplete or unsuccessful surgery, since a meaningful proportion of post-cholecystectomy symptoms ultimately prove unrelated to the biliary system altogether. A detailed timeline of when symptoms began relative to the surgery, whether they represent a continuation of preoperative symptoms, a new symptom pattern, or a delayed onset well after an initial asymptomatic recovery period, provides important diagnostic clues that a general symptom inventory alone would not capture as clearly. Empiric reassurance without adequate evaluation, offered simply because the surgery is presumed to have been technically successful, similarly risks missing a genuine, treatable cause of ongoing symptoms and should be avoided in favor of the systematic differential approach described here. Systematic beats reflexive reassurance.

### Bile Duct Injury Recognition and Management

Bile duct injury, an uncommon but serious complication of cholecystectomy, most often resulting from misidentification of anatomy during laparoscopic dissection, should be suspected in a patient with unexplained abdominal pain, jaundice, bile leak, or sepsis in the days following cholecystectomy, and prompt cross-sectional imaging and, where indicated, MRCP or ERCP to define the injury's location and extent is essential before definitive management is planned, since the specific injury classification directly determines whether endoscopic, percutaneous, or surgical repair is the appropriate approach. Early referral to a hepatobiliary surgery center with specific expertise in complex bile duct reconstruction, rather than attempting definitive repair at a center without this specialized experience, improves long-term outcomes substantially, and this referral threshold should be applied even when the injury is recognized at the index operation, since immediate, well-planned referral for definitive repair generally produces better outcomes than a repair attempted without this specific expertise, even when performed promptly. Documenting the specific injury classification, using a recognized system such as the Strasberg classification, in the medical record supports clear communication between the referring surgeon and the receiving hepatobiliary specialist, ensuring the full clinical picture is transmitted accurately rather than requiring the receiving center to reconstruct this information from incomplete records. Psychosocial support for the patient, who is often experiencing significant fear and distrust following an unexpected complication of what they understood to be a routine, low-risk procedure, should accompany the technical evaluation and treatment plan, since bile duct injury carries substantial emotional as well as physical burden that deserves explicit acknowledgment. Words matter here too.

**Figure 13.3 Percutaneous Cholecystostomy Tube Placement**

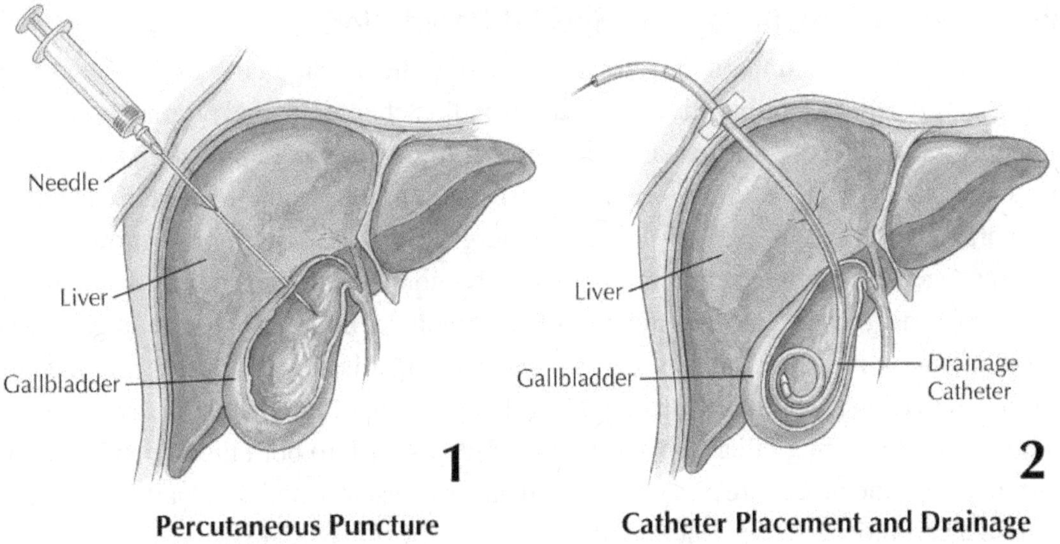


Case Presentation: A 68-year-old man presents with fever, jaundice, and right upper quadrant pain, and initial evaluation reveals hypotension and altered mental status. Applying the reasoning developed in this chapter, broad-spectrum antibiotics are initiated immediately upon clinical suspicion of cholangitis, without waiting for confirmatory imaging, given his hemodynamic instability. Ultrasound confirms a dilated common bile duct with a visualized stone, and his presentation meets criteria for severe cholangitis given his altered mental status and hypotension. Per the threshold developed in this chapter, the on-call advanced endoscopy team is mobilized emergently rather than deferring to the next routine procedural slot, and he undergoes ERCP with stone extraction and sphincterotomy within several hours of presentation, with clinical stabilization following decompression. He subsequently undergoes cholecystectomy once fully recovered. This case illustrates the chapter's central severity-based urgency principle: his Reynolds' pentad features defined an emergent, not routine, decompression timeline, and the emergent mobilization achieved was the key determinant of his favorable outcome.

Case Presentation: A 45-year-old woman undergoes abdominal ultrasound for an unrelated indication, which incidentally identifies a 6-millimeter gallbladder polyp without gallstones. Applying the reasoning developed in this chapter, this polyp falls below the one-centimeter threshold generally warranting cholecystectomy, and in the absence of additional risk factors, age under fifty, no concurrent gallstones, and no rapid growth on this single assessment, surveillance ultrasound rather than immediate cholecystectomy is the appropriate initial approach. She is scheduled for repeat ultrasound at a defined interval, and at follow-up, the polyp has grown to 9 millimeters over eighteen months. Given this growth trajectory, even though the polyp remains below the one-centimeter threshold in absolute size, the additional risk factor of documented interval growth is applied per the reasoning developed in this chapter, and she is referred for cholecystectomy given the meaningfully increased malignant potential this growth pattern suggests despite the polyp's current size still being just under the traditional threshold. This case illustrates that polyp size alone, assessed only at a single point in time, is an incomplete risk assessment, and growth trajectory on serial imaging independently informs the threshold for intervention.

## Gallstone Disease in Pregnancy and Special Populations

Gallstone disease is more common in pregnancy given the hormonally mediated changes in bile composition and gallbladder motility discussed earlier in this chapter, and symptomatic gallstone disease during pregnancy is managed with the same threshold-based reasoning applied elsewhere in this book, favoring laparoscopic cholecystectomy, generally performed in the second trimester when feasible given the more favorable balance of fetal and maternal surgical risk during this window, over prolonged conservative management that risks recurrent, potentially more severe episodes as pregnancy progresses. ERCP during pregnancy, when a clear indication such as choledocholithiasis or cholangitis exists, follows the same radiation-minimization and shielding precautions discussed in the previous chapter for pancreatitis, and deferring a genuinely indicated ERCP purely out of pregnancy-related radiation concern, when the alternative is ongoing biliary obstruction or infection risk to both mother and fetus, is generally the wrong choice once the procedure's true indication has been established. Postpartum resolution of some pregnancy-associated biliary sludge and small stones does occur, which is why asymptomatic findings identified incidentally during pregnancy, absent the symptomatic threshold discussed above, do not necessarily require intervention during the pregnancy itself and can reasonably be reassessed after delivery. Multidisciplinary coordination among gastroenterology, surgery, obstetrics, and anesthesia is essential when intervention is pursued during pregnancy, ensuring all relevant specialties contribute to timing and technique decisions that account for both maternal and fetal considerations simultaneously.

### Gallstone Disease in Patients With Cirrhosis

Cholecystectomy in patients with cirrhosis, particularly decompensated cirrhosis discussed in a later chapter, carries substantially elevated perioperative risk from coagulopathy, portal hypertension-related bleeding, and impaired hepatic reserve, and this elevated risk should prompt careful, individualized surgical risk assessment, often incorporating a formal hepatic risk stratification score, before proceeding with elective cholecystectomy in this population, with percutaneous or endoscopic alternatives, including endoscopic gallbladder drainage where locally available, considered preferentially over surgery in patients whose hepatic reserve makes surgical risk prohibitive. Preoperative correction of coagulopathy, where feasible, and careful attention to volume status given the hemodynamic sensitivity of decompensated cirrhosis, should be addressed proactively when surgery is ultimately pursued in this population, applying the same careful, individualized preoperative optimization principle relevant across other high-risk surgical populations discussed elsewhere in this book. Coordinating this evaluation with the patient's hepatologist, where one is already involved in their care, ensures the surgical risk assessment incorporates the most current, complete picture of their liver disease severity rather than relying solely on data available to the surgical team in isolation.

| Condition | Key Distinguishing Feature | First-Line Management |
|---|---|---|
| Biliary colic | Episodic, self-limited pain | Elective cholecystectomy |
| Acute cholecystitis | Persistent pain, fever, positive Murphy sign | Early laparoscopic cholecystectomy |
| Choledocholithiasis | Elevated bilirubin, dilated duct, visualized stone | Risk-stratified ERCP or MRCP/EUS |
| Acute cholangitis | Charcot triad ± Reynolds pentad | Antibiotics + severity-based urgent decompression |
| Acalculous cholecystitis | Critically ill patient, no stones | Percutaneous cholecystostomy |

### THE GI THRESHOLD DECISION SYSTEM — Biliary Disease Thresholds

**Presentation Signature:** This chapter's threshold instances addressed surgical timing in acute cholecystitis and severity-based urgency of decompression in acute cholangitis.

**Threshold Point:** Symptom duration and surgical fitness gate early versus delayed cholecystectomy timing; cholangitis severity criteria gate emergent versus urgent decompression timing.

**The Call:** Both thresholds replace a uniform, one-size-fits-all timeline with a specific, criteria-based urgency assessment that matches intervention timing to the actual clinical risk profile of the individual patient.

**Trap Logic:** Defaulting to delayed cholecystectomy out of outdated practice habit, and treating cholangitis as suitable for routine next-day scheduling regardless of severity, are this chapter's most consequential threshold misapplications.

**Decision Anchor:** Pursue early cholecystectomy within the appropriate window for fit candidates with acute cholecystitis, and classify cholangitis severity explicitly to determine whether emergent or urgent decompression timing is warranted.

## Summary and Key Concepts

Asymptomatic gallstones generally do not require prophylactic cholecystectomy, while biliary colic, once it develops, warrants elective cholecystectomy given the substantial risk of recurrence or progression to a complication.

Early laparoscopic cholecystectomy within 72 hours of symptom onset, rather than delayed surgery, is preferred for acute cholecystitis in fit surgical candidates given evidence of shorter hospital stays and fewer complications.

Choledocholithiasis risk stratification, using clinical, laboratory, and imaging findings, determines whether a patient proceeds directly to therapeutic ERCP, further noninvasive imaging, or cholecystectomy alone.

Acute cholangitis requires immediate antibiotics upon clinical suspicion, and severity, particularly Reynolds pentad features, determines whether biliary decompression must be emergent or can proceed on a somewhat less urgent timeline.

Acalculous cholecystitis should be considered in critically ill patients with unexplained sepsis even without gallstones, and gallbladder polyps are risk-stratified by both size and growth trajectory on serial imaging.

Post-cholecystectomy syndrome has a heterogeneous differential spanning biliary and nonbiliary causes, and suspected bile duct injury warrants prompt imaging and referral to a center with specific hepatobiliary reconstruction expertise.

# CHAPTER 14: PANCREATIC AND BILIARY NEOPLASIA

**Learning Objectives**

1. Describe the epidemiology, risk factors, and screening approach for pancreatic adenocarcinoma in high-risk individuals.
2. Apply a diagnostic and staging workup for suspected pancreatic adenocarcinoma and determine resectability status.
3. Classify pancreatic cystic neoplasms and apply risk-stratified surveillance and surgical referral criteria.
4. Distinguish functional from nonfunctional pancreatic neuroendocrine tumors and apply an appropriate evaluation and management approach.
5. Describe the staging and management of cholangiocarcinoma and ampullary neoplasia.

**Chapter Outline**

This chapter develops pancreatic and biliary neoplasia from pancreatic adenocarcinoma, its risk factors, diagnostic and staging workup, and treatment approach, through the pancreatic cystic neoplasms and their risk-stratified surveillance, pancreatic neuroendocrine tumors, and closes with cholangiocarcinoma and ampullary neoplasia. Each section connects a specific risk, imaging, or staging threshold to a defined management pathway.

## Pancreatic Adenocarcinoma

### Epidemiology, Risk Factors, and Screening in High-Risk Individuals

Pancreatic adenocarcinoma carries a poor overall prognosis given its tendency toward late-stage diagnosis, and established risk factors include smoking, the single most significant modifiable risk factor, chronic pancreatitis discussed in the twelfth chapter, particularly hereditary pancreatitis, obesity and long-standing type 2 diabetes, and a family history meeting defined hereditary pancreatic cancer criteria, including specific germline pathogenic variants in genes such as BRCA1, BRCA2, PALB2, and the Lynch syndrome genes introduced in the eleventh chapter, each of which confers an elevated lifetime pancreatic cancer risk beyond their more commonly recognized associated cancer types. Screening for pancreatic cancer in the general population is not recommended given the disease's relatively low overall incidence and the absence of an adequately sensitive, specific, and cost-effective screening test, but structured surveillance using endoscopic ultrasound and MRI, alternating or combined at defined intervals, is recommended in confirmed high-risk individuals meeting specific genetic or strong family history criteria, applying the same risk-stratified screening principle already established throughout this book for other malignancies. The magnitude of risk conferred by each of these genetic and clinical factors varies considerably, and genetic counseling should present this individualized risk estimate rather than a single generic elevated-risk statement, since a patient's specific gene and family history combination meaningfully shapes both their absolute risk and the resulting surveillance recommendations they receive. The false-positive and overdiagnosis risk from even a well-designed surveillance program is not negligible, and this should be discussed openly with high-risk individuals before they enter a surveillance program, since some detected findings will ultimately prove benign despite prompting further, sometimes invasive, evaluation.

**Figure 14.1:** Pancreatic Adenocarcinoma Resectability Criteria on CT

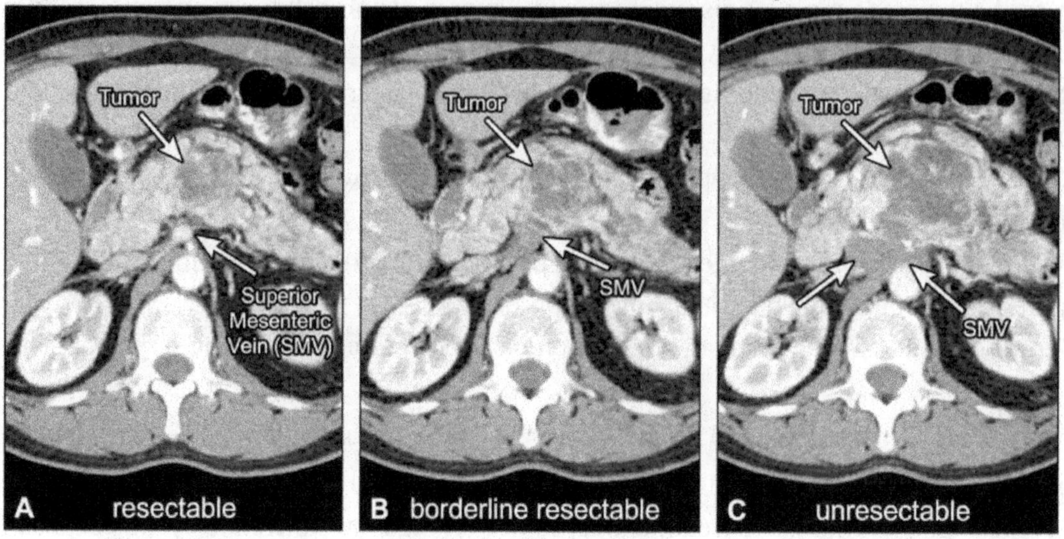


Resectable Borderline Resectable Unresectable

## Clinical Presentation and Diagnostic Workup

Pancreatic adenocarcinoma presents differently depending on tumor location: head-of-pancreas tumors, the most common location, frequently produce painless jaundice from biliary obstruction, discussed in the previous chapter, often accompanied by pale stools, dark urine, and pruritus, while body and tail tumors more often present later with vague abdominal or back pain, weight loss, and new-onset diabetes, since these tumors lack the early biliary obstruction warning sign that head tumors provide. New-onset diabetes in a patient over 50, particularly when accompanied by unexplained weight loss rather than the weight gain typically associated with new type 2 diabetes, is a recognized, underappreciated early clue to occult pancreatic adenocarcinoma, and this specific atypical presentation, weight loss with new hyperglycemia rather than the more expected weight gain, should prompt consideration of pancreatic imaging in an appropriately selected patient rather than assuming routine new-onset type 2 diabetes. Diagnostic workup integrates cross-sectional imaging, most commonly pancreatic protocol CT optimized specifically for pancreatic and vascular visualization, with endoscopic ultrasound-guided tissue sampling providing definitive histologic confirmation, and CA 19-9, while not sufficiently sensitive or specific for screening or diagnosis, provides a useful baseline for later treatment response monitoring, applying the same baseline-for-trending-rather-than-diagnostic-use principle already established for tumor markers in earlier chapters. Migratory thrombophlebitis, historically termed Trousseau syndrome, an unexplained, recurrent venous thromboembolism affecting unusual or migratory sites, is a recognized, if uncommon, paraneoplastic presentation of pancreatic adenocarcinoma, and this association is worth remembering in a patient with recurrent, otherwise unexplained thromboembolic events, since it can occasionally represent the presenting clue that leads to the underlying cancer diagnosis. Primary care clinicians, who most often encounter new-onset diabetes as an isolated finding without the broader gastrointestinal context this book provides, may benefit from specific education about this atypical presentation pattern, since they are typically the first point of contact for a patient whose new diabetes diagnosis might, in a minority of cases, herald an underlying malignancy rather than represent routine type 2 diabetes. CA 19-9 interpretation also requires awareness of a specific pitfall: a small subset of the population lacks the Lewis antigen required to produce CA 19-9 at all, meaning these patients will have a persistently low or undetectable CA 19-9 even with extensive disease, a pitfall worth remembering before relying too heavily on serial CA 19-9 trending as the sole marker of treatment response or recurrence.

**Staging and Resectability Assessment**

Resectability assessment, determined primarily by the tumor's relationship to key peripancreatic vasculature, the superior mesenteric artery, celiac axis, and superior mesenteric and portal veins, on dedicated pancreatic protocol imaging, classifies tumors as resectable, borderline resectable, with limited vascular involvement potentially amenable to resection after response to neoadjuvant therapy, or unresectable due to locally advanced vascular involvement or the presence of distant metastatic disease, and this three-tier classification directly determines whether a patient proceeds to upfront surgery, neoadjuvant therapy followed by reassessment, or systemic therapy alone without surgical intent. Distant metastatic disease, most commonly to the liver, peritoneum, or lung, should be actively searched for during staging workup even when locoregional imaging suggests a technically resectable primary tumor, since finding occult metastatic disease changes management entirely toward systemic therapy alone, and this staging thoroughness prevents an unnecessary surgical attempt in a patient whose disease has already spread beyond the reach of curative-intent local therapy.

**THE GI THRESHOLD DECISION SYSTEM — Pancreatobiliary Thresholds — Resectability Classification and Treatment Sequencing**

---

**Presentation Signature:** A patient with newly diagnosed pancreatic adenocarcinoma requires staging to determine whether upfront surgery, neoadjuvant therapy, or systemic therapy alone is the appropriate initial treatment pathway.

**Threshold Point:** The specific degree of tumor contact with the superior mesenteric artery, celiac axis, and mesenteric-portal venous confluence on dedicated imaging defines the threshold separating resectable, borderline resectable, and unresectable disease, and this vascular relationship, not tumor size alone, is the determining factor.

**The Call:** Resectable disease proceeds to surgery, often with neoadjuvant therapy increasingly favored even in this group given evolving evidence; borderline resectable disease receives neoadjuvant chemotherapy with restaging before a resection decision is finalized; unresectable, non-metastatic disease receives systemic therapy, with resection reconsidered only if a favorable response converts the tumor to a resectable category.

**Trap Logic:** Assessing resectability by tumor size or general impression rather than the specific vascular relationship criteria risks both understaging a technically unresectable tumor as resectable, leading to an incomplete or futile surgical attempt, and overstaging a genuinely resectable tumor as unresectable, denying a patient their best chance at surgical cure.

**Decision Anchor:** Classify resectability using the specific vascular contact criteria on dedicated pancreatic protocol imaging, reviewed by radiology and surgery together, rather than a general size-based or subjective impression of the tumor's extent.

### Treatment Overview: Surgical, Neoadjuvant, and Adjuvant Therapy

Pancreaticoduodenectomy, the Whipple procedure, removing the pancreatic head, duodenum, distal common bile duct, and gallbladder with reconstruction of pancreatic, biliary, and gastrointestinal continuity, is the standard surgical approach for resectable head-of-pancreas tumors, while distal pancreatectomy, often with splenectomy, addresses body and tail tumors, and both operations carry substantial perioperative morbidity even at high-volume centers, reinforcing why referral to a center with high procedural volume specifically for this operation, rather than a lower-volume center, is associated with meaningfully better perioperative outcomes and should be a routine referral consideration. Adjuvant chemotherapy following resection reduces recurrence risk and is now standard practice for essentially all patients able to tolerate it, and the increasing use of neoadjuvant, rather than purely adjuvant, chemotherapy even in resectable disease reflects evolving evidence that early systemic treatment addresses micrometastatic disease before surgery and may improve the likelihood of a margin-negative resection, representing a meaningful evolution in treatment sequencing philosophy for this specific malignancy. Postoperative complications, including delayed gastric emptying, pancreatic fistula, and postpancreatectomy hemorrhage, require specific institutional protocols and experienced multidisciplinary postoperative management, further reinforcing why referral to a high-volume center, with the accumulated experience to both prevent and manage these specific complications effectively, meaningfully affects patient outcomes beyond the operation itself. Adequate recovery time before initiating adjuvant chemotherapy, generally requiring several weeks after major pancreatic surgery, must be balanced against the risk that excessive delay reduces the treatment's ultimate benefit, requiring close, individualized coordination between surgery and medical oncology.

## Pancreatic Cystic Neoplasms

### Classification: IPMN, MCN, Serous Cystadenoma, and Solid Pseudopapillary Neoplasm

Intraductal papillary mucinous neoplasm, the most commonly encountered pancreatic cystic neoplasm given the frequency of incidental cyst detection on cross-sectional imaging obtained for other indications, is classified by ductal involvement as main-duct, branch-duct, or mixed-type, and this distinction carries substantial prognostic weight, since main-duct involvement carries a significantly higher malignant transformation risk than branch-duct disease alone, directly informing the surveillance intensity and surgical threshold discussed below. Mucinous cystic neoplasm, distinguished from intraductal papillary mucinous neoplasm by its characteristic ovarian-type stroma on histology and its strong predilection for the pancreatic body and tail in middle-aged women, similarly carries malignant potential warranting surgical consideration in most cases given the difficulty reliably excluding malignancy preoperatively. Serous cystadenoma, in contrast, is essentially always benign and does not require surveillance once confidently diagnosed by its characteristic microcystic, honeycomb imaging appearance, and correctly distinguishing this benign entity from the malignant-potential cysts discussed above prevents both unnecessary surveillance burden and unnecessary surgical referral for a lesion that poses no meaningful cancer risk. Solid pseudopapillary neoplasm, an uncommon entity occurring predominantly in young women, has low but genuine malignant potential and is generally treated with surgical resection given both its malignant potential and its tendency to grow to a substantial size if left untreated. The distinction between branch-duct and main-duct involvement is not always perfectly clear-cut on imaging alone, and MRCP, with its superior ductal visualization compared to standard cross-sectional imaging, is generally the preferred modality for this specific classification determination when the distinction is not already obvious on the initial imaging study that identified the cyst. The strong female predominance and characteristic body-tail location of mucinous cystic neoplasm, distinct from the more variable location seen with IPMN, can itself be a useful clinical clue supporting this diagnosis even before histologic confirmation, though imaging and clinical features alone are not always sufficient to distinguish these two entities with complete confidence preoperatively. A small subset of serous cystadenomas can grow large enough to produce mass-effect symptoms, and surgical resection remains an option in this specific symptomatic scenario despite the lesion's benign nature, illustrating that surgical decision-making is not driven by malignant potential alone but also by symptom burden when present. Recurrence after resection of solid pseudopapillary neoplasm is uncommon but recognized, and long-term follow-up imaging, though the required duration and interval are less well established for this rarer entity than for the more common cystic lesions discussed above, is a reasonable component of postoperative surveillance.

Figure 14.2: IPMN Classification: Main-Duct, Branch-Duct, and Mixed-Type

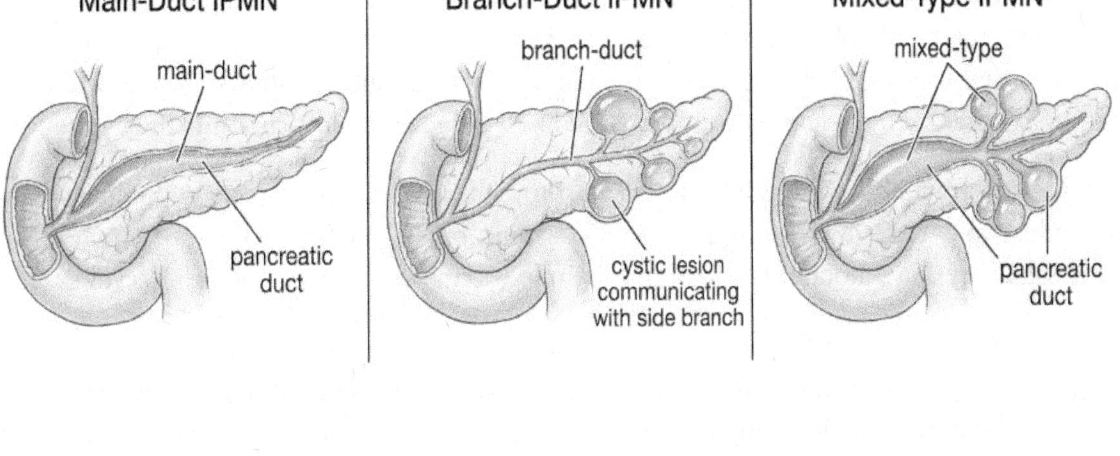

### Risk Stratification and Surveillance

Worrisome features and high-risk stigmata, standardized imaging and clinical findings including cyst size, main pancreatic duct dilation, the presence of a mural nodule or solid component, and, most concerning, obstructive jaundice arising from a cystic lesion in the pancreatic head, stratify intraductal papillary mucinous neoplasm and mucinous cystic neoplasm management, and this graded system, rather than cyst size alone, determines whether continued surveillance, endoscopic ultrasound with fine-needle aspiration for cyst fluid analysis, or surgical referral is the appropriate next step. Cyst fluid analysis, obtained via endoscopic ultrasound-guided fine-needle aspiration, measuring carcinoembryonic antigen level, which helps distinguish mucinous from nonmucinous cysts, amylase, elevated in cysts communicating with the pancreatic ductal system, and, increasingly, molecular analysis for mutations characteristic of mucinous neoplasia, adds diagnostic specificity beyond imaging characteristics alone in cases where the cyst classification remains genuinely uncertain after standard cross-sectional and endoscopic ultrasound imaging. Applying this framework consistently requires the same standardized reporting language across radiology and endoscopy reports that has been emphasized for other risk-stratification systems throughout this book, since inconsistent terminology between reports can otherwise obscure whether a specific finding truly meets a defined worrisome feature or high-risk stigmata criterion. The procedural risk of endoscopic ultrasound-guided fine-needle aspiration, including pancreatitis and, rarely, bleeding or infection, though generally low, should be weighed against the added diagnostic certainty it provides, and this procedure is reserved for cases where the additional information would genuinely change management rather than performed routinely on every incidentally identified cyst regardless of its baseline risk profile.

### THE GI THRESHOLD DECISION SYSTEM — Pancreatobiliary Thresholds — Surgical Referral in Branch-Duct IPMN

---

**Presentation Signature:** A patient with a confirmed branch-duct intraductal papillary mucinous neoplasm is undergoing periodic surveillance imaging, and the clinician must determine whether continued surveillance or surgical referral is appropriate at each reassessment.

**Threshold Point:** The presence of any high-risk stigmata, including obstructive jaundice from the cyst, an enhancing mural nodule of significant size, or main pancreatic duct dilation above a defined threshold, defines the threshold for surgical referral; worrisome features without high-risk stigmata define a threshold for endoscopic ultrasound evaluation and intensified surveillance rather than immediate surgery.

**The Call:** Cysts with high-risk stigmata are referred for surgical resection; cysts with worrisome features undergo endoscopic ultrasound with fine-needle aspiration to further risk-stratify before a surgical decision is made; cysts without either feature continue routine surveillance at an interval determined by cyst size.

**Trap Logic:** Applying a uniform surveillance interval regardless of cyst size or feature evolution, or conversely referring every incidentally discovered cyst for surgery reflexively regardless of risk features, both fail to match intervention intensity to the actual, individualized malignancy risk a given cyst presents.

**Decision Anchor:** Apply the standardized worrisome-feature and high-risk-stigmata framework at every surveillance reassessment, and escalate to endoscopic ultrasound or surgical referral specifically when these defined criteria are met rather than through a size-only or uniformly conservative or uniformly aggressive default approach.

## Pancreatic Neuroendocrine Tumors

### Functional Versus Nonfunctional Tumors

Pancreatic neuroendocrine tumors are classified as functional, producing a clinical hormone-excess syndrome from active hormone secretion, or nonfunctional, the majority of cases, in which the tumor does not produce a recognizable hormone-excess syndrome despite sometimes retaining hormone-staining characteristics on pathology, and this functional status, rather than tumor grade alone, substantially shapes the clinical presentation and initial diagnostic approach. Insulinoma, the most common functional subtype, produces Whipple's triad, hypoglycemic symptoms, a documented low glucose at the time of symptoms, and symptom resolution with glucose administration, while gastrinoma produces the severe, treatment-refractory peptic ulcer disease and secretory diarrhea characteristic of Zollinger-Ellison syndrome, and recognizing these specific hormone-excess presentations, rather than a generic mass-related symptom complex, is essential for timely diagnosis given how differently these functional tumors present compared to nonfunctional disease. Multiple endocrine neoplasia type 1 syndrome should be considered specifically in a patient with multiple pancreatic neuroendocrine tumors, or a single tumor accompanied by concurrent parathyroid or pituitary abnormalities, since this syndrome's characteristic combination of endocrine tumors across multiple organ systems provides an important diagnostic and family-counseling clue that a solitary sporadic tumor would not carry. Less common functional subtypes, including glucagonoma, presenting with a characteristic migratory necrolytic erythema rash alongside new diabetes, VIPoma, producing profuse secretory diarrhea and electrolyte derangement, and somatostatinoma, producing a triad of diabetes, gallstones, and steatorrhea, each present with their own distinctive hormone-excess syndrome that, once recognized, points directly toward the underlying functional tumor subtype responsible.

### Diagnostic Evaluation and Management

Diagnostic evaluation of a suspected functional tumor centers on biochemical confirmation of the specific hormone-excess syndrome, a supervised fasting test with serial glucose and insulin measurement for suspected insulinoma, or fasting serum gastrin, ideally after withholding proton pump inhibitor therapy for an adequate washout period, for suspected gastrinoma, before proceeding to localization imaging, since biochemical confirmation should generally precede the search for the tumor itself rather than the reverse. Somatostatin receptor imaging, exploiting the high somatostatin receptor expression characteristic of most neuroendocrine tumors, provides both localization and, in some cases, prognostic information beyond conventional cross-sectional imaging alone, and surgical resection remains the primary treatment for localized disease, while somatostatin analogue therapy, targeting the same receptor pathway used diagnostically, provides both symptomatic hormone-excess control and, in appropriately selected patients, antiproliferative benefit in unresectable or metastatic disease. Tumor grading, based on proliferative index measured by Ki-67 staining and mitotic count, provides important prognostic information independent of functional status, and low-grade, well-differentiated tumors, even when metastatic, can follow a substantially more indolent course than the grading terminology might otherwise suggest to a patient unfamiliar with neuroendocrine tumor biology specifically. Peptide receptor radionuclide therapy, delivering targeted radiation directly to somatostatin-receptor-expressing tumor cells, offers an additional treatment option for progressive, unresectable neuroendocrine tumors that continue to express somatostatin receptors on imaging, representing a targeted radiotherapeutic approach reserved for patients whose disease has progressed despite somatostatin analogue therapy.

**Figure 14.3. Somatostatin receptor imaging in neuroendocrine tumors**

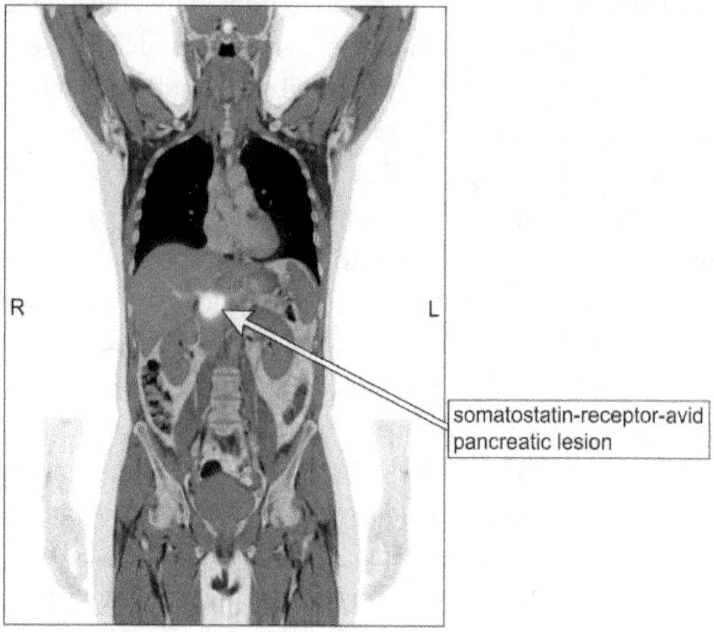


## Palliative Care and Symptom Management in Advanced Pancreatobiliary Malignancy

Biliary obstruction in unresectable pancreatic or biliary malignancy is palliated with endoscopic stenting, generally preferred over percutaneous or surgical bypass given its lower morbidity, and stent selection, self-expanding metal stents for patients with a longer anticipated survival given their greater patency duration compared to plastic stents, which are more appropriate for a shorter anticipated survival or when a subsequent surgical intervention might alter the biliary anatomy, should be individualized to the patient's overall prognosis and treatment plan rather than a single default stent type applied uniformly. Duodenal obstruction, a common complication of advanced pancreatic head malignancy from local tumor extension, is palliated with either endoscopic duodenal stenting or surgical gastrojejunostomy bypass, and the choice between these approaches depends on the patient's overall prognosis and performance status, with endoscopic stenting generally favored in patients with more limited life expectancy given its lower procedural burden, while surgical bypass may be preferred in patients with better prognosis given its greater durability. Stent occlusion presenting as recurrent jaundice or cholangitis in a patient with an existing biliary stent should prompt prompt stent exchange rather than an extensive re-evaluation for other causes, since this is by far the most common explanation for recurrent biliary symptoms in this specific clinical context. A careful assessment for concurrent biliary obstruction before pursuing duodenal stenting is essential, since placing a duodenal stent across the ampulla can complicate future biliary access, making the sequence and coordination of these two interventions, when both are needed, an important planning consideration best addressed collaboratively between the involved specialists.

### Pain Management and Celiac Plexus Neurolysis

Pain from locally advanced or metastatic pancreatic cancer, often severe and refractory to standard oral analgesic escalation, can be addressed with celiac plexus neurolysis, chemically ablating the celiac plexus nerve fibers that transmit visceral pain signals from the pancreas, performed under endoscopic ultrasound guidance, and this procedure, while not curative, can meaningfully reduce opioid requirements and improve quality of life in appropriately selected patients, representing an important palliative tool that should be considered proactively rather than only after maximal oral analgesic therapy has already failed to control pain adequately. Referral to an endoscopist with specific experience in this technique, given its specialized nature, and coordination with the patient's oncology and palliative care team ensures this intervention is integrated appropriately into their broader pain management plan rather than pursued in isolation. Coordination beats isolated care.

## Psychosocial Impact and Multidisciplinary Care in Pancreatic Cancer

Pancreatic cancer carries a uniquely severe psychosocial burden given its typically poor prognosis, the physically demanding nature of both the disease and its treatment, and the specific weight loss, pain, and exocrine insufficiency symptoms discussed elsewhere in this book that compound the emotional burden of the diagnosis itself, and integrating palliative care early, alongside rather than only after disease-directed treatment has been exhausted, applying the same early-integration principle increasingly recognized across oncology more broadly, improves quality of life and, in some studies, may even modestly improve survival compared with palliative care introduced only late in the disease course. Screening for anxiety and depression, applying the same routine screening standard already established throughout this book, deserves particular emphasis in this population given both the severity of the diagnosis and the physical symptom burden that can compound psychological distress, and coordinating this mental health support alongside oncology, palliative care, and nutrition services within a genuinely multidisciplinary program provides more comprehensive support than any single specialty could offer independently. Caregiver burden in pancreatic cancer is also substantial given the disease's typically rapid trajectory and intensive care needs, and screening caregivers themselves for burnout and distress, not only the patient, is a reasonable component of comprehensive supportive care that is sometimes overlooked when clinical attention is understandably focused primarily on the patient. Timing this integration explicitly at diagnosis, rather than waiting for a formal referral trigger later in the disease course, sets the expectation from the outset that palliative care is a collaborative partner throughout treatment, not a marker of treatment failure introduced only near the end of life.

### Nutritional Support in Pancreatic Cancer

Exocrine pancreatic insufficiency, whether from the tumor itself obstructing pancreatic secretory flow or from surgical resection of a substantial portion of the gland, is common in pancreatic cancer and should be proactively screened for and treated with pancreatic enzyme replacement therapy, applying the same principles developed in the twelfth chapter for chronic pancreatitis-related exocrine insufficiency, since untreated malabsorption compounds the weight loss and nutritional decline that independently worsen both quality of life and treatment tolerance in this already vulnerable population. Dietitian involvement early in the treatment course, rather than only after significant weight loss has already occurred, supports more proactive nutritional management and may help preserve treatment tolerance by maintaining better overall nutritional status throughout an often physically demanding treatment course. Regular reassessment of nutritional status, not a single evaluation at diagnosis alone, captures the evolving needs of a patient whose disease and treatment tolerance change over the course of illness. Always.

## Rare Pancreatic Neoplasms and Metastatic Disease to the Pancreas

Acinar cell carcinoma, an uncommon pancreatic malignancy distinct histologically and biologically from the far more common ductal adenocarcinoma, occasionally produces a distinctive paraneoplastic syndrome from excess lipase secretion, causing subcutaneous fat necrosis and polyarthralgia, and recognizing this specific paraneoplastic presentation, though rare, can provide an important diagnostic clue in a patient presenting with these unusual systemic findings alongside a pancreatic mass. Pancreatoblastoma, occurring predominantly in children, and metastatic disease to the pancreas from a distant primary malignancy, most commonly renal cell carcinoma given its recognized tendency for delayed, sometimes solitary pancreatic metastasis even many years after treatment of the original kidney tumor, round out the differential for a pancreatic mass and should be considered specifically when the clinical history includes a prior malignancy, particularly renal cell carcinoma, that might explain an atypically presenting pancreatic lesion. Correctly identifying this rare paraneoplastic syndrome prevents a potentially prolonged and unproductive rheumatologic or dermatologic workup pursued in isolation from the underlying pancreatic diagnosis, when in fact both the skin and joint findings would be expected to resolve once the underlying malignancy is definitively treated. A structured review of the patient's full oncologic history, not just their current symptoms, should be part of the initial evaluation of any new pancreatic mass, since a distant prior malignancy years earlier can easily be overlooked or considered unrelated if it is not specifically elicited during history-taking. Rare presentations deserve documentation for future learning. Yes.

### The Value of Tissue Diagnosis Before Treatment

Given the substantial differences in prognosis and treatment approach among these various pancreatic mass etiologies, adenocarcinoma, neuroendocrine tumor, acinar cell carcinoma, lymphoma, and metastatic disease from a distant primary, obtaining tissue diagnosis before committing to a treatment plan, rather than presuming ductal adenocarcinoma based on imaging appearance and clinical context alone, is essential in any case where the diagnosis is not already unambiguous, since a pancreatic mass that turns out to be lymphoma, for example, would be treated with an entirely different, chemotherapy-based approach rather than the surgical-first pathway appropriate for ductal adenocarcinoma. Communicating with the patient about the reason for a delay in finalizing their treatment plan, when tissue diagnosis takes additional time to complete, helps manage the understandable anxiety that accompanies any delay between an initial concerning finding and a definitive treatment start date. Patience here protects patients from mistreatment. Truly.

## Pancreatic Lymphoma and Metastasis-Mimicking Presentations

Primary pancreatic lymphoma, an uncommon but important diagnosis to exclude given its dramatically different, chemotherapy-based treatment approach compared with ductal adenocarcinoma, should be specifically considered when a pancreatic mass presents with a bulky, relatively homogeneous appearance without the ductal obstruction or vascular encasement more typical of adenocarcinoma, and endoscopic ultrasound-guided biopsy with adequate tissue for flow cytometry and immunohistochemistry, rather than the more limited sampling sometimes adequate for adenocarcinoma diagnosis alone, is essential when this diagnosis is genuinely being considered, since a definitive lymphoma diagnosis requires this more extensive tissue characterization. Autoimmune pancreatitis, discussed in detail in the twelfth chapter, remains an important entity to reconsider whenever a pancreatic mass workup is pursued, since its imaging mimicry of pancreatic adenocarcinoma means this diagnosis should be actively revisited, not simply assumed excluded, whenever a mass lesion's biopsy or clinical course raises any doubt about a straightforward adenocarcinoma diagnosis. Staging for lymphoma, once diagnosed, differs substantially from the pancreatic-adenocarcinoma-specific staging system discussed earlier in this chapter, following the standard lymphoma staging framework instead, which further underscores why an accurate tissue diagnosis at the outset is essential to selecting the correct staging and treatment pathway from the start. This active reconsideration is especially important given the framework this book has emphasized throughout: an initial working diagnosis, however reasonable at the time, should always remain open to revision when subsequent findings do not fully align with the expected clinical course. This distinction changes everything downstream.

### Multidisciplinary Tumor Board Review for Diagnostic Uncertainty

Genuinely uncertain pancreatic mass cases, where imaging, biopsy, and clinical context do not converge cleanly on a single diagnosis, benefit substantially from dedicated multidisciplinary tumor board discussion involving radiology, pathology, gastroenterology, and surgical oncology together, applying the same collaborative diagnostic model already established in earlier chapters for other complex gastrointestinal malignancies, since this collective review can identify diagnostic possibilities or additional testing needs that might be overlooked when a single specialty manages a complex case in relative isolation from the others. Even when a case does not initially seem to require this level of collaborative discussion, a low threshold for requesting tumor board input, rather than waiting until a case has already become genuinely difficult, allows earlier course correction if the working diagnosis proves incorrect. Collective wisdom outperforms isolated judgment. Indeed.

## Pancreatic Cancer Chemotherapy Regimens and Emerging Therapies

Combination chemotherapy regimens, most commonly FOLFIRINOX, combining fluorouracil, leucovorin, irinotecan, and oxaliplatin, or gemcitabine plus nab-paclitaxel, form the backbone of systemic therapy for pancreatic adenocarcinoma across the neoadjuvant, adjuvant, and metastatic treatment settings, and regimen selection is individualized based on performance status, comorbidities, and treatment goals, since FOLFIRINOX, while generally more effective, carries a substantially higher toxicity burden that limits its use to patients with adequate functional reserve to tolerate this more intensive regimen. Molecular profiling of the tumor, increasingly performed alongside the germline testing discussed earlier in this chapter, can identify actionable somatic alterations in a subset of patients, including microsatellite instability predicting response to immune checkpoint inhibition, applying the same biomarker-directed therapy principle already established in the eleventh chapter for colorectal cancer, and specific fusion alterations that may respond to targeted therapy, reinforcing why comprehensive molecular characterization, not just germline testing alone, is increasingly incorporated into the initial workup of newly diagnosed pancreatic cancer. Dose modification and supportive care, including growth factor support and antiemetic optimization, allow many patients with borderline functional status to tolerate more intensive regimens than might initially seem feasible, and this individualized dose adjustment approach, rather than a binary decision between full-intensity and no chemotherapy at all, better serves patients across a range of baseline fitness levels. Turnaround time for comprehensive molecular profiling can be several weeks, and this timeline should be factored into treatment planning so that starting systemic therapy is not unnecessarily delayed while awaiting results that, in most cases, will not change the initial treatment recommendation. Individualized dosing serves patients better than rigid protocols.

### Clinical Trial Enrollment and Access to Emerging Therapies

Given the persistent limitations of current standard therapy for pancreatic adenocarcinoma, clinical trial enrollment should be actively considered and discussed with every eligible patient at diagnosis and at each major treatment decision point, rather than reserved as a last resort only after all standard options have been exhausted, since many of the most promising emerging therapies, including novel targeted agents and immunotherapy combinations, are accessible only through trial participation, and referral to a center with an active pancreatic cancer clinical trials program, even when the patient's primary care continues locally, can meaningfully expand their treatment options without requiring them to transfer their entire care to that center. Even a brief, direct mention of trial availability, rather than a lengthy separate conversation, plants the idea and gives the patient permission to ask more questions if interested, without requiring the primary treating team to become experts in every open trial themselves.

## Incidental Pancreatic Findings and Duodenal Subepithelial Lesions

An incidentally discovered solid pancreatic lesion, identified on imaging obtained for an unrelated indication, warrants a systematic evaluation rather than immediate biopsy or dismissal, beginning with dedicated pancreatic protocol imaging to characterize the lesion's specific features, since a small, incidentally discovered solid lesion could represent anything from a benign entity such as focal fatty infiltration or an accessory spleen mimicking a mass, to a small, early-stage pancreatic neuroendocrine tumor, to early adenocarcinoma, and each of these possibilities requires a different subsequent evaluation pathway. Multidisciplinary discussion, particularly for small, indeterminate lesions where the balance between overdiagnosis and missing a genuine early malignancy is genuinely difficult to judge from imaging characteristics alone, supports a more considered approach than either reflexive biopsy of every small incidental finding or reflexive dismissal of findings that might represent clinically significant early disease. Documenting the specific rationale for the chosen follow-up interval or investigation strategy in the medical record supports continuity of care if the patient is subsequently evaluated by a different clinician who was not present for the original discussion. Good documentation is a gift to future clinicians.

### Ampullary and Periampullary Subepithelial Lesions

Subepithelial lesions identified near the ampulla during upper endoscopy, distinct from the mucosal ampullary adenomas discussed earlier in this chapter, require careful characterization with endoscopic ultrasound to determine the layer of origin and likely histology, since this anatomic location can harbor a range of entities from benign lipomas and leiomyomas to gastrointestinal stromal tumors carrying their own malignant potential, and accurate characterization before any biopsy attempt is particularly important in this specific location given the technical difficulty and complication risk of biopsying lesions in close proximity to both the pancreatic and bile ducts. Referral to an endoscopist with specific experience in this anatomically complex region, rather than pursuing an unfamiliar biopsy attempt without this specialized background, meaningfully reduces the risk of an avoidable complication in this technically demanding location. Expertise matters most in tight anatomic spaces.

## Age-Related Considerations Across Pancreatobiliary Neoplasia

Pancreatic and biliary malignancies in younger patients, while less common overall than in older adults, carry particular diagnostic challenges since these conditions are less anticipated by clinicians in this age group, and unexplained pancreatobiliary symptoms in a younger patient should not be dismissed simply because malignancy is statistically less likely, particularly when a hereditary predisposition syndrome, discussed earlier in this chapter, might explain an earlier-than-typical age of onset. Older adults, conversely, require careful individualized assessment of overall functional status and treatment tolerance before committing to an intensive multimodality treatment approach, since chronologic age alone is an imperfect predictor of a patient's ability to tolerate major pancreatic surgery or intensive chemotherapy, and a formal geriatric assessment, incorporating functional status, cognition, and comorbidity burden, provides a more complete picture than age alone when planning treatment intensity in this population. Explaining this diagnostic uncertainty honestly to a younger patient, rather than either dismissing symptoms prematurely or alarming them unnecessarily, supports a balanced, appropriately paced evaluation that neither delays a genuine diagnosis nor subjects a young patient to excessive worry. Balance protects patients emotionally too.

### Treatment Decision-Making in Frail or Elderly Patients

A frail or elderly patient with newly diagnosed pancreatic or biliary malignancy benefits from the same explicit, values-based goals-of-care conversation already emphasized elsewhere in this book for other populations with limited physiologic reserve, weighing the potential benefit of aggressive, curative-intent treatment against its considerable burden in a patient whose overall life expectancy or functional status may substantially limit the realistic benefit achievable, and this conversation should be revisited as treatment proceeds and the patient's actual tolerance becomes clearer, rather than fixed permanently based on an initial assessment made before treatment has even begun. Involving family members appropriately, with the patient's consent, in these goals-of-care discussions can provide valuable additional perspective while still keeping the patient's own values and wishes central to the final decision. Values should always guide the plan.

## Cholangiocarcinoma and Ampullary Neoplasia

### Cholangiocarcinoma Staging and Management

Cholangiocarcinoma, introduced in the previous chapter, is anatomically classified as intrahepatic, arising within the liver parenchyma and often presenting as a mass lesion rather than with the biliary obstruction more typical of the other subtypes, perihilar, arising at or near the confluence of the right and left hepatic ducts and historically termed a Klatskin tumor, or distal, arising in the extrahepatic bile duct closer to the ampulla, and this anatomic classification directly determines surgical approach, since perihilar tumors often require extensive hepatic resection alongside biliary reconstruction while distal tumors are managed with the same pancreaticoduodenectomy approach used for pancreatic head adenocarcinoma given their shared anatomic location. Preoperative biliary drainage in a patient with resectable perihilar cholangiocarcinoma and significant jaundice is individualized rather than routine, since drainage can reduce surgical risk from severe cholestasis but also carries its own infection and stent-related complication risk, and this decision should be made collaboratively between hepatobiliary surgery and interventional endoscopy or radiology based on the specific severity of jaundice and planned surgical timeline rather than a uniform default practice applied to every jaundiced surgical candidate. Bismuth-Corlette classification further subdivides perihilar cholangiocarcinoma by the specific extent of ductal involvement at the hepatic hilum, and this classification directly informs the extent of hepatic resection required, since more extensive ductal involvement generally necessitates more extensive concurrent liver resection to achieve an adequate margin. Future liver remnant volume assessment, calculating the anticipated functional liver volume remaining after the planned resection, is another essential preoperative planning step specific to perihilar cholangiocarcinoma surgery, since an inadequate remnant volume risks postoperative liver failure regardless of how technically successful the resection itself proves to be.

**Ampullary Adenoma and Carcinoma**

Ampullary adenomas, benign precursor lesions arising at the ampulla of Vater, carry malignant potential following an adenoma-to-carcinoma progression pathway similar to the colorectal sequence discussed in the eleventh chapter, and endoscopic ampullectomy, removing the lesion endoscopically during a specialized procedure distinct from standard polypectomy given the ampulla's unique anatomic relationship to both the pancreatic and bile ducts, is an effective, less invasive alternative to surgical resection for appropriately selected adenomas without evidence of invasive carcinoma, performed at centers with specific expertise given the technical demands and complication risks, including pancreatitis and bleeding, that this specific procedure carries. Ampullary adenomas occurring in the context of familial adenomatous polyposis, introduced in the eleventh chapter, warrant the same syndrome-specific surveillance intensity already established for duodenal polyposis in that condition, reinforcing the value of recognizing when an ampullary finding is an isolated, sporadic lesion versus a manifestation of an underlying hereditary polyposis syndrome requiring its own dedicated, ongoing surveillance program. Endoscopic surveillance after ampullectomy is essential given the recognized recurrence risk even after apparently complete resection, and this ongoing surveillance commitment, following a defined interval protocol, should be discussed with the patient explicitly at the time the ampullectomy is planned rather than presented only afterward as an unanticipated additional requirement.

Case Presentation: A 64-year-old man presents with painless jaundice, and workup reveals a 2.5-centimeter mass in the pancreatic head. Endoscopic ultrasound-guided biopsy confirms pancreatic adenocarcinoma, and dedicated pancreatic protocol CT demonstrates the tumor abutting less than 180 degrees of the superior mesenteric vein circumference without arterial involvement. Applying the resectability criteria developed in this chapter, this vascular relationship classifies the tumor as resectable, and he is presented at multidisciplinary tumor board where increasingly favored neoadjuvant chemotherapy, rather than immediate surgery, is recommended given evolving evidence supporting this sequencing even in resectable disease. He completes neoadjuvant chemotherapy with a favorable radiographic response and undergoes pancreaticoduodenectomy at a high-volume center, achieving a margin-negative resection. He completes adjuvant chemotherapy per current standard practice. This case illustrates the chapter's central resectability principle: precise vascular relationship assessment, not tumor size or a general impression of extent, determined his treatment pathway, and referral to a high-volume surgical center for his ultimately curative-intent operation reflected the same access-to-expertise principle emphasized throughout this book for complex, high-risk procedures.

Case Presentation: A 61-year-old woman has a 2.8-centimeter branch-duct intraductal papillary mucinous neoplasm in the pancreatic tail, followed with annual surveillance imaging for three years without change. At her most recent surveillance MRI, the cyst has grown to 3.4 centimeters, and a new 9-millimeter enhancing mural nodule is identified within the cyst. Applying the reasoning developed in this chapter, this enhancing mural nodule meets high-risk stigmata criteria, defining the threshold for surgical referral rather than continued surveillance or even endoscopic ultrasound reassessment alone. She is referred to hepatobiliary surgery and undergoes distal pancreatectomy, with final pathology demonstrating high-grade dysplasia without invasive carcinoma. This case illustrates the chapter's core surveillance principle:

a specific, defined high-risk stigmata finding, not simply cyst growth in isolation, is what crossed the threshold to surgical referral, and the favorable pathologic outcome, high-grade dysplasia caught before progression to invasive cancer, reflects the value of consistent, structured surveillance in identifying this transition at an actionable point.

## Genetic Counseling and Hereditary Pancreatic Cancer Syndromes

Germline genetic testing is now recommended for essentially all patients newly diagnosed with pancreatic adenocarcinoma regardless of family history, reflecting the same universal testing philosophy already established in the eleventh chapter for colorectal cancer, given evidence that a meaningful proportion of pancreatic cancer patients carry a clinically actionable germline pathogenic variant even without a suggestive family history, and identifying such a variant carries both treatment implications, since certain variants, particularly in BRCA1 and BRCA2, predict enhanced sensitivity to platinum-based chemotherapy and PARP inhibitor maintenance therapy, and family counseling implications for at-risk relatives. Cascade testing for identified relatives, applying the same structured process already developed in the eleventh chapter for hereditary colorectal cancer syndromes, allows at-risk family members to access the high-risk pancreatic cancer surveillance program discussed earlier in this chapter, converting a single patient's diagnosis into an opportunity for earlier detection across their extended family. Insurance coverage for this testing has generally improved as it has become more standard of care, though coverage variability still exists across different payers and regions, and awareness of local coverage patterns helps clinicians counsel patients accurately about potential out-of-pocket costs before testing is pursued. Providing the index patient with clear written information about their specific genetic finding, suitable for sharing directly with relatives, supports this cascade process practically rather than relying solely on the patient's own recollection of a complex genetic counseling conversation. Clarity helps families.

### Structuring the High-Risk Surveillance Program

High-risk individuals entering a pancreatic cancer surveillance program should have this care coordinated at a center with specific expertise in this relatively specialized surveillance protocol, given the technical demands of endoscopic ultrasound interpretation in this context and the psychological burden of ongoing surveillance for a malignancy that, even when caught through surveillance, often still carries significant treatment complexity; providing these patients with realistic expectations about both the benefits and the genuine limitations of current surveillance technology supports informed, sustained engagement with what is typically a lifelong surveillance commitment. A dedicated care coordinator or nurse navigator for this specific surveillance population can meaningfully improve adherence to the recommended imaging schedule, particularly given the alternating multi-modality protocol these programs often use, which can be more complex to track than a single-test, single-interval screening protocol. Peer support connecting these high-risk individuals with others navigating the same surveillance journey can also provide valuable practical and emotional support beyond what the medical team alone typically offers. Support matters deeply.

| Cystic Lesion | Malignant Potential | Key Distinguishing Feature |
|---|---|---|
| Branch-duct IPMN | Low to moderate | Cyst communicating with a side branch duct |
| Main-duct IPMN | High | Main pancreatic duct dilation |
| Mucinous cystic neoplasm | Moderate to high | Ovarian-type stroma; body/tail, middle-aged women |
| Serous cystadenoma | Essentially none | Microcystic, honeycomb appearance |
| Solid pseudopapillary neoplasm | Low but present | Young women; solid and cystic components |

### THE GI THRESHOLD DECISION SYSTEM — Pancreatobiliary Neoplasia Thresholds

**Presentation Signature:** This chapter's threshold instances addressed resectability classification in pancreatic adenocarcinoma and surgical referral criteria in branch-duct IPMN surveillance.

**Threshold Point:** Specific vascular contact criteria on dedicated imaging gate resectability classification; specific worrisome features and high-risk stigmata gate surgical referral in IPMN.

**The Call:** Both thresholds replace size-based or subjective impression with standardized, criteria-based classification that directly determines the treatment pathway pursued.

**Trap Logic:** Assessing resectability by general impression rather than specific vascular criteria, and applying a uniform surveillance or surgical-referral approach to IPMN regardless of the standardized risk-feature framework, are this chapter's most consequential threshold misapplications.

**Decision Anchor:** Classify pancreatic adenocarcinoma resectability using specific vascular contact criteria reviewed collaboratively, and apply the standardized worrisome-feature and high-risk-stigmata framework at every IPMN surveillance reassessment rather than defaulting to a size-only or uniform approach.

## Summary and Key Concepts

Pancreatic adenocarcinoma screening is reserved for confirmed high-risk individuals meeting genetic or strong family history criteria, and new-onset diabetes with weight loss in a patient over 50 is an underappreciated early clue warranting consideration of pancreatic imaging.

Resectability is determined by the tumor's specific relationship to peripancreatic vasculature, not size alone, and this classification directs the choice among upfront surgery, neoadjuvant therapy, or systemic therapy alone.

Referral to a high-volume surgical center for pancreaticoduodenectomy or distal pancreatectomy is associated with meaningfully better perioperative outcomes than lower-volume centers.

Pancreatic cystic neoplasms are classified by type, IPMN, MCN, serous cystadenoma, or solid pseudopapillary neoplasm, and worrisome features and high-risk stigmata, not cyst size alone, determine surveillance intensity and surgical referral in IPMN and MCN.

Functional pancreatic neuroendocrine tumors, including insulinoma and gastrinoma, present with recognizable hormone-excess syndromes, and biochemical confirmation should generally precede localization imaging in suspected functional disease.

Cholangiocarcinoma's anatomic classification, intrahepatic, perihilar, or distal, directly determines surgical approach, and ampullary adenomas can often be managed with endoscopic ampullectomy rather than surgical resection in appropriately selected cases.

# CHAPTER 15: EVALUATION OF ABNORMAL LIVER CHEMISTRIES AND ACUTE LIVER INJURY

**Learning Objectives**

1. Classify abnormal liver chemistries into hepatocellular, cholestatic, and mixed patterns and apply a structured diagnostic approach to each.
2. Distinguish acute liver injury from acute liver failure and identify the specific criteria defining each.
3. Recognize and manage acetaminophen-induced liver injury, including the specific threshold for N-acetylcysteine therapy.
4. Apply a structured diagnostic approach to suspected drug-induced liver injury beyond acetaminophen.
5. Recognize ischemic hepatitis and apply appropriate criteria for liver transplant referral in acute liver failure.

**Chapter Outline**

This chapter develops a systematic approach to abnormal liver chemistries, beginning with pattern recognition, hepatocellular, cholestatic, or mixed, and the specific diagnostic pathway each pattern implies, before addressing acute liver injury and acute liver failure, acetaminophen and other drug-induced liver injury, the standard diagnostic workup, and ischemic hepatitis. Each section connects a specific biochemical pattern or severity threshold to a defined diagnostic or management pathway.

## Approach to Abnormal Liver Chemistries

### Patterns of Liver Injury: Hepatocellular, Cholestatic, and Mixed

Abnormal liver chemistries are classified by pattern using the R-value, calculated as the ratio of the alanine aminotransferase elevation relative to its upper limit of normal divided by the alkaline phosphatase elevation relative to its upper limit of normal, with a value above 5 indicating a hepatocellular pattern, a value below 2 indicating a cholestatic pattern, and an intermediate value indicating a mixed pattern, and this calculated ratio, rather than simply noting that both enzymes are elevated, should be the first analytic step in any new abnormal liver chemistry evaluation since the resulting pattern fundamentally redirects the entire subsequent diagnostic workup. A hepatocellular pattern points toward the differential developed later in this chapter, including viral hepatitis, drug-induced injury, and ischemic hepatitis, while a cholestatic pattern points toward the biliary obstruction and cholestatic liver disease differential developed in the previous chapter and a later chapter of this book, and applying the wrong differential to a given pattern, for example pursuing an extensive viral hepatitis workup in a patient whose R-value actually indicates a cholestatic process, wastes time and resources while delaying the correct diagnostic pathway. Recalculating the R-value at each subsequent liver chemistry reassessment, rather than relying on a single initial classification, captures cases where the injury pattern evolves over the course of an evaluation, which can itself provide additional diagnostic information about the underlying process. This first step sets the entire evaluation on the right track.

**Figure 15.1:** R-Value Calculation and Liver Injury Pattern Classification

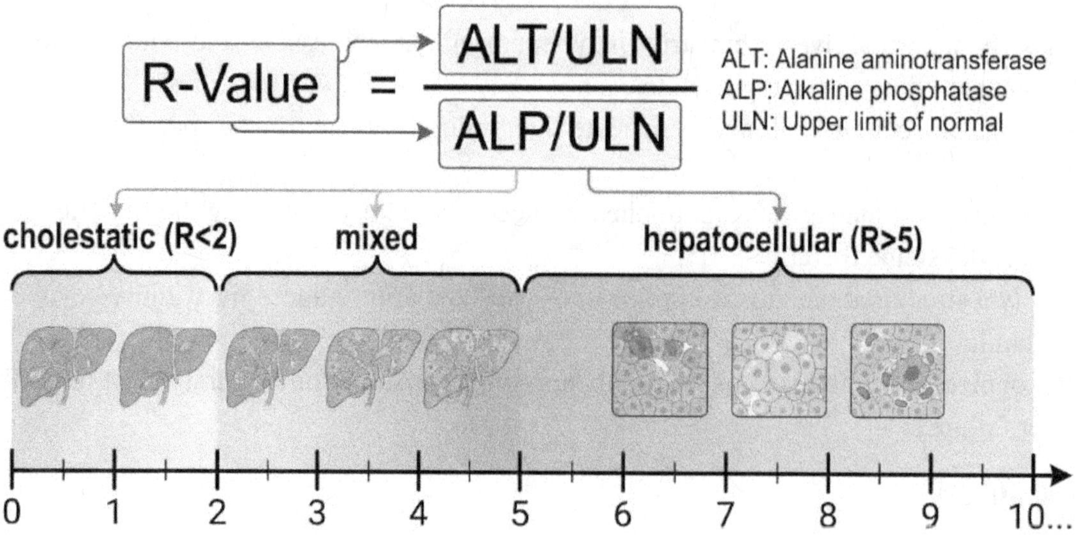


### Interpreting Elevated Aminotransferases

The magnitude of aminotransferase elevation itself carries diagnostic information: mild elevations, generally less than five times the upper limit of normal, are compatible with a broad range of causes including chronic viral hepatitis, metabolic dysfunction-associated steatotic liver disease discussed in the following chapter, and medication effect, while marked elevations, often exceeding ten to twenty times the upper limit of normal or more, narrow the differential substantially toward acute viral hepatitis, ischemic hepatitis, acetaminophen toxicity, or autoimmune hepatitis, each of which is capable of producing this degree of acute hepatocellular injury. The relative magnitude of aspartate aminotransferase compared to alanine aminotransferase also carries diagnostic weight, with an aspartate-to-alanine ratio greater than 2, particularly when both values are only modestly elevated, suggestive of alcohol-related liver injury, reflecting the specific pattern of mitochondrial enzyme release characteristic of alcohol-mediated hepatocyte injury discussed further in the following chapter. A very markedly elevated aminotransferase level, particularly when accompanied by a disproportionately modest bilirubin elevation, should specifically prompt consideration of ischemic hepatitis or acute viral or toxic injury discussed throughout this chapter, since these acute processes are more likely to produce the most dramatic elevations compared to the more gradual, sustained elevations typical of chronic liver disease. Magnitude alone, however, is never sufficient without the clinical context.

## Interpreting Elevated Alkaline Phosphatase and Bilirubin

Elevated alkaline phosphatase, before being attributed to liver disease, should be confirmed as hepatobiliary in origin using gamma-glutamyl transferase or an alkaline phosphatase isoenzyme panel, since alkaline phosphatase is also produced by bone, placenta, and intestine, and an elevated value without this confirmatory step risks pursuing an unnecessary hepatobiliary workup for what may instead reflect bone turnover, pregnancy, or another nonhepatic source entirely. Bilirubin elevation is further classified as predominantly unconjugated, most commonly reflecting increased bilirubin production from hemolysis or a benign conjugation disorder such as Gilbert syndrome, or predominantly conjugated, reflecting impaired hepatocellular excretion or biliary obstruction, and this fractionation, rather than total bilirubin alone, should guide the subsequent workup, since an isolated unconjugated hyperbilirubinemia in an otherwise well patient with normal other liver chemistries generally requires reassurance and confirmation of Gilbert syndrome rather than the more extensive workup an elevated conjugated bilirubin would warrant. A concurrently elevated gamma-glutamyl transferase alongside the alkaline phosphatase supports a hepatobiliary source, while a normal gamma-glutamyl transferase in the setting of an isolated alkaline phosphatase elevation should prompt consideration of a bone or other nonhepatic source before pursuing further liver-directed testing. Gilbert syndrome, an extremely common, benign genetic conjugation disorder producing mild, fluctuating unconjugated hyperbilirubinemia often exacerbated by fasting, illness, or stress, requires no treatment and does not progress to liver disease, and confirming this diagnosis clinically, without further invasive testing, in a patient with the classic isolated, mild, unconjugated pattern and otherwise normal liver chemistries provides significant reassurance and avoids an unnecessary extensive workup. This confirmation step is simple but often skipped. Reassurance grounded in evidence beats vague reassurance alone.

## THE GI THRESHOLD DECISION SYSTEM — Hepatic Thresholds — Pattern-Based Triage of Abnormal Liver Chemistries

**Presentation Signature:** A patient presents with newly identified abnormal liver chemistries, and the clinician must determine the appropriate diagnostic pathway before pursuing further testing.

**Threshold Point:** The calculated R-value, using the alanine aminotransferase and alkaline phosphatase elevations relative to their respective upper limits of normal, defines the threshold separating hepatocellular, cholestatic, and mixed injury patterns, and this classification must be established before selecting subsequent diagnostic tests.

**The Call:** A hepatocellular pattern directs the workup toward viral hepatitis serologies, autoimmune markers, and a medication and toxin history; a cholestatic pattern directs the workup toward biliary imaging and the cholestatic liver disease differential; a mixed pattern requires a broader initial evaluation encompassing both differentials until the picture clarifies.

**Trap Logic:** Ordering a broad, undifferentiated panel of liver-related tests without first calculating the injury pattern wastes resources on tests poorly matched to the actual underlying process and can produce misleading incidental findings that complicate rather than clarify the diagnostic picture.

**Decision Anchor:** Calculate the R-value as the first analytic step for any new abnormal liver chemistry finding, and let the resulting pattern, not an undifferentiated broad panel, determine which subsequent tests are ordered.

## Acute Liver Injury and Acute Liver Failure

### Definitions and Initial Evaluation

Acute liver injury describes new-onset hepatocellular dysfunction without the encephalopathy or coagulopathy that define the more severe entity, acute liver failure, and this distinction, encephalopathy and an international normalized ratio above a defined threshold in a patient without preexisting chronic liver disease, is not merely academic but defines a categorically different management pathway, since acute liver failure carries a specific, time-sensitive transplant evaluation urgency that acute liver injury alone does not. Initial evaluation of significant acute liver injury should proceed efficiently rather than sequentially, obtaining viral hepatitis serologies, acetaminophen level regardless of reported history given the frequency of unrecognized or denied acetaminophen exposure, autoimmune markers, and a detailed medication, supplement, and toxin history simultaneously rather than working through this differential one test at a time, since the specific cause identified directly determines the availability of a targeted antidote or treatment, most critically for acetaminophen toxicity discussed next. Grading encephalopathy severity systematically, using a standardized clinical grading scale from mild confusion through deep coma, rather than a vague, subjective description, provides the objective, reproducible documentation this specific threshold-based classification requires and supports consistent communication among the multiple clinicians typically involved in managing a critically ill acute liver failure patient. Ordering these tests as a coordinated panel at the time of initial presentation, rather than sequentially adding tests over subsequent days as each prior result returns unrevealing, reflects the same efficient, parallel diagnostic approach already emphasized throughout this book whenever a time-sensitive differential must be worked through rapidly. This coordinated approach also reduces the number of separate blood draws the patient must undergo. Reassessing grade at each nursing shift change, rather than only once daily, catches rapid neurologic changes earlier. Precision here saves lives.

### Acetaminophen-Induced Liver Injury

Acetaminophen toxicity, the most common cause of acute liver failure in many populations, follows a predictable, dose-dependent toxicity mechanism mediated by a reactive metabolite that depletes hepatic glutathione stores once the normal, non-toxic metabolic pathways are saturated, and the Rumack-Matthew nomogram, plotting serum acetaminophen concentration against time since a single, acute ingestion, defines the specific threshold above which N-acetylcysteine therapy, replenishing glutathione and providing the primary antidote for this specific toxicity, is indicated. N-acetylcysteine should be initiated without waiting for the acetaminophen level to return in a patient with a clearly toxic ingestion history or a presentation strongly suggestive of acetaminophen toxicity, since the treatment's efficacy diminishes significantly with delay and its safety profile is favorable enough that empiric initiation while awaiting confirmatory results is the appropriate default rather than a treatment reserved only after laboratory confirmation. Chronic, supratherapeutic acetaminophen ingestion, occurring over days rather than as a single acute overdose, produces a distinct toxicity pattern not well captured by the Rumack-Matthew nomogram, which applies specifically to single, acute ingestions with a known ingestion time, and clinical judgment, rather than nomogram-based calculation, guides treatment decisions in this specific chronic ingestion scenario, generally favoring a lower threshold for treatment initiation given the nomogram's inapplicability. Both oral and intravenous N-acetylcysteine formulations are available, and selection between them is generally guided by the patient's ability to tolerate oral intake, severity of presentation, and institutional protocol, with intravenous administration generally preferred when significant nausea, vomiting, or altered mental status would compromise reliable oral dosing. Anaphylactoid reactions to intravenous N-acetylcysteine, while uncommon, are a recognized adverse effect requiring prompt recognition, typically resolving with a temporary infusion pause and antihistamine administration rather than permanent treatment discontinuation. Consulting a poison control center or medical toxicologist is reasonable whenever this specific chronic ingestion scenario complicates a straightforward treatment decision. Documenting the specific point plotted relative to the treatment line supports clear team communication. Yes indeed.

### Drug-Induced Liver Injury Beyond Acetaminophen

Drug-induced liver injury from agents other than acetaminophen follows an idiosyncratic, dose-independent mechanism in most cases, making it substantially less predictable than acetaminophen toxicity, and its diagnosis depends heavily on establishing a temporal relationship between a new medication or supplement and the onset of liver injury alongside exclusion of other causes, since no specific confirmatory test exists for most drug-induced liver injury cases beyond this careful causality assessment. A comprehensive medication and supplement history, explicitly including herbal and dietary supplements that patients frequently do not volunteer or consider relevant to disclose, applying the same systematic medication-review discipline emphasized throughout this book, is essential, and online causality assessment tools, incorporating the temporal relationship, the specific drug's known hepatotoxicity profile, and exclusion of alternative causes, provide a structured framework for this otherwise challenging diagnostic determination. Certain medication classes carry disproportionately high, well-documented hepatotoxicity risk, including specific antibiotics, antiepileptics, and antituberculosis agents, and maintaining familiarity with this higher-risk medication list allows a clinician to raise suspicion more readily when a patient on one of these specific agents develops otherwise unexplained liver chemistry abnormalities. Rechallenge with a suspected causative agent, deliberately reintroducing the medication to confirm the diagnosis, is generally avoided given the risk of provoking more severe recurrent injury, meaning most drug-induced liver injury diagnoses are established through careful exclusionary and temporal reasoning rather than direct confirmatory rechallenge testing. Regularly updated reference resources on drug hepatotoxicity, given how frequently new medications enter clinical use, help keep this awareness current rather than static. Vigilance never goes out of style.

**Figure 15.2:** Rumack-Matthew Nomogram for Acetaminophen Toxicity

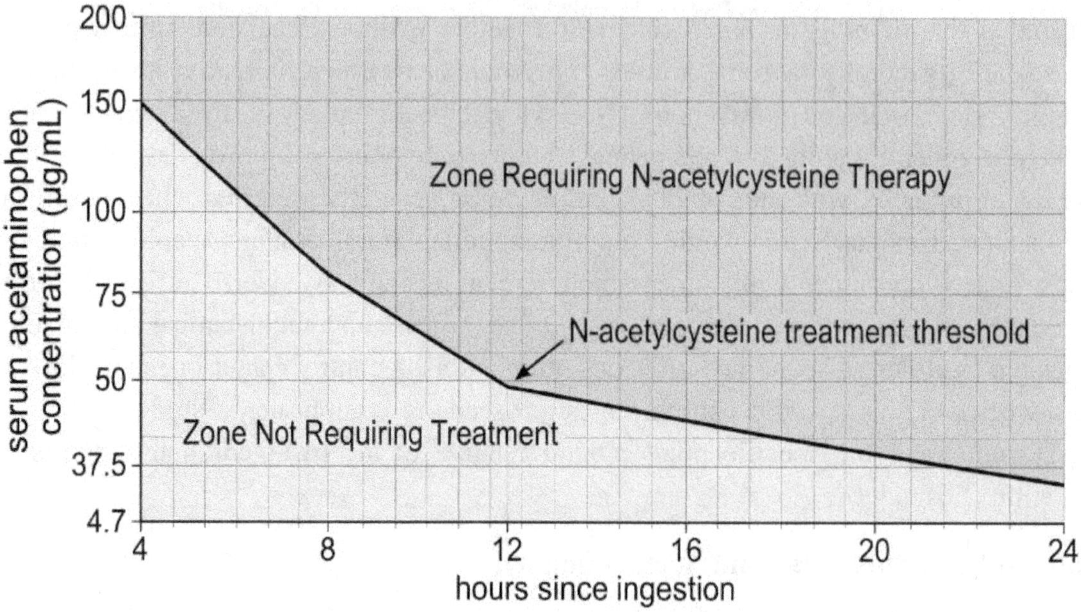


**THE GI THRESHOLD DECISION SYSTEM — Hepatic Thresholds — Transplant Referral Criteria in Acute Liver Failure**

**Presentation Signature:** A patient with acute liver failure is being managed, and the clinician must determine whether and when to initiate liver transplant evaluation.

**Threshold Point:** Established prognostic criteria, incorporating the specific etiology, degree of coagulopathy, and grade of encephalopathy, define the threshold predicting a low likelihood of spontaneous recovery without transplantation, and this threshold, not a general clinical impression of severity, should trigger transplant center referral.

**The Call:** Patients meeting these established prognostic criteria are referred to a transplant center immediately, ideally before the patient has deteriorated to a point where transfer itself becomes clinically hazardous, while patients with a favorable predicted spontaneous recovery trajectory continue supportive management with close monitoring for any deterioration that would cross this threshold.

**Trap Logic:** Delaying transplant center referral until a patient has deteriorated to an unambiguously critical state risks both a clinically hazardous transfer and a missed window for timely listing, since acute liver failure can progress rapidly and transplant evaluation and organ allocation take time that a late referral does not allow.

**Decision Anchor:** Apply established prognostic criteria promptly in every acute liver failure patient, and refer to a transplant center as soon as these criteria are met rather than waiting for further clinical deterioration to confirm the severity already indicated by the prognostic assessment.

## Diagnostic Workup of Elevated Liver Chemistries

### Standard Initial Workup

The standard initial workup for unexplained hepatocellular pattern liver chemistry elevation includes hepatitis A, B, and C serologies, autoimmune markers including antinuclear antibody, anti-smooth muscle antibody, and immunoglobulin G level, iron studies to screen for hereditary hemochromatosis, ceruloplasmin in appropriately selected younger patients to screen for Wilson disease, and alpha-1 antitrypsin level, and this panel, applied systematically rather than piecemeal across multiple visits, efficiently narrows the differential before more invasive testing is considered. Abdominal imaging, generally ultrasound as the initial modality given its low cost, wide availability, and lack of radiation exposure, assesses hepatic parenchymal appearance, biliary anatomy, and vascular patency, and should be obtained early in the workup rather than reserved only for cases where the biochemical evaluation has failed to identify a clear cause, since imaging can identify or support several diagnoses, including steatotic liver disease and vascular causes of liver injury, that complement rather than duplicate the biochemical workup. Ordering this panel as a coordinated set at the time of the initial visit, rather than adding individual tests reactively across multiple subsequent appointments as each prior test returns unrevealing, respects the patient's time and reaches a diagnosis more efficiently than a sequential, one-test-at-a-time approach. Doppler evaluation of hepatic vascular flow, included as part of a complete ultrasound examination, can identify vascular causes of liver injury, including portal or hepatic vein thrombosis, that would otherwise be missed on standard grayscale imaging alone and that carry their own distinct, urgent management implications once identified. Efficiency respects the patient.

### When to Pursue Liver Biopsy

Liver biopsy is reserved for cases where the noninvasive workup has not yielded a clear diagnosis, where the specific diagnosis remains uncertain despite a compatible biochemical and serologic picture, or where the biopsy itself would provide additional information beyond diagnosis, most notably staging fibrosis severity in a confirmed chronic liver disease, and this selective, rather than routine, use of biopsy reflects the same diagnostic-yield-driven reasoning already established throughout this book for other invasive procedures. Noninvasive fibrosis assessment, including elastography techniques introduced in later chapters and validated serum fibrosis panels, has substantially reduced the need for biopsy specifically for fibrosis staging in many chronic liver disease contexts, reserving biopsy more specifically for genuine diagnostic uncertainty rather than routine staging, a meaningful evolution in practice that has reduced the overall invasive procedure burden for many chronic liver disease patients.

## Wilson Disease and Acute Presentations of Chronic Liver Disease

Wilson disease, a genetic disorder of copper metabolism, can present with acute liver failure, particularly in younger patients, and this presentation carries a distinctive, recognizable pattern including a disproportionately low alkaline phosphatase relative to the degree of hyperbilirubinemia, Coombs-negative hemolytic anemia from copper-mediated red cell injury, and a low serum ceruloplasmin, though ceruloplasmin can be normal in a subset of cases including acute presentations, meaning a normal ceruloplasmin does not fully exclude the diagnosis when clinical suspicion remains high. Recognizing

Wilson disease specifically in a younger patient presenting with acute liver failure matters urgently, since this specific presentation carries an extremely poor prognosis without transplantation and standard medical therapy is generally inadequate once this fulminant presentation has developed, meaning that transplant evaluation should be pursued expeditiously rather than attempting an extended trial of medical copper-chelation therapy in this specific acute presentation. A serum ceruloplasmin-to-alkaline phosphatase ratio and a serum bilirubin-to-alkaline phosphatase ratio have both been proposed as additional supportive diagnostic tools in this specific acute presentation, reflecting ongoing efforts to improve early recognition of this rare but highly treatable-if-caught-early, and otherwise rapidly fatal, presentation.

### Autoimmune Hepatitis Presenting Acutely

Autoimmune hepatitis, discussed in greater detail in a later chapter, can present acutely with severe, even fulminant, hepatocellular injury rather than the more commonly recognized indolent, chronic course, and this acute presentation should be actively considered in the differential for acute liver failure or severe acute liver injury of unclear etiology, since a favorable response to corticosteroid therapy, when this diagnosis is confirmed and treatment is not further delayed, can meaningfully alter the clinical course and potentially avoid the need for transplantation in appropriately selected patients. A liver biopsy, when the patient's coagulation status and overall clinical stability permit safe performance, is often pursued even in this acute setting to confirm the diagnosis before committing to corticosteroid therapy, since the diagnosis of autoimmune hepatitis carries specific histologic features that support confidence in this diagnosis before exposing an already critically ill patient to the additional risks of immunosuppressive therapy.

## Supportive Management of Acute Liver Failure

Beyond the etiology-specific treatments discussed earlier in this chapter, acute liver failure management requires intensive, protocol-driven supportive care addressing the multi-organ complications this condition characteristically produces, including cerebral edema, monitored clinically and, in severe cases, with more invasive intracranial pressure assessment, since untreated elevated intracranial pressure is a major cause of mortality independent of the underlying liver injury itself. Coagulopathy management in acute liver failure differs meaningfully from coagulopathy management in other clinical contexts, since prophylactic correction of an elevated international normalized ratio in the absence of active bleeding or a planned invasive procedure is generally avoided, both because the international normalized ratio serves as an important prognostic and monitoring marker that correction would obscure, and because evidence does not support that prophylactic correction reduces bleeding risk in this specific population, a nuance that differs from more reflexive coagulopathy correction practices applied in other clinical contexts. Early recognition of subtle neurologic changes, monitored with frequent, standardized assessment rather than infrequent, informal checks, allows earlier detection of evolving cerebral edema before it progresses to a more advanced, harder-to-manage stage, reinforcing the value of a structured, protocol-driven monitoring schedule in this rapidly evolving condition. Communicating this specific, counterintuitive management approach to colleagues from other specialties less familiar with acute liver failure, who might otherwise instinctively want to correct an elevated INR reflexively, prevents unnecessary and potentially harmful blood product administration in this specific clinical context. Clarity prevents harm.

### Renal and Metabolic Support

Acute kidney injury frequently complicates acute liver failure through a combination of the underlying etiology's direct nephrotoxic effects, when present, hepatorenal physiology, and the hemodynamic instability that severe liver failure itself produces, and renal replacement therapy, when required, should be provided using continuous rather than intermittent modalities in hemodynamically unstable patients, given the more favorable hemodynamic tolerance continuous therapy offers in this specific critically ill population. Hypoglycemia, from impaired hepatic gluconeogenesis, and electrolyte derangements, particularly hypophosphatemia and hypokalemia which can themselves impair hepatocyte regeneration if uncorrected, require frequent monitoring and proactive correction throughout the acute liver failure course, reflecting the same close, protocol-driven monitoring standard already established throughout this book for other critically ill, rapidly evolving clinical presentations. Nephrotoxic medications should be reviewed and minimized wherever possible in this population given their already elevated baseline acute kidney injury risk, applying the same systematic medication-review discipline emphasized throughout this book specifically to renal protection in this vulnerable, critically ill population. Standardized order sets incorporating scheduled glucose and electrolyte checks at defined intervals, rather than relying on ad hoc ordering by individual clinicians, help ensure this frequent monitoring is applied consistently across every acute liver failure admission regardless of which team member is managing the patient at any given time. Consistency saves lives.

## Infectious and Toxin-Related Causes Beyond Viral Hepatitis

Non-hepatotropic viral infections, including Epstein-Barr virus, cytomegalovirus, and herpes simplex virus, can produce significant, occasionally severe hepatitis, particularly in immunocompromised patients, and herpes simplex virus hepatitis specifically deserves urgent recognition given its potential for rapid, life-threatening progression and its specific antiviral treatment, meaning that empiric acyclovir should be considered in an appropriately compatible clinical scenario, disseminated illness with fever and marked transaminase elevation in an immunocompromised or peripartum patient, while confirmatory testing is pending, applying the same time-sensitive empiric treatment principle already established in this chapter for acetaminophen toxicity. Mushroom poisoning, most notably from Amanita phalloides and related species, produces a distinctive delayed-onset hepatotoxicity syndrome, with gastrointestinal symptoms appearing hours after ingestion followed by a deceptive symptom-free interval before severe hepatotoxicity manifests days later, and recognizing this specific toxidrome in a patient with a foraging history or ingestion of wild mushrooms is essential given the specific, though imperfect, treatment options available and the otherwise high mortality of untreated severe cases. Specific PCR-based testing for these viruses, rather than the standard hepatitis A, B, and C serologies alone, must be specifically requested when this broader differential is being considered, since these tests are not included in a routine viral hepatitis panel and will be missed entirely if not ordered explicitly based on clinical suspicion. Poison control center consultation should be obtained promptly whenever mushroom poisoning is suspected, given the specialized, evolving treatment recommendations for this specific toxidrome and the value of expert guidance in a condition few clinicians encounter with any regularity in routine practice. Early liver transplant center notification, even before the full toxicity picture has developed, is reasonable in a confirmed or strongly suspected severe Amanita ingestion given how rapidly this specific toxidrome can progress to liver failure once symptoms begin in earnest. Always.

### Heat Stroke and Other Systemic Causes

Heat stroke, producing liver injury through a combination of direct thermal hepatocyte injury and the same hypoperfusion mechanism responsible for ischemic hepatitis discussed earlier in this chapter, should be considered in the appropriate clinical context, extreme environmental heat exposure or exertional heat illness, and this cause, like ischemic hepatitis, generally resolves with treatment of the underlying systemic process rather than requiring liver-specific intervention beyond supportive care. Recognizing these less common but clinically important causes of acute liver injury, systematically considered alongside the more familiar viral, drug-induced, and autoimmune causes developed earlier in this chapter, prevents diagnostic delay in a patient whose presentation does not fit the most commonly encountered etiologies. Rapid, aggressive cooling remains the cornerstone of heat stroke management overall, and the associated liver injury, like the other systemic causes discussed here, generally does not require any liver-specific intervention beyond the supportive monitoring already established as standard practice throughout this chapter for acute liver injury from any cause. Screening for other heat-related organ dysfunction, including rhabdomyolysis and acute kidney injury, should proceed in parallel with monitoring the liver injury, since heat stroke characteristically produces multi-organ involvement rather than an isolated hepatic effect.

## Psychosocial Considerations and Communication in Acute Liver Injury

Acute liver injury, particularly when caused by an intentional acetaminophen overdose as in the first case presentation developed later in this chapter, requires the same compassionate, nonjudgmental approach to underlying mental health and substance use concerns already emphasized throughout this book, and psychiatric evaluation should be arranged for every patient presenting after an intentional overdose regardless of the ultimate severity of the resulting liver injury, since the underlying psychiatric crisis that prompted the overdose requires its own dedicated attention independent of the medical outcome. Patients and families facing a new diagnosis of acute liver failure experience substantial acute distress given the condition's potential severity and rapid trajectory, and clear, honest, and frequently updated communication about prognosis and the transplant evaluation process, delivered by a consistent point of contact whenever possible, supports this family through what is often one of the most acutely stressful periods they will experience, applying the same crisis-communication principles relevant across other rapidly evolving, high-stakes medical situations. A one-to-one, private conversation, separate from the medical team's discussion of the liver injury itself, communicates that this psychiatric evaluation is taken seriously as its own priority rather than treated as a secondary formality appended to the primary medical concern. Written summaries of key updates, provided alongside verbal conversations, can help family members retain and process information that is easy to forget or misremember during a period of acute stress and rapidly changing clinical status.

### Communicating Uncertainty in Evolving Acute Liver Injury

Acute liver injury and failure can evolve rapidly and unpredictably in either direction, toward recovery or toward the need for transplantation, and communicating this genuine uncertainty honestly to patients and families, rather than either false reassurance or premature worst-case framing, respects their need for accurate information while acknowledging that the clinical trajectory may not be fully clear for several days, a communication challenge that requires ongoing, updated conversation rather than a single definitive prognostic statement delivered once at initial presentation. Scheduling brief, regular update conversations at predictable intervals, rather than only in response to a major change in status, gives families a consistent touchpoint they can anticipate and reduces the anxiety of wondering when the next piece of information will arrive.

## Alpha-1 Antitrypsin Deficiency and Hereditary Hemochromatosis in the Acute Chemistry Workup

Alpha-1 antitrypsin deficiency, screened for as part of the standard initial workup discussed earlier in this chapter, produces liver disease through an accumulation mechanism distinct from most other causes discussed in this chapter, in which misfolded alpha-1 antitrypsin protein accumulates within hepatocytes and triggers progressive liver injury, and a low alpha-1 antitrypsin level should prompt confirmatory genotyping to identify the specific allelic variant, since the degree of liver disease risk varies meaningfully by genotype, with the homozygous PiZZ genotype carrying the highest risk of clinically significant liver disease among the recognized variants. Hereditary hemochromatosis, similarly screened for via iron studies in the standard workup, more commonly produces a chronic, insidious rather than acute liver injury pattern, though genetic confirmation with HFE gene testing in a patient with elevated transferrin saturation and ferritin supports early diagnosis before advanced fibrosis or cirrhosis develops, and identifying this treatable, genetic cause of liver injury carries family-counseling implications for at-risk relatives paralleling the cascade-testing principle already developed in earlier chapters for other hereditary conditions. Family members of a confirmed PiZZ homozygous patient should be offered testing given the inheritance pattern this genotype implies, applying the same cascade testing principle already established in earlier chapters for other hereditary conditions with actionable implications for at-risk relatives. Therapeutic phlebotomy, the primary treatment for confirmed hereditary hemochromatosis, is generally well tolerated and highly effective at reducing iron burden when initiated before advanced organ damage has occurred, reinforcing why early identification through this screening pathway carries meaningful, actionable treatment implications.

### Integrating Metabolic Screening Into the Initial Workup

Both alpha-1 antitrypsin deficiency and hereditary hemochromatosis are relatively uncommon causes of any individual patient's abnormal liver chemistries but carry sufficiently important treatment and family-counseling implications, and sufficiently low-cost, low-burden screening tests, that their inclusion in the standard initial hepatocellular pattern workup represents an efficient, evidence-based screening strategy rather than an excessive or low-yield addition to the diagnostic evaluation.

## Statin-Associated Liver Chemistry Elevation and Common Outpatient Scenarios

Mild, asymptomatic aminotransferase elevation in a patient on statin therapy is a common outpatient scenario that generates disproportionate clinical concern given the historical, now largely outdated, practice of routine liver chemistry monitoring for all statin users, and current evidence supports that clinically significant statin-induced liver injury is rare, that routine liver chemistry monitoring is no longer recommended for most patients on stable statin therapy, and that statins can generally be continued even in patients with pre-existing mild chronic liver disease, including metabolic dysfunction-associated steatotic liver disease discussed in the following chapter, since statins are not associated with the disease progression some clinicians historically feared and cardiovascular risk reduction benefits generally outweigh the minimal hepatotoxicity risk in this population. When statin discontinuation is genuinely warranted, generally reserved for aminotransferase elevations exceeding three times the upper limit of normal with symptoms, or higher thresholds in asymptomatic patients per current guidance, this decision should be made deliberately rather than reflexively, given the cardiovascular risk of unnecessary statin discontinuation in a patient who does not actually have clinically significant statin-associated liver injury. Communicating this updated, reassuring evidence directly to patients who may have heard the older, more cautious guidance from a prior clinician or from general public awareness supports continued statin adherence and prevents unnecessary discontinuation of a cardiovascular-protective medication out of an outdated safety concern. Substituting an alternative statin at a lower dose, rather than abandoning statin therapy entirely, is a reasonable next step in a patient who genuinely requires discontinuation, since cross-reactivity between different statins is not universal and a lower-intensity regimen may still provide meaningful cardiovascular benefit. Shared decision-making, informed by this current evidence, should guide the conversation rather than a unilateral decision made without discussing the updated risk-benefit picture with the patient directly.

### Isolated Mild Aminotransferase Elevation in Otherwise Asymptomatic Patients

Mild, isolated aminotransferase elevation discovered incidentally in an asymptomatic patient, a common scenario given the frequency of liver chemistry testing performed as part of routine health maintenance panels, warrants a measured, stepwise approach beginning with confirmation on repeat testing, since transient, self-resolving elevations are common and do not necessarily warrant an extensive immediate workup, followed by the standard evaluation developed throughout this chapter only if the elevation persists on repeat testing, applying the same avoid-overreacting-to-a-single-value principle already emphasized elsewhere in this book for other laboratory findings subject to normal biological variability. Setting a specific, defined timeframe for repeat testing, generally within a few weeks to a few months depending on the degree of initial elevation, rather than leaving the follow-up interval vague or open-ended, ensures this reassessment actually occurs rather than being lost to follow-up in a patient who otherwise feels well and has no immediate reason to return. Communicating the reasoning behind this measured approach to the patient, rather than leaving them to wonder why an abnormal result is not being acted upon immediately, supports trust in the overall diagnostic process.

## Acetaminophen Co-Ingestion and Combination Product Awareness

Acetaminophen is a common ingredient in numerous combination over-the-counter and prescription products, including many cold, flu, and pain medications, and patients frequently do not recognize these combination products as containing acetaminophen, creating a genuine risk of inadvertent cumulative overdose when a patient takes a standalone acetaminophen product alongside a combination product without realizing both contain the same active ingredient, and specifically asking about all over-the-counter medications, not only prescription drugs, during a medication history is essential to capturing this risk. This combination-product awareness is particularly important in patients with chronic pain who may be taking a prescribed opioid-acetaminophen combination product alongside additional standalone acetaminophen for breakthrough symptoms, a scenario that can produce cumulative supratherapeutic dosing over time without any single acute overdose event, and this chronic, cumulative pattern, discussed earlier in this chapter as distinct from the single-ingestion pattern the standard nomogram addresses, requires the same clinical vigilance regardless of whether the excess intake was intentional or an inadvertent consequence of combination product use. Pharmacists are well positioned to reinforce this specific counseling point at the time a combination product is dispensed, and collaborating with pharmacy colleagues on standardized counseling messaging around acetaminophen-containing combination products extends this safety message beyond what any single prescribing clinician can accomplish alone. Reviewing a pain management plan explicitly for this specific overlap risk, ideally with pharmacy involvement, should be a routine part of managing any patient on a chronic combination opioid-acetaminophen regimen, rather than an afterthought considered only after a concerning liver chemistry result has already prompted investigation. This same awareness applies to caregivers managing medications for children or elderly family members, who may inadvertently double-dose across multiple combination products without recognizing the shared active ingredient.

### Patient Education on Acetaminophen Dosing Limits

Proactive patient education about maximum daily acetaminophen dosing limits, delivered at the time any acetaminophen-containing product is prescribed or recommended, and specifically addressing the combination-product risk described above, is a simple, low-cost preventive intervention that can meaningfully reduce the incidence of inadvertent acetaminophen toxicity, particularly in patients managing chronic pain with multiple concurrent over-the-counter and prescription products who may not have received this specific counseling previously.

## Immune Checkpoint Inhibitor Hepatotoxicity

Immune checkpoint inhibitor therapy, an increasingly widely used oncologic treatment class, produces a distinct form of drug-induced liver injury mediated by immune activation rather than the direct or idiosyncratic hepatotoxicity mechanisms discussed earlier in this chapter, and recognizing this specific etiology in a patient on active checkpoint inhibitor therapy who develops new liver chemistry abnormalities is essential given its specific, immunosuppression-based treatment approach, generally corticosteroids, which differs fundamentally from the supportive-care-and-discontinuation approach appropriate for most other drug-induced liver injury. Grading the severity of immune-related hepatitis using an oncology-specific toxicity grading system, rather than the general hepatocellular injury severity framework used elsewhere in this chapter, determines whether checkpoint inhibitor therapy can continue with close monitoring, requires temporary interruption, or must be permanently discontinued, and this decision should be made collaboratively with the treating oncologist given the need to balance ongoing cancer treatment against the hepatotoxicity risk in a population where the underlying malignancy itself carries serious, independent mortality risk. As checkpoint inhibitor use continues to expand into an increasing range of cancer types, this specific hepatotoxicity pattern will be encountered more frequently across general gastroenterology and hepatology practice, making familiarity with its recognition and management increasingly relevant even for clinicians without a primary oncology focus. Documenting this grading and the specific rationale for the treatment decision reached, whether continuation, interruption, or permanent discontinuation, supports clear communication between the involved specialties and provides a reference point if the patient's clinical course subsequently changes. Patient education about symptoms warranting prompt reporting, including jaundice, dark urine, or unusual fatigue, empowers patients on active checkpoint inhibitor therapy to seek evaluation early rather than delaying until symptoms have become severe. Indeed. Truly.

### Coordinating Care With Oncology in Checkpoint Inhibitor Hepatotoxicity

Given the relatively specialized, oncology-specific management this condition requires, gastroenterology or hepatology involvement should be sought promptly once immune-related hepatitis is suspected or confirmed, both to confirm the diagnosis by excluding alternative causes of the liver chemistry abnormality and to guide corticosteroid dosing and tapering, applying the same collaborative, cross-specialty management model already established throughout this book for other complex conditions spanning multiple areas of expertise. Establishing this collaborative referral pathway proactively, before the first case is encountered, rather than improvising an ad hoc consultation process at the time of an acute presentation, supports a smoother, faster response when a patient does develop this specific complication. Preparation matters.

## Ischemic Hepatitis and Other Acute Causes

### Ischemic Hepatitis

Ischemic hepatitis, also termed shock liver despite frequently occurring without overt hypotension, results from acute hepatic hypoperfusion, most commonly in the setting of cardiogenic shock, severe sepsis, or another acute hemodynamic insult, and produces a characteristic pattern of dramatically elevated aminotransferases, often exceeding a thousand units per liter, that rise and fall rapidly in parallel with the underlying hemodynamic event, distinguishing it from the more sustained elevations typical of viral hepatitis or drug-induced injury. Recognizing ischemic hepatitis correctly, rather than pursuing an extensive viral or autoimmune workup for a dramatic aminotransferase elevation that actually reflects a recent hemodynamic insult evident from the clinical context, the concurrent hypotensive episode, cardiac arrest, or severe sepsis, prevents unnecessary testing and correctly redirects management toward addressing the underlying hemodynamic cause, since the liver injury itself typically resolves rapidly once perfusion is restored without requiring liver-directed treatment.

Case Presentation: A 24-year-old woman is brought to the emergency department twenty hours after an intentional acetaminophen overdose, reporting she took the medication the previous evening. She is alert without evidence of encephalopathy. Applying the reasoning developed in this chapter, N-acetylcysteine is initiated immediately upon her arrival, before her acetaminophen level or liver chemistries return, given the clear history of a toxic ingestion and the time-sensitive nature of this antidote's efficacy. Her acetaminophen level returns markedly elevated, and her aminotransferases, initially normal on arrival, rise substantially over the following 24 hours before beginning to trend downward with continued N-acetylcysteine therapy. Her coagulation studies remain normal throughout, and she does not develop encephalopathy, meeting criteria for acute liver injury without progression to acute liver failure. She completes her N-acetylcysteine course with full biochemical recovery and is transferred to psychiatric care for the underlying intentional overdose. This case illustrates the chapter's central acetaminophen-toxicity principle: N-acetylcysteine initiated promptly, without waiting for confirmatory laboratory results, and continued through the expected trajectory of injury and recovery, achieved a favorable outcome that delayed treatment might not have.

Case Presentation: A 56-year-old man presents with fatigue and jaundice three weeks after starting a new herbal supplement for joint pain, with no other new medications and no significant alcohol use. Liver chemistries demonstrate an R-value consistent with a hepatocellular pattern, and the standard initial workup for viral hepatitis, autoimmune markers, and metabolic causes is unrevealing. Applying the reasoning developed in this chapter, the temporal relationship between supplement initiation and symptom onset, combined with exclusion of other causes through the standard workup, supports a diagnosis of drug-induced liver injury from the herbal supplement, which he had not initially mentioned during his medication history until specifically asked about supplements and herbal products directly. The supplement is discontinued, and his liver chemistries improve progressively over the following weeks with supportive care alone. This case illustrates the chapter's core drug-induced liver injury principle: a comprehensive history explicitly including herbal and dietary supplements, not assumed to be volunteered spontaneously, was essential to identifying the causative agent that a medication history limited to prescription drugs alone would have missed entirely.

## Pregnancy-Related Acute Liver Disease

Acute liver disease in pregnancy encompasses several distinct entities requiring rapid recognition given the risk to both mother and fetus, including hyperemesis gravidarum-associated mild liver chemistry elevation, intrahepatic cholestasis of pregnancy, producing pruritus and a cholestatic biochemical pattern typically in the third trimester, and the more severe preeclampsia-spectrum conditions, HELLP syndrome and acute fatty liver of pregnancy, both of which can progress rapidly and require prompt delivery as the primary, definitive treatment regardless of gestational age once these diagnoses are confirmed. Distinguishing HELLP syndrome and acute fatty liver of pregnancy from one another, while both requiring the same urgent delivery-focused management, matters for maternal monitoring and counseling about recurrence risk in future pregnancies, since acute fatty liver of pregnancy specifically has an associated genetic metabolic defect in a subset of cases with implications for the fetus as well as maternal recurrence risk. Distinguishing these pregnancy-specific liver disorders from acute viral hepatitis or other causes unrelated to pregnancy itself, while pursuing the standard workup discussed earlier in this chapter in parallel, ensures a pregnancy-specific diagnosis is not overlooked simply because pregnancy naturally shifts diagnostic attention toward obstetric causes. Ursodeoxycholic acid, the primary treatment for intrahepatic cholestasis of pregnancy, improves maternal pruritus and, in some studies, reduces adverse fetal outcomes, and its use should be initiated promptly once this diagnosis is confirmed rather than delayed while the more severe conditions in this differential are further excluded. Genetic testing for the associated fatty acid oxidation defect, when acute fatty liver of pregnancy is confirmed, should be offered given its implications for the affected infant's own metabolic screening and management, extending the diagnostic workup beyond the mother alone in this specific condition. Yes.

### Multidisciplinary Coordination in Pregnancy-Related Liver Disease

Given the maternal and fetal stakes involved, any pregnant patient presenting with acute liver chemistry abnormalities warrants prompt, coordinated evaluation involving obstetrics, maternal-fetal medicine, and hepatology or gastroenterology together, applying the same collaborative, multidisciplinary decision-making model already established throughout this book for other complex, time-sensitive presentations, and this coordination should be initiated immediately upon recognition of the abnormality rather than after a delay while awaiting additional, potentially unnecessary testing that could otherwise be pursued in parallel with specialist involvement. Anesthesia and neonatology should also be looped into this coordination once delivery becomes imminent, ensuring the full care team is aligned on both the timing and the specific delivery approach best suited to the maternal condition and fetal status. Anesthesia and neonatology should also be looped in once delivery becomes imminent, ensuring the full care team is aligned on both timing and the specific delivery approach best suited to the maternal condition and fetal status.

| Pattern | R-Value | Representative Differential |
|---|---|---|
| Hepatocellular | > 5 | Viral hepatitis, DILI, ischemic hepatitis, autoimmune hepatitis |
| Cholestatic | < 2 | Biliary obstruction, PBC, PSC, cholestatic DILI |
| Mixed | 2-5 | Overlap presentations; broader initial workup needed |

**THE GI THRESHOLD DECISION SYSTEM — Acute Liver Injury Thresholds**

**Presentation Signature:** This chapter's threshold instances addressed pattern-based triage of abnormal liver chemistries and transplant referral criteria in acute liver failure.

**Threshold Point:** The calculated R-value gates the diagnostic pathway pursued for abnormal liver chemistries; established prognostic criteria gate the timing of transplant center referral in acute liver failure.

**The Call:** Both thresholds replace an undifferentiated, reactive approach with an early, criteria-based classification that directs subsequent testing or referral efficiently and proactively.

**Trap Logic:** Ordering a broad, undifferentiated liver panel without first calculating the injury pattern, and delaying transplant referral until a patient has already deteriorated to an unambiguously critical state, are this chapter's most consequential threshold misapplications.

**Decision Anchor:** Calculate the R-value as the first step for any new abnormal liver chemistry finding, and apply established prognostic criteria promptly in acute liver failure to trigger timely, rather than delayed, transplant center referral.

## Summary and Key Concepts

The R-value, calculated from the relative elevations of alanine aminotransferase and alkaline phosphatase, classifies liver injury as hepatocellular, cholestatic, or mixed, and this pattern determines the subsequent diagnostic pathway.

Elevated alkaline phosphatase should be confirmed as hepatobiliary in origin before pursuing a liver workup, and bilirubin fractionation into unconjugated and conjugated components guides the subsequent evaluation.

Acute liver failure, defined by encephalopathy and coagulopathy in a patient without preexisting chronic liver disease, is categorically distinct from acute liver injury and requires urgent transplant center evaluation using established prognostic criteria.

N-acetylcysteine should be initiated empirically in suspected acetaminophen toxicity without waiting for confirmatory laboratory results, given the treatment's time-sensitive efficacy and favorable safety profile.

Drug-induced liver injury from non-acetaminophen agents relies on temporal relationship and exclusion of other causes, and a comprehensive history must explicitly include herbal and dietary supplements that patients often do not volunteer.

Ischemic hepatitis produces dramatic, rapidly rising and falling aminotransferase elevations correlating with a recent hemodynamic insult, and recognizing this pattern prevents unnecessary additional workup and correctly redirects management toward the underlying hemodynamic cause.

# CHAPTER 16: VIRAL HEPATITIS, ALCOHOL-ASSOCIATED LIVER DISEASE, AND METABOLIC DYSFUNCTION-ASSOCIATED STEATOTIC LIVER DISEASE

**Learning Objectives**

1. Describe the natural history and management of hepatitis A, B, C, and E, including specific treatment thresholds for chronic hepatitis B.
2. Apply current hepatitis C screening, diagnosis, and direct-acting antiviral treatment principles.
3. Classify the spectrum of alcohol-associated liver disease and apply severity assessment and treatment criteria for severe alcohol-associated hepatitis.
4. Apply current diagnostic criteria and nomenclature for metabolic dysfunction-associated steatotic liver disease.
5. Apply fibrosis risk stratification and evidence-based management, including emerging pharmacotherapy, for metabolic dysfunction-associated steatotic liver disease.

**Chapter Outline**

This chapter develops the three most common causes of chronic liver disease worldwide: viral hepatitis, including hepatitis A, B, C, and E and the specific treatment thresholds and cure strategies each requires, alcohol-associated liver disease across its spectrum from steatosis through severe alcohol-associated hepatitis, and metabolic dysfunction-associated steatotic liver disease, its evolving nomenclature, fibrosis risk stratification, and emerging pharmacotherapy. Each section connects a specific diagnostic or severity threshold to a defined management pathway.

## Viral Hepatitis

### Hepatitis A and E

Hepatitis A, transmitted via the fecal-oral route, produces an acute, generally self-limited illness that does not progress to chronic infection, and management is primarily supportive, though fulminant hepatitis A, while uncommon, can occur, particularly in patients with underlying chronic liver disease, and this population should be specifically counseled about hepatitis A vaccination given their elevated risk of severe acute infection superimposed on already compromised hepatic reserve. Hepatitis E, similarly transmitted via the fecal-oral route and typically self-limited in immunocompetent hosts, carries a distinct, well-recognized risk of severe, even fulminant disease in pregnant women, particularly during the third trimester, and can also produce chronic infection in immunocompromised patients, including solid organ transplant recipients, a distinction from the acute-only course typical of immunocompetent hosts that changes both the surveillance and treatment approach required in this specific population. Postexposure prophylaxis with either vaccine or immunoglobulin, depending on the specific timing and the exposed individual's age and health status, can prevent clinical infection when administered promptly after a known exposure, and this option should be considered in any household or close contact of a confirmed hepatitis A case. Ribavirin therapy has shown efficacy in treating chronic hepatitis E in immunocompromised patients, including reducing or, when feasible, transitioning immunosuppression alongside antiviral therapy in transplant recipients, addressing both the viral infection itself and the underlying immunosuppressed state permitting its chronicity. Vaccination should also be considered for household contacts of a patient with chronic liver disease of any etiology, extending this protective recommendation beyond the affected patient alone to reduce the risk of introducing a superimposed acute infection into the household.

**Hepatitis B: Natural History and Treatment**

Chronic hepatitis B progresses through recognized phases, defined by the relationship between viral replication, measured by HBV DNA level and hepatitis B e-antigen status, and host immune response, measured by aminotransferase levels and liver histology, and this phase classification, rather than HBV DNA level or aminotransferase elevation considered in isolation, determines whether antiviral treatment is indicated, since not every phase of chronic hepatitis B infection warrants treatment despite the presence of detectable viral replication. The immune-active phases, characterized by elevated aminotransferases alongside significant viral replication, generally warrant antiviral therapy, most commonly with a potent, high-genetic-barrier nucleos(t)ide analogue such as tenofovir or entecavir, while the immune-tolerant and inactive carrier phases, despite sometimes showing substantial HBV DNA levels or a positive hepatitis B surface antigen respectively, do not require treatment but do require ongoing monitoring for phase transition, since a patient can move between these phases over time and treatment decisions must be reassessed accordingly rather than fixed permanently based on an initial classification. Applying this phase classification consistently requires periodic reassessment, generally every six to twelve months in an untreated patient, since a single snapshot of viral and biochemical markers cannot capture the dynamic, sometimes fluctuating nature of the host-virus relationship that defines this condition's natural history. Treatment duration in hepatitis B is generally indefinite for most patients started on therapy, distinct from the finite, curative treatment course achievable in hepatitis C discussed below, and this expectation should be communicated clearly at the time treatment is initiated, since a patient anticipating a short, curative course analogous to hepatitis C treatment may otherwise be confused or frustrated by the different treatment paradigm hepatitis B requires. Explaining these phases to the patient using accessible language, avoiding excessive technical jargon while still conveying the genuine clinical nuance involved, supports the patient's understanding of why treatment recommendations might change over time as their own phase classification evolves. Clarity here builds lasting trust with patients.

## Figure 16.1: Chronic Hepatitis B Phases and Treatment Indications

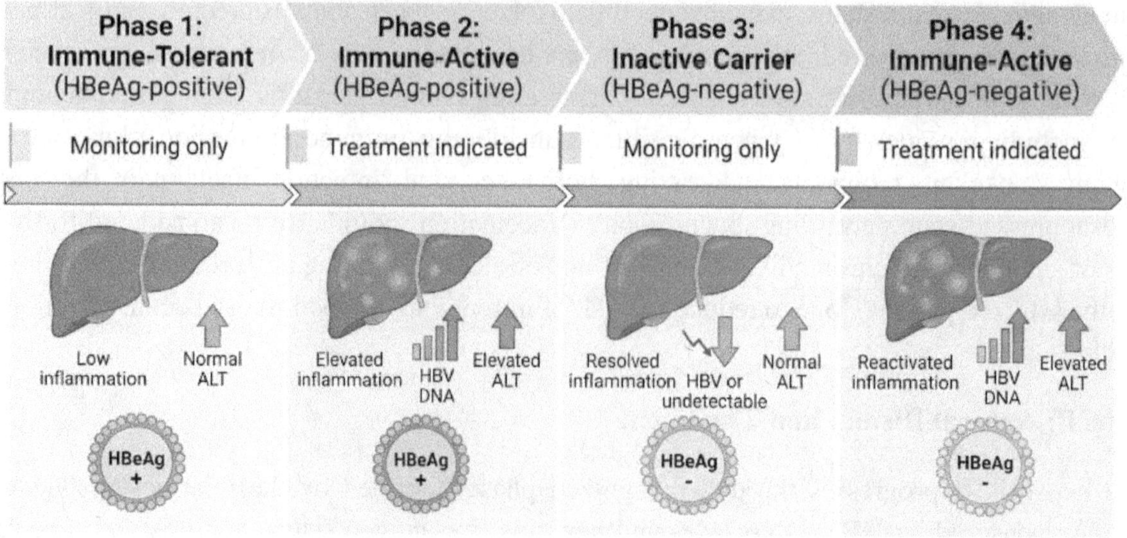


**THE GI THRESHOLD DECISION SYSTEM — Hepatic Thresholds — Treatment Initiation in Chronic Hepatitis B**

**Presentation Signature:** A patient with chronic hepatitis B infection is undergoing routine monitoring, and the clinician must determine whether antiviral treatment is indicated at the current assessment.

**Threshold Point:** The combination of HBV DNA level, aminotransferase elevation, and evidence of significant fibrosis on noninvasive assessment or biopsy defines the threshold for antiviral treatment initiation, with treatment generally indicated in the immune-active phases or in any patient with significant fibrosis regardless of phase classification.

**The Call:** Patients meeting treatment criteria are started on a potent, high-genetic-barrier antiviral agent with a long-term, generally indefinite treatment course; patients in the immune-tolerant or inactive carrier phase without significant fibrosis continue monitoring at defined intervals, with treatment initiated promptly if reassessment reveals phase transition or fibrosis progression.

**Trap Logic:** Treating every patient with detectable HBV DNA regardless of phase, or conversely withholding treatment indefinitely from a patient who has transitioned to an immune-active phase simply because they were previously classified as inactive, both misapply this threshold and produce either unnecessary treatment or missed opportunity for disease-modifying therapy.

**Decision Anchor:** Reassess phase classification, not a single HBV DNA or aminotransferase value in isolation, at each monitoring visit, and initiate antiviral therapy promptly once immune-active phase criteria or significant fibrosis is identified, rather than treating an initial classification as permanent.

## Hepatitis C: Screening, Diagnosis, and Direct-Acting Antiviral Therapy

Universal one-time hepatitis C screening is now recommended for all adults regardless of specific risk factors, reflecting both the substantial proportion of infected individuals who do not report a recognized risk factor and the transformative efficacy of current treatment, and this universal approach, rather than risk-factor-based screening alone, applies the same broadened screening philosophy already established in earlier chapters for other conditions where risk-factor-based screening alone was found to miss a meaningful proportion of affected individuals. Diagnosis requires a positive antibody screen followed by confirmatory HCV RNA testing, since antibody positivity alone reflects prior exposure and does not distinguish active infection from spontaneously cleared or previously treated infection, and this two-step confirmatory sequence should be completed in a single specimen or coordinated visit whenever possible rather than requiring the patient to return separately for confirmatory testing, a practical step that meaningfully improves linkage to care. Periodic repeat screening beyond the one-time baseline is recommended for individuals with ongoing risk factors, including active injection drug use, since a single lifetime negative screen does not protect against subsequent acquisition in a patient whose risk exposure continues after that initial test. Integrating this universal screening into routine order sets for adult preventive care, rather than relying on individual clinician memory to order it as a discretionary test, supports consistent application across a large patient population regardless of any individual clinician's awareness of the current universal recommendation. Reflex testing protocols, in which a laboratory automatically performs confirmatory RNA testing on any antibody-positive specimen without requiring a separate clinician order, further streamline this process and reduce the number of patients lost between the initial screen and confirmatory diagnosis. This coordinated approach reduces missed diagnoses substantially.

Direct-acting antiviral therapy, combining agents targeting different steps of the hepatitis C viral replication cycle, achieves sustained virologic response, the functional cure endpoint measured twelve weeks after treatment completion, in the substantial majority of patients across nearly all genotypes and disease stages with a short, well-tolerated oral treatment course, representing one of the most dramatic treatment transformations in the recent history of gastroenterology and hepatology, and this high cure rate means that a hepatitis C diagnosis should now be framed to patients as a highly treatable, generally curable condition rather than the more guarded prognosis appropriate in the earlier interferon-based treatment era many patients or their family members may still associate with this diagnosis. Drug interaction screening before initiating therapy remains an essential step given the number of concurrent medications many patients take, and consulting a reliable, regularly updated interaction resource, rather than relying on memory of interactions that may have applied to older, now less commonly used regimens, ensures the selected regimen is genuinely safe for the individual patient's full medication list.

## Alcohol-Associated Liver Disease

### Spectrum of Disease: Steatosis, Steatohepatitis, and Cirrhosis

Alcohol-associated liver disease progresses through a recognized spectrum, beginning with simple hepatic steatosis, generally reversible with alcohol cessation, through alcohol-associated steatohepatitis, characterized by inflammation and hepatocyte injury alongside steatosis, to progressive fibrosis and eventually cirrhosis in a subset of affected individuals, and the amount and duration of alcohol consumption required to produce this progression varies considerably between individuals, reflecting genetic and other host susceptibility factors that are not yet fully characterized, meaning that a specific consumption threshold cannot reliably predict which individual patient will progress to advanced disease. Sustained alcohol cessation is the single most impactful intervention at every stage of this spectrum, capable of producing meaningful histologic improvement even in patients with established fibrosis, reinforcing why alcohol cessation counseling, applying the same nonjudgmental, direct communication principle emphasized throughout this book, should be a central, ongoing component of management regardless of the specific stage of disease a patient has reached at presentation. Patients with concurrent MASLD risk factors, discussed later in this chapter, appear to experience accelerated alcohol-associated liver disease progression at lower alcohol consumption thresholds than patients without these metabolic risk factors, illustrating how these two increasingly common liver disease processes can interact and compound one another rather than existing as entirely independent conditions in a given patient. Even a partial reduction in consumption, when complete cessation is not immediately achievable, confers meaningful benefit and should be encouraged and supported as a reasonable intermediate goal rather than treated as an unacceptable compromise relative to complete abstinence alone. Framing this progression as a continuum rather than a series of fixed, discrete categories helps patients understand that intervention at any point along this spectrum, not only at an early or a late stage specifically, offers genuine benefit. Hope, grounded in evidence, motivates lasting change more effectively than fear alone.

### Alcohol-Associated Hepatitis: Diagnosis and Severity Assessment

Alcohol-associated hepatitis presents with the acute onset of jaundice in a patient with heavy, sustained alcohol use, typically accompanied by an aspartate-to-alanine aminotransferase ratio greater than 2, with both values usually only modestly elevated, a laboratory pattern discussed in the previous chapter, and severity assessment using a validated score, most commonly the Maddrey discriminant function or the model for end-stage liver disease score, distinguishes severe from non-severe disease and directly determines whether specific pharmacologic treatment, discussed below, is warranted. Liver biopsy, while not required for diagnosis in a patient with a classic clinical presentation, is considered when the diagnosis remains uncertain or when an alternative or additional cause of liver injury is suspected, since a confident clinical diagnosis based on history, laboratory pattern, and exclusion of other causes is sufficient in most straightforward presentations without requiring routine invasive confirmation. The model for end-stage liver disease score offers an advantage over the older Maddrey discriminant function in that it is already familiar to clinicians from its broader use in liver transplant allocation and general cirrhosis severity assessment, discussed further in a later chapter, allowing a single scoring framework to serve multiple purposes across a patient's overall liver disease management. When biopsy is pursued in this population, coagulopathy from underlying liver dysfunction may necessitate a transjugular rather than percutaneous approach, applying the same procedural safety consideration already established in earlier chapters for biopsy in patients with an elevated bleeding risk profile. Consistent application of one of these validated scores at initial presentation, rather than an informal clinical severity impression alone, ensures that the treatment threshold discussed throughout this section is applied systematically rather than left to variable individual clinician judgment. Structured, systematic assessment protects patients from inconsistent, ad hoc decision-making.

Figure 16.2: Histologic Spectrum of Alcohol-Associated Liver Disease

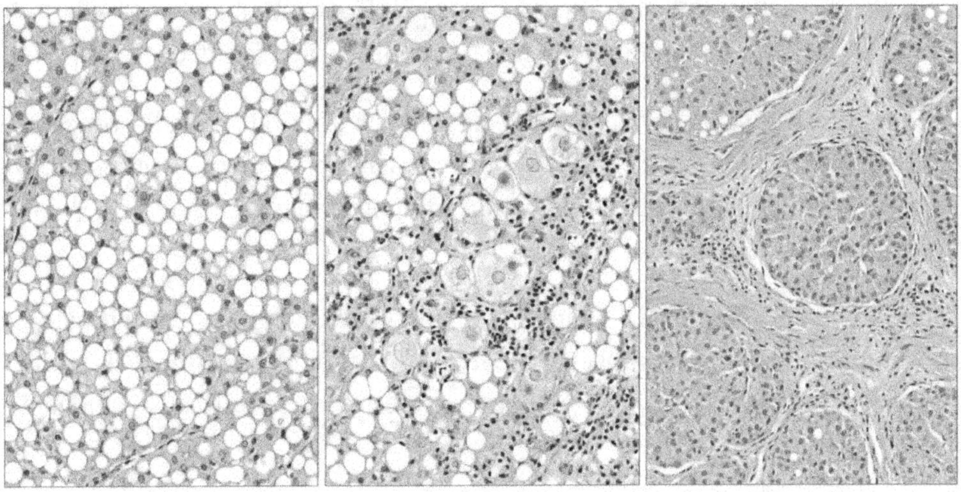


## Treatment of Severe Alcohol-Associated Hepatitis

Corticosteroid therapy, generally prednisolone, is the primary pharmacologic treatment for severe alcohol-associated hepatitis meeting the severity threshold discussed above, and treatment response is formally reassessed at day seven using the Lille score, which incorporates the trajectory of bilirubin change from baseline, with a favorable Lille score indicating meaningful mortality benefit from continued corticosteroid therapy and an unfavorable score indicating corticosteroid futility, at which point continued treatment should be discontinued rather than persisted with in hope of delayed benefit that the scoring system's validation studies do not support. Infection screening, given the immunosuppressive effect of corticosteroid therapy layered onto an already immunologically vulnerable population, should be completed before initiating corticosteroids, and active, untreated infection is a contraindication to corticosteroid therapy until adequately treated, reinforcing why this screening step must precede rather than follow treatment initiation in a condition where corticosteroid therapy is otherwise clearly indicated by severity criteria. Pentoxifylline, an older alternative therapy for severe alcohol-associated hepatitis, has largely fallen out of favor given more limited evidence of mortality benefit compared to corticosteroids, though it may still be considered in a patient with a contraindication to corticosteroid therapy, such as active, uncontrolled infection, where corticosteroid-associated immunosuppression risk would be unacceptable.

**THE GI THRESHOLD DECISION SYSTEM — Hepatic Thresholds — The Day-Seven Lille Score Reassessment in Severe Alcohol-Associated Hepatitis**

**Presentation Signature:** A patient with severe alcohol-associated hepatitis has been started on corticosteroid therapy, and the clinician must determine whether to continue or discontinue treatment at the planned reassessment point.

**Threshold Point:** The Lille score, calculated at day seven of corticosteroid therapy using the trajectory of bilirubin change from baseline, defines the threshold separating corticosteroid responders, who derive meaningful mortality benefit from continued therapy, from nonresponders, in whom continued corticosteroid therapy provides no additional benefit and only prolongs infection risk exposure.

**The Call:** A favorable Lille score at day seven supports continuing the full corticosteroid course; an unfavorable score defines corticosteroid futility and treatment should be discontinued, with the patient's overall management, including transplant evaluation in appropriately selected candidates, reconsidered based on this nonresponse.

**Trap Logic:** Continuing corticosteroid therapy beyond day seven in a patient with an unfavorable Lille score, hoping for delayed response, exposes the patient to ongoing infection risk without the mortality benefit that would justify this risk, since the scoring system was specifically validated to identify this futility point.

**Decision Anchor:** Calculate the Lille score formally at day seven of corticosteroid therapy in every treated patient, and discontinue therapy promptly upon an unfavorable result rather than continuing treatment based on clinical impression alone.

## Hepatitis D and Coinfection Considerations

Hepatitis D, a defective virus requiring hepatitis B surface antigen for its own viral assembly and therefore occurring exclusively as either a simultaneous coinfection or a superinfection in a patient already chronically infected with hepatitis B, produces a more aggressive disease course than hepatitis B monoinfection alone, with accelerated progression to cirrhosis and higher rates of hepatocellular carcinoma, and screening for hepatitis D should be considered in any patient with chronic hepatitis B who has risk factors for this coinfection or who demonstrates an unexpectedly severe or atypical disease course relative to their hepatitis B markers alone. Treatment options for hepatitis D have historically been limited, with pegylated interferon representing the mainstay for many years despite modest efficacy, though newer targeted antiviral agents specifically developed for hepatitis D have recently become available in some regions, representing a meaningful advance for a condition that has lagged behind the treatment progress achieved for hepatitis B and C individually. Hepatitis D prevalence varies substantially by geographic region, with certain areas demonstrating considerably higher rates than others, and this geographic variation should inform the threshold for screening in a patient with a relevant travel or immigration history from a higher-prevalence region.

### HIV Coinfection With Viral Hepatitis

HIV coinfection with hepatitis B or C accelerates liver disease progression and requires coordinated management between hepatology and infectious disease given the specific drug interaction considerations between antiretroviral and hepatitis-directed therapy, and patients with HIV should be specifically screened for both hepatitis B and C given their shared transmission routes and the substantially worse liver-related outcomes this coinfection produces if unrecognized and untreated. Sequencing of treatment initiation between the two infections, when both require simultaneous therapy, should be planned collaboratively rather than assuming a default order, since certain drug interactions and the risk of immune reconstitution-related hepatic flares can influence the optimal timing in a given patient's specific clinical situation.

## Hepatitis B and C in Pregnancy and Vertical Transmission Prevention

Hepatitis B screening is a standard, universal component of prenatal care, and infants born to hepatitis B surface antigen-positive mothers require both hepatitis B immunoglobulin and initiation of the hepatitis B vaccine series within a specific window after birth, generally within twelve hours, to effectively prevent vertical transmission, and mothers with high viral loads late in pregnancy may additionally receive antiviral therapy specifically to further reduce transmission risk beyond what neonatal immunoprophylaxis alone achieves, reflecting a layered prevention strategy tailored to maternal viral load. Hepatitis C, in contrast, has no available immunoprophylaxis or vaccine, and vertical transmission prevention currently relies on avoiding unnecessary invasive obstetric procedures during delivery when feasible, though the overall vertical transmission rate is relatively low even without a specific preventive intervention, and infants born to hepatitis C-positive mothers should be tested using an appropriately timed strategy that accounts for the persistence of maternal antibody in the infant's circulation for many months after birth. Confirming this immunoprophylaxis was actually administered and completed on schedule, rather than assuming it occurred simply because the protocol exists, requires deliberate follow-up given the serious consequences of a missed dose in this specific, time-sensitive prevention window. Breastfeeding is not contraindicated in hepatitis C-positive mothers under most circumstances, a reassurance worth communicating explicitly given the understandable concern many new mothers have about potential transmission through breast milk, since current evidence does not support meaningful transmission risk through this route in the absence of cracked or bleeding nipples.

### Treatment Timing Considerations in Reproductive-Age Patients

Direct-acting antiviral therapy for hepatitis C is not currently recommended during pregnancy given limited safety data in this population, meaning that treatment is generally deferred until after delivery in a woman who becomes pregnant while infected or is diagnosed during pregnancy, while hepatitis B antiviral therapy, when indicated for the mother's own disease control independent of the transmission-prevention indication discussed above, uses agents with an established pregnancy safety profile, illustrating how treatment timing and agent selection in reproductive-age patients require this hepatitis-B-versus-hepatitis-C-specific consideration rather than a uniform approach applied across both viral hepatitis types. Discussing this deferral plan explicitly with the patient, including realistic timing for treatment initiation after delivery, prevents the misunderstanding that the pregnancy diagnosis somehow disqualifies the patient from ever receiving curative treatment rather than simply postponing it to a safer time.

## Alcohol Use Disorder Screening and Treatment Integration

Screening for alcohol use disorder using a brief, validated instrument should be a routine, standardized component of every encounter with a patient presenting with any stage of alcohol-associated liver disease, applying the same universal, nonjudgmental screening standard already emphasized throughout this book, rather than relying on the patient to volunteer their consumption pattern accurately, since underreporting of alcohol use is common and well documented across clinical settings for reasons including stigma, denial, and simple underestimation of actual intake. Pharmacologic therapy for alcohol use disorder, including naltrexone, acamprosate, and, in appropriately selected patients without significant hepatic impairment precluding its use, disulfiram, should be considered alongside behavioral interventions for patients with alcohol-associated liver disease, and the presence of liver disease itself should not automatically preclude pharmacologic treatment for the underlying alcohol use disorder, since certain agents are safe even in the setting of significant hepatic impairment, with agent selection individualized based on the specific degree of liver disease severity and other patient-specific factors. Integrating this screening directly into the standard intake or vital-signs workflow, rather than treating it as an optional add-on dependent on individual clinician initiative, improves consistency of application across a busy practice managing many competing priorities during any given visit. Consulting with addiction medicine or a hepatologist experienced in this specific population, when significant hepatic impairment makes agent selection genuinely uncertain, supports safe, individualized prescribing rather than either withholding pharmacotherapy entirely out of excessive caution or selecting an agent without adequately considering the patient's specific degree of hepatic impairment.

### Integrated Hepatology-Addiction Medicine Care Models

Integrated care models combining hepatology and addiction medicine within the same clinical encounter or closely coordinated visits have demonstrated improved outcomes compared with the traditional, more fragmented approach of separate, uncoordinated referrals, and establishing or referring to such an integrated program, where available, represents a meaningful improvement over managing the liver disease and the underlying alcohol use disorder as separate, parallel processes without deliberate coordination between the treating teams. Building such a program requires deliberate institutional investment and leadership support, and even without a fully integrated clinic, informal, proactive coordination between the involved specialties, initiated by whichever clinician first encounters the patient, achieves much of this benefit without requiring a formal, resource-intensive program to be established first. Yes.

## Early Transplant Referral in Severe Alcohol-Associated Hepatitis

Early liver transplantation, before the traditional six-month sobriety requirement historically applied uniformly to all liver transplant candidates, has emerged as an evidence-based option for carefully selected patients with severe alcohol-associated hepatitis not responding to corticosteroid therapy, based on outcomes data demonstrating meaningful survival benefit in appropriately selected patients evaluated by experienced, multidisciplinary transplant teams using structured psychosocial assessment tools rather than an arbitrary, fixed sobriety duration applied uniformly regardless of individual circumstances. This represents a significant evolution from historical transplant practice, and patients and referring clinicians unfamiliar with this evolving evidence and practice pattern may not realize this option exists, making explicit discussion of early transplant referral appropriate in a corticosteroid-nonresponsive severe alcohol-associated hepatitis patient who would otherwise be presumed ineligible under the older, uniform sobriety-duration standard. Post-transplant relapse rates in this early-transplant population, while a legitimate consideration, have not proven prohibitively high in the studies supporting this practice shift, and this outcome data, rather than an intuitive assumption that early transplant necessarily carries excessive relapse risk, should inform the clinical decision-making and patient counseling around this option. Truly.

### Psychosocial Assessment for Early Transplant Candidacy

Structured psychosocial assessment tools used to evaluate early transplant candidacy in this population incorporate factors beyond simple sobriety duration alone, including insight into the alcohol use disorder, social support, and commitment to post-transplant treatment engagement, and this more nuanced, multidimensional assessment approach reflects growing recognition that a fixed sobriety duration alone is an imperfect predictor of post-transplant outcomes, including relapse risk, compared to this more comprehensive evaluation framework. Involving family members in this assessment, with the patient's consent, provides additional context about social support that the patient's own self-report alone might not fully capture, supporting a more complete, accurate evaluation of the multiple factors this assessment framework considers. Yes.

## Pediatric and Lean MASLD Considerations

Metabolic dysfunction-associated steatotic liver disease is increasingly recognized in children and adolescents, paralleling rising pediatric obesity rates, and its evaluation and management in this population requires specific pediatric expertise given differences in disease presentation, the histologic pattern of injury, which can differ from the typical adult pattern, and the family-centered behavioral intervention approach required for meaningful, sustained lifestyle modification in a pediatric patient whose dietary and activity patterns are substantially influenced by household and family factors beyond the patient's own individual control. Lean MASLD, occurring in patients without obesity by conventional body mass index criteria but who nonetheless meet the cardiometabolic risk factor criteria discussed earlier in this chapter, represents an important and increasingly recognized phenotype, particularly in certain ethnic populations with a predisposition toward visceral adiposity and metabolic dysfunction at a lower body mass index threshold than more traditional risk stratification models were originally developed to capture, and clinicians should not dismiss the possibility of clinically significant MASLD in a patient who does not appear overweight by simple visual assessment or standard body mass index calculation alone. Coordinating care with a pediatric hepatologist or gastroenterologist, where available, provides more targeted expertise than an adult-focused approach applied without modification to this distinct population, and this specialized referral should be considered proactively rather than only after standard adult-oriented counseling has already failed to produce meaningful change. Waist circumference, rather than body mass index alone, may better capture the visceral adiposity pattern driving risk in this specific phenotype, and incorporating this simple, low-cost measurement into routine assessment can help identify at-risk patients who would otherwise be overlooked by body mass index screening alone.

### Ethnic and Population-Specific Risk Variation

Genetic variants, most notably in the PNPLA3 gene, contribute to differential MASLD risk and severity across different ethnic populations independent of body mass index or other conventional metabolic risk factors, and awareness of this genetic contribution helps explain why some patients develop significant liver disease despite seemingly modest conventional risk factor burden, reinforcing why cardiometabolic risk factor assessment, rather than body habitus alone, should drive the decision to evaluate for MASLD in any given patient. Genetic testing for these specific variants is not currently recommended as routine clinical practice given limited actionable implications at the individual patient level beyond the risk-factor-based assessment already established in this chapter, and this research finding should be understood as informing population-level risk variation rather than serving as an indication for individual genetic testing at this time. Population science informs individual care indirectly.

## Occupational and Public Health Considerations in Viral Hepatitis

Healthcare workers with occupational exposure to blood or body fluids require a structured post-exposure evaluation protocol addressing hepatitis B, hepatitis C, and HIV simultaneously, and hepatitis B immune status should be documented and, where indicated, boosted proactively as part of routine occupational health screening for healthcare workers, given that the availability of an effective vaccine makes hepatitis B, unlike hepatitis C, a preventable occupational exposure risk when immunity is properly established and maintained before any exposure occurs. Public health reporting requirements for viral hepatitis vary by jurisdiction but generally require timely notification of newly diagnosed cases to support contact tracing and, where relevant, outbreak investigation, and clinicians should be familiar with their local reporting obligations rather than assuming this responsibility falls entirely to the laboratory or another party, since delayed or missed reporting can meaningfully hamper public health efforts to identify and interrupt ongoing transmission chains, particularly in the setting of a recognized local outbreak. Timely, standardized post-exposure protocols, ideally accessible through a dedicated occupational health service available around the clock, ensure that healthcare workers who sustain an exposure receive appropriate risk assessment and, where indicated, prophylaxis without delay, since some interventions carry meaningfully reduced efficacy the longer they are delayed after the exposure event. Building this reporting step into the standard workflow used when a positive result is received, rather than relying on the ordering clinician to separately remember this obligation, reduces the likelihood a report is inadvertently missed amid other clinical priorities. Prevention is always preferable.

### Harm Reduction Approaches for Injection Drug Use-Related Transmission

Harm reduction services, including needle and syringe exchange programs and medication-assisted treatment for opioid use disorder, meaningfully reduce hepatitis B and C transmission in populations with injection drug use, and gastroenterologists and hepatologists, even when not directly providing these services themselves, should be familiar with locally available harm reduction resources and make referrals proactively for patients whose ongoing injection drug use places them at continued risk of both new infection and reinfection after successful hepatitis C treatment, since treatment success alone does not address the underlying risk behavior that led to the initial infection. Approaching this referral conversation without judgment, framing it as a practical, protective step rather than a moral commentary on the patient's substance use, supports the same nonjudgmental communication standard emphasized throughout this book for other sensitive topics. Always.

## Reinfection After Hepatitis C Cure and Post-Treatment Monitoring

Sustained virologic response following direct-acting antiviral therapy represents a functional cure with an extremely low relapse rate, but patients with ongoing risk factors, most notably continued injection drug use, remain susceptible to reinfection with a new hepatitis C exposure, and this distinction, reinfection from a new exposure rather than relapse of the originally treated infection, should be communicated clearly to patients, since a positive HCV RNA test after prior confirmed cure years later most likely represents this new infection rather than a failure of the original treatment, an important point for accurate patient counseling and appropriate management planning. Post-treatment monitoring beyond confirming sustained virologic response is generally limited in patients without significant fibrosis at the time of treatment, since the liver-related risk in this population becomes quite low following successful cure, while patients with advanced fibrosis or cirrhosis at the time of treatment continue to require the same hepatocellular carcinoma surveillance program discussed earlier in this chapter, since successful viral cure reduces but does not entirely eliminate the elevated cancer risk that established advanced fibrosis or cirrhosis confers, even after the underlying viral driver has been eliminated. Counseling patients about reinfection risk at the time of treatment completion, rather than only if a subsequent positive test raises the concern, proactively sets expectations and supports continued engagement with any relevant harm reduction resources discussed earlier in this chapter. Clearly documenting each patient's specific fibrosis stage at the time of treatment, rather than a general note that treatment was successful, ensures this critical distinction, whether ongoing hepatocellular carcinoma surveillance is indicated, remains clear to any clinician reviewing the record in the future. Truly.

### Communicating the Distinction Between Cure and Ongoing Risk

This nuanced message, that hepatitis C is curable but that advanced fibrosis-related cancer risk persists even after cure, and that ongoing risk behavior can still result in a new infection despite prior successful treatment, requires careful, clear communication to avoid either of two problematic extremes: a patient who believes cure eliminates all future liver-related risk and therefore discontinues appropriate surveillance, or a patient who becomes discouraged believing that treatment success was somehow incomplete or meaningless given these ongoing considerations. A brief, structured explanation delivered at the treatment-completion visit, ideally reinforced in writing, provides a durable reference the patient can revisit later if questions arise well after the treatment course has concluded and the details of this initial conversation have faded from memory. Indeed.

## Metabolic Dysfunction-Associated Steatotic Liver Disease

### Diagnostic Criteria and Nomenclature Evolution

Metabolic dysfunction-associated steatotic liver disease, the current preferred terminology replacing the previously used nonalcoholic fatty liver disease nomenclature, requires evidence of hepatic steatosis on imaging or histology alongside at least one cardiometabolic risk factor, including obesity, type 2 diabetes, hypertension, or dyslipidemia, and this updated nomenclature and diagnostic framework reflects a deliberate shift away from a diagnosis defined primarily by exclusion, the absence of significant alcohol use, toward a diagnosis defined positively by the presence of specific metabolic risk factors, a change intended to reduce diagnostic stigma and more accurately reflect the disease's underlying metabolic pathophysiology. This condition represents the hepatic manifestation of the broader metabolic syndrome and has become the most common cause of chronic liver disease in many populations, paralleling rising rates of obesity and type 2 diabetes, and clinicians should recognize this condition as a systemic metabolic disorder with hepatic manifestations rather than an isolated liver disease, since its management, discussed below, extends well beyond liver-directed therapy alone. This nomenclature transition has occurred relatively recently, and clinicians, patients, and the broader medical literature will continue to reference the older terminology for some time, making familiarity with both naming conventions, and the ability to communicate the equivalence between them, a practical necessity during this transitional period. Screening for MASLD in patients with established cardiometabolic risk factors, such as type 2 diabetes, applying the same proactive rather than reactive screening philosophy already established throughout this book, allows earlier identification and intervention before significant fibrosis has developed, rather than waiting for symptoms or incidentally discovered abnormal liver chemistries to prompt evaluation. Both terms will likely appear side by side in clinical documentation, patient education materials, and the broader literature for the foreseeable future, and clinicians should be prepared to use either term fluently depending on their audience. Reassessing cardiometabolic risk factors periodically over time, since they can develop or worsen after an initial evaluation, ensures this screening indication is not overlooked in a patient whose risk profile evolves. Precision in language reduces confusion across the care team. Nothing about this is static.

## Risk Stratification and Fibrosis Assessment

Most patients with metabolic dysfunction-associated steatotic liver disease have simple steatosis without significant fibrosis and a relatively favorable long-term liver-related prognosis, while a meaningful minority progress to metabolic dysfunction-associated steatohepatitis with fibrosis and, in a smaller subset, to cirrhosis, and identifying this higher-risk minority is the central goal of the risk stratification approach developed throughout this section, since liver-related mortality risk correlates most strongly with fibrosis stage rather than with the presence or severity of steatosis or inflammation alone. The fibrosis-4 index, calculated from age, aminotransferases, and platelet count, and available at essentially no additional cost using values already present in routine laboratory testing, serves as an efficient first-line risk stratification tool, with a low score providing reassurance against significant fibrosis and a high or indeterminate score prompting further evaluation with vibration-controlled transient elastography or another validated noninvasive fibrosis assessment technique, reserving liver biopsy, as established in the previous chapter, for cases where noninvasive assessment remains genuinely inconclusive. Communicating this risk-stratification concept directly to patients, that the presence of fatty liver alone is not the primary concern but rather the degree of fibrosis it may or may not have caused, helps patients understand why some are managed with lifestyle counseling alone while others require more intensive fibrosis-focused evaluation and treatment. The fibrosis-4 index has recognized limitations in certain populations, including reduced accuracy at the extremes of age, and clinicians should be aware of these specific limitations rather than applying the tool uncritically without considering whether they might apply to the individual patient being assessed. This message, that fibrosis stage matters far more than the presence of fat alone, is worth repeating at multiple points during a patient's ongoing care. Repetition, delivered warmly, aids retention.

## Management: Lifestyle and Emerging Pharmacotherapy

Weight loss, generally targeting a specific percentage of total body weight loss depending on disease severity, with greater weight loss required to achieve fibrosis regression than to achieve steatosis or inflammation improvement alone, remains the cornerstone of management, achieved through structured dietary modification, increased physical activity, and, in appropriately selected patients with more severe disease or obesity, pharmacologic weight loss therapy or bariatric surgery, and this graded weight-loss target, rather than a single generic recommendation to lose weight, helps set realistic, disease-severity-matched expectations for the degree of change required to achieve meaningful histologic benefit. Pharmacotherapy specifically targeting metabolic dysfunction-associated steatohepatitis has expanded meaningfully in recent years, with an approved agent, resmetirom, a thyroid hormone receptor beta agonist, now available for patients with biopsy-confirmed steatohepatitis and significant fibrosis, and glucagon-like peptide-1 receptor agonists, developed and initially approved for diabetes and weight management, demonstrating benefit for liver-related endpoints as well, reflecting the increasingly integrated, multi-system treatment approach this condition's metabolic underpinnings support, and coordination with endocrinology or obesity medicine specialists is increasingly a valuable component of comprehensive management given this expanding, overlapping pharmacologic landscape. Referral to a structured, multidisciplinary weight management program, incorporating dietary counseling, behavioral support, and, where appropriate, pharmacologic or surgical options together, generally achieves more sustained weight loss than generic dietary advice delivered in isolation during a routine clinic visit, and this referral should be considered proactively in patients with more advanced disease where the required weight loss target is substantial. Patient selection for resmetirom specifically requires the biopsy-confirmed fibrosis stage this agent's approval was based on, meaning noninvasive fibrosis assessment alone, while adequate for general risk stratification, may not currently be sufficient to determine eligibility without biopsy confirmation, an important practical distinction to communicate to interested patients. Gradual, sustained weight loss over months rather than rapid weight loss carries the additional benefit of avoiding the rare but recognized paradoxical liver injury that can accompany extremely rapid weight reduction. Staying current with this rapidly evolving pharmacologic landscape, including newly approved agents and expanding indications, is essential given the pace of recent progress in this area. Small, sustained changes outperform dramatic, short-lived ones. Standing still is not an option.

FIGURE 16.3: FIBROSIS-4 INDEX AND NONINVASIVE RISK STRATIFICATION PATHWAY

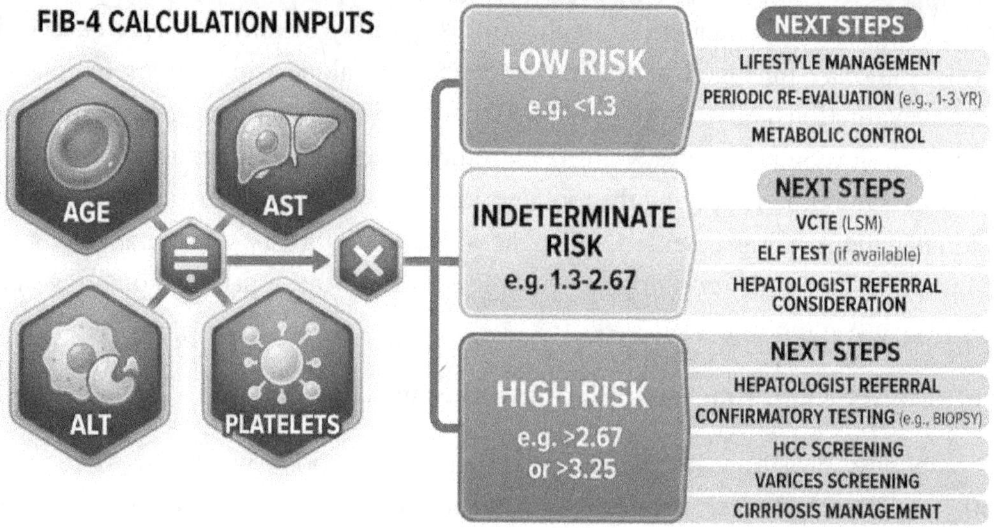


Case Presentation: A 52-year-old man is identified through universal screening to have chronic hepatitis C infection, confirmed with positive HCV RNA testing, genotype 1, and noninvasive fibrosis assessment demonstrates no significant fibrosis. Applying the reasoning developed in this chapter, he is counseled that his infection is highly treatable with a short course of oral direct-acting antiviral therapy, addressing his initial anxiety based on an outdated understanding of hepatitis C treatment from years ago when a family member underwent unsuccessful, poorly tolerated interferon-based therapy. He completes an 8-week direct-acting antiviral regimen without significant side effects, and HCV RNA testing twelve weeks after treatment completion confirms sustained virologic response, meeting criteria for cure. This case illustrates the chapter's central hepatitis C treatment principle: current direct-acting antiviral therapy achieves cure in the substantial majority of patients with a short, well-tolerated course, and communicating this transformed prognosis explicitly counters outdated perceptions that might otherwise create unnecessary anxiety or treatment hesitancy.

Case Presentation: A 48-year-old woman with a long history of heavy alcohol use presents with jaundice, and laboratory evaluation demonstrates an aspartate-to-alanine aminotransferase ratio of 2.8 with both values modestly elevated, alongside a Maddrey discriminant function score meeting criteria for severe alcohol-associated hepatitis. Infection screening is completed and is negative, and corticosteroid therapy is initiated. Applying the reasoning developed in this chapter, the Lille score is formally calculated at day seven, demonstrating a favorable response based on her bilirubin trajectory. She completes her full corticosteroid course with continued clinical improvement and is engaged with addiction medicine for structured alcohol treatment before discharge. This case illustrates the chapter's central severe alcohol-associated hepatitis principle: the day-seven Lille score reassessment, rather than clinical impression alone, confirmed that continued corticosteroid therapy was warranted, and infection screening completed before treatment initiation ensured this immunosuppressive therapy could be given safely.

## Hepatocellular Carcinoma Surveillance Across Etiologies

Hepatocellular carcinoma surveillance, generally performed with ultrasound at defined intervals, with or without serum alpha-fetoprotein, is recommended for patients with cirrhosis from any etiology and for a subset of noncirrhotic patients with chronic hepatitis B who meet specific age, ethnicity, or family history criteria that confer elevated risk even in the absence of cirrhosis, reflecting hepatitis B's distinct oncogenic potential through direct viral integration into the host genome rather than solely through the cirrhosis pathway that drives hepatocellular carcinoma risk in most other chronic liver disease etiologies. This distinction matters practically, since a clinician might reasonably assume, incorrectly, that surveillance is unnecessary in a noncirrhotic hepatitis B patient given the absence of the advanced fibrosis that typically triggers surveillance in other liver diseases, when in fact specific hepatitis B patient subgroups warrant surveillance independent of fibrosis stage. Adherence to surveillance in this specific noncirrhotic hepatitis B subgroup tends to be lower than in cirrhotic patients across most practice settings, likely reflecting the less intuitive rationale for surveillance in a patient without the more visible marker of advanced liver disease that cirrhosis represents, making explicit patient and clinician education about this specific indication particularly valuable.

### Surveillance Adherence and Systems-Level Support

Surveillance adherence across all eligible patient populations remains suboptimal in many practice settings, and systems-level interventions, including automated recall reminders built into the electronic health record and dedicated nursing or care coordinator support for scheduling, meaningfully improve adherence beyond what relying on individual clinician or patient initiative alone typically achieves, applying the same systems-based quality improvement principle already emphasized throughout this book for other surveillance programs requiring sustained, longitudinal engagement. Tracking surveillance completion rates at the practice or health system level, similar to other quality metrics tracked throughout medicine, can identify gaps and drive targeted improvement efforts rather than relying solely on individual clinician vigilance across a large, dispersed patient population.

| Disease | Key Diagnostic Step | First-Line Treatment |
|---|---|---|
| Chronic hepatitis B | Phase classification (HBV DNA, HBeAg, ALT) | Tenofovir or entecavir if immune-active |
| Chronic hepatitis C | Antibody screen + confirmatory HCV RNA | Direct-acting antiviral therapy (8-12 weeks) |
| Severe alcohol-associated hepatitis | Maddrey discriminant function or MELD | Corticosteroids with day-7 Lille reassessment |
| MASLD | Cardiometabolic risk factor + steatosis on imaging | Weight loss; resmetirom or GLP-1 RA if indicated |

**THE GI THRESHOLD DECISION SYSTEM — Chronic and Acute Liver Disease Treatment Thresholds**

**Presentation Signature:** This chapter's threshold instances addressed treatment initiation criteria in chronic hepatitis B and the day-seven Lille score reassessment in severe alcohol-associated hepatitis.

**Threshold Point:** Phase classification, not a single viral load or aminotransferase value, gates hepatitis B treatment initiation; the day-seven Lille score, not clinical impression, gates continuation or discontinuation of corticosteroid therapy in severe alcohol-associated hepatitis.

**The Call:** Both thresholds convert an evolving clinical picture into a structured, criteria-based decision point rather than leaving treatment initiation or continuation to informal, momentary clinical judgment.

**Trap Logic:** Treating hepatitis B based on a single value without phase reassessment, and continuing corticosteroids in severe alcohol-associated hepatitis beyond an unfavorable day-seven Lille score, are this chapter's most consequential threshold misapplications.

**Decision Anchor:** Reassess hepatitis B phase classification at each monitoring visit before deciding on treatment, and calculate the Lille score formally at day seven in every corticosteroid-treated severe alcohol-associated hepatitis patient, discontinuing therapy promptly upon an unfavorable result.

## Summary and Key Concepts

Hepatitis A and E are generally self-limited in immunocompetent hosts, though hepatitis E can cause severe disease in pregnancy and chronic infection in immunocompromised patients.

Chronic hepatitis B treatment is determined by phase classification, incorporating HBV DNA, HBeAg status, and aminotransferase levels, reassessed at each visit rather than fixed permanently.

Universal one-time hepatitis C screening is now recommended for all adults, and current direct-acting antiviral therapy achieves cure in the substantial majority of patients with a short oral course.

Alcohol-associated liver disease progresses through steatosis, steatohepatitis, and fibrosis, with sustained cessation capable of producing meaningful improvement at every stage, and severe alcohol-associated hepatitis is treated with corticosteroids reassessed using the day-seven Lille score.

Metabolic dysfunction-associated steatotic liver disease, the updated nomenclature reflecting a positive, metabolic-risk-factor-based diagnostic approach, requires steatosis alongside at least one cardiometabolic risk factor.

Fibrosis stage, assessed efficiently using the FIB-4 index as a first-line tool, correlates most strongly with liver-related mortality in MASLD, and management combines graded weight-loss targets with emerging pharmacotherapy including resmetirom and GLP-1 receptor agonists.

# CHAPTER 17: AUTOIMMUNE, CHOLESTATIC, AND GENETIC LIVER DISEASE

**Learning Objectives**

1. Apply diagnostic criteria for autoimmune hepatitis and describe its induction and maintenance treatment approach, including the treatment withdrawal threshold.
2. Diagnose primary biliary cholangitis and apply a response-based treatment escalation pathway.
3. Diagnose primary sclerosing cholangitis and describe its association with inflammatory bowel disease and cholangiocarcinoma risk.
4. Apply surveillance and management strategies specific to primary sclerosing cholangitis.
5. Describe the diagnosis and management of hereditary hemochromatosis, Wilson disease, and alpha-1 antitrypsin deficiency in their chronic presentations.

**Chapter Outline**

This chapter develops the immune-mediated and genetic liver diseases that produce chronic, often insidious liver injury: autoimmune hepatitis and its diagnostic scoring and treatment withdrawal threshold, primary biliary cholangitis and its response-based treatment escalation pathway, primary sclerosing cholangitis and its distinctive inflammatory bowel disease association and cholangiocarcinoma risk, and the genetic and metabolic liver diseases, hereditary hemochromatosis, Wilson disease, and alpha-1 antitrypsin deficiency, in their chronic presentations. Each section connects a specific diagnostic or treatment-response threshold to a defined management pathway.

## Autoimmune Hepatitis

### Diagnosis and Diagnostic Scoring

Autoimmune hepatitis, introduced briefly in an earlier chapter as a cause of acute severe liver injury, more commonly presents with an indolent, chronic course, and diagnosis integrates elevated aminotransferases, positive autoantibodies, most commonly antinuclear antibody or anti-smooth muscle antibody in type 1 disease and anti-liver-kidney microsomal antibody in the less common type 2 disease, elevated immunoglobulin G, and characteristic histologic findings including interface hepatitis and plasma cell infiltration, with a validated diagnostic scoring system available to standardize this integration when the diagnosis remains uncertain based on individual features alone. Liver biopsy is generally recommended before finalizing the diagnosis and initiating treatment, since histologic confirmation both supports diagnostic certainty and provides a baseline against which future treatment response and, eventually, potential treatment withdrawal can be assessed, and this baseline biopsy, rather than a diagnosis established on serologic and biochemical grounds alone, provides essential information for the long-term management decisions developed later in this section. Type 1 disease is far more common overall, while type 2 disease, defined by anti-liver-kidney microsomal antibody positivity, tends to present at a younger age and, in some studies, follows a somewhat more aggressive course, information that can inform both prognostic counseling and the intensity of initial monitoring for a given patient. In rare cases where coagulopathy or another contraindication makes percutaneous biopsy unsafe, empiric treatment based on strong clinical and serologic evidence, with a plan to obtain biopsy once safely feasible, is a reasonable pragmatic alternative rather than delaying treatment indefinitely in a patient whose presentation otherwise strongly supports the diagnosis. Testing for both antibody types should be pursued together at initial evaluation, rather than sequentially, given the practical efficiency of a combined panel and the diagnostic importance of correctly classifying which subtype a given patient has from the outset.

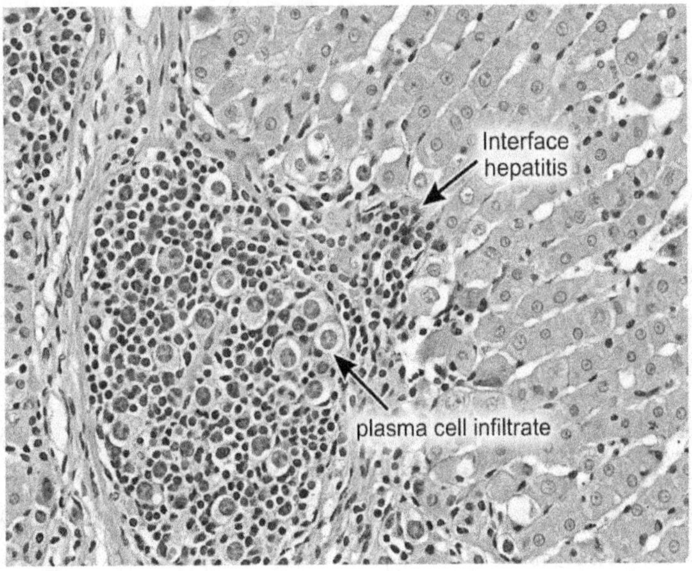


**Treatment: Induction and Maintenance**

Corticosteroid therapy, generally combined with azathioprine as a steroid-sparing agent introduced once initial response is established, induces remission in the substantial majority of patients, and treatment response is monitored using aminotransferase normalization and, ultimately, histologic remission on repeat biopsy, since biochemical remission alone can precede or, in some cases, lag behind genuine histologic resolution of the underlying inflammatory process. Maintenance therapy, typically with azathioprine alone once corticosteroids have been tapered and discontinued, is generally continued for a minimum of two to three years of sustained biochemical and, where available, histologic remission before treatment withdrawal is even considered, reflecting the substantial relapse risk this condition carries and the corresponding need for a cautious, evidence-based approach to eventually discontinuing therapy rather than withdrawing treatment prematurely based on biochemical improvement alone. Thiopurine methyltransferase testing before initiating azathioprine identifies patients at elevated risk of severe azathioprine-related toxicity, particularly myelosuppression, and this testing, applying the same pharmacogenomic screening principle used for other thiopurine-based therapies discussed in earlier chapters, supports safer, more individualized dosing than a uniform starting dose applied without this genetic information. Patients who relapse after an unsuccessful treatment withdrawal attempt generally require reinitiation of the full induction-maintenance sequence, and this relapse, while disappointing, does not indicate treatment failure in the broader sense but rather confirms that the withdrawal attempt was made before the underlying disease process had genuinely resolved. In settings where thiopurine methyltransferase testing is not readily available, close initial monitoring for cytopenia, particularly during the first several weeks of azathioprine therapy, provides a reasonable alternative safeguard, though it does not offer the same pre-treatment risk stratification that genetic testing affords. Precision here compounds over years.

**THE GI THRESHOLD DECISION SYSTEM — Hepatic Thresholds — Treatment Withdrawal in Autoimmune Hepatitis**

**Presentation Signature:** A patient with autoimmune hepatitis has maintained biochemical remission on maintenance therapy for an extended period, and the clinician must determine whether treatment withdrawal can be safely attempted.

**Threshold Point:** Sustained biochemical remission for a minimum duration, generally at least two to three years, combined with histologic remission confirmed on repeat biopsy, defines the threshold below which treatment withdrawal carries an acceptably low relapse risk to attempt; withdrawal attempted before this threshold, based on biochemical improvement alone without histologic confirmation, carries a substantially higher relapse risk.

**The Call:** Patients meeting both the duration and histologic remission criteria may attempt a carefully monitored treatment withdrawal, with close biochemical follow-up to detect early relapse; patients not yet meeting this threshold continue maintenance therapy, with withdrawal reconsidered at a future reassessment once the threshold is met.

**Trap Logic:** Withdrawing treatment based on biochemical remission alone, without the histologic confirmation this threshold requires, risks a relapse that a repeat biopsy might have predicted and prevented by identifying persistent subclinical inflammation despite normalized liver chemistries.

**Decision Anchor:** Require both sustained biochemical remission of adequate duration and histologic confirmation before attempting treatment withdrawal in autoimmune hepatitis, rather than withdrawing therapy based on biochemical normalization alone.

## Primary Biliary Cholangitis

### Diagnosis and Natural History

Primary biliary cholangitis, predominantly affecting middle-aged women, produces a cholestatic biochemical pattern, discussed in an earlier chapter, and diagnosis is established through the combination of this cholestatic pattern with a positive antimitochondrial antibody, present in the substantial majority of cases, without requiring liver biopsy in most straightforward presentations, reserving biopsy for cases where antimitochondrial antibody is negative despite a compatible clinical picture or where an overlapping condition, most notably autoimmune hepatitis, is suspected. Pruritus, often disproportionate to the degree of biochemical cholestasis and sometimes the presenting or most functionally limiting symptom, and fatigue are common and should be specifically assessed and addressed as part of comprehensive management, since these symptoms, while not directly reflecting disease severity, substantially affect quality of life and deserve dedicated attention independent of the liver-directed treatment discussed below. Antinuclear antibody positivity with specific staining patterns, including anti-gp210 and anti-centromere patterns, can occur in primary biliary cholangitis independent of antimitochondrial antibody status and may carry additional prognostic information in some studies, though antimitochondrial antibody remains the primary diagnostic marker relied upon in routine clinical practice. Fatigue in this population, similarly, does not correlate reliably with liver biochemical severity and should be validated as a genuine, disease-related symptom rather than dismissed or attributed reflexively to an unrelated cause simply because it does not track with the objective disease markers a clinician might otherwise expect to explain it. Consultation with a hepatopathologist experienced in interpreting these specific staining patterns can add value in genuinely ambiguous cases, particularly when the standard antimitochondrial antibody result is negative despite a clinical picture otherwise strongly suggestive of primary biliary cholangitis.

### Treatment and Response Assessment

Ursodeoxycholic acid is first-line therapy for essentially all patients with confirmed primary biliary cholangitis, and treatment response is formally assessed after approximately one year using validated biochemical response criteria incorporating alkaline phosphatase and bilirubin trajectory, since an adequate response to ursodeoxycholic acid alone predicts a favorable long-term prognosis approaching that of the general population, while an inadequate response identifies patients at meaningfully elevated risk of disease progression who require treatment escalation. Second-line therapy, most commonly obeticholic acid or a fibrate, is added for patients with an inadequate ursodeoxycholic acid response at this one-year assessment, and this response-based escalation pathway, rather than continuing ursodeoxycholic acid monotherapy indefinitely regardless of response, reflects the same treat-to-target philosophy already established in earlier chapters for other chronic conditions where objective response assessment, rather than treatment duration alone, determines whether escalation is warranted. Weight-based dosing of ursodeoxycholic acid, rather than a fixed dose applied uniformly regardless of patient size, is standard practice, and confirming adequate dosing at the outset prevents an apparent nonresponse that actually reflects underdosing rather than a genuine biological lack of response to this first-line therapy. Obeticholic acid carries a specific labeled warning regarding use in patients with more advanced cirrhosis given a recognized risk of hepatic decompensation in this specific population, and this restriction should be reviewed before initiating second-line therapy, reserving the fibrate-based alternative for patients in whom obeticholic acid carries this contraindication. Documenting the calculated weight-based dose explicitly in the chart, rather than a generic instruction, supports accurate dose verification at subsequent visits and prevents an inadvertent underdosing error from persisting unnoticed over time. Small details of dosing matter more than they might initially seem.

**THE GI THRESHOLD DECISION SYSTEM — Hepatic Thresholds — Treatment Escalation in Primary Biliary Cholangitis**

**Presentation Signature:** A patient with primary biliary cholangitis has completed approximately one year of ursodeoxycholic acid therapy, and the clinician must determine whether to continue monotherapy or escalate to second-line treatment.

**Threshold Point:** Formal biochemical response criteria, incorporating alkaline phosphatase and bilirubin values at the one-year assessment, define the threshold separating adequate responders, who continue favorable long-term prognosis on ursodeoxycholic acid alone, from inadequate responders, who face meaningfully elevated progression risk without treatment escalation.

**The Call:** Adequate responders continue ursodeoxycholic acid monotherapy with ongoing periodic reassessment; inadequate responders are escalated to second-line therapy, most commonly obeticholic acid or a fibrate, added to continued ursodeoxycholic acid rather than substituted for it.

**Trap Logic:** Continuing ursodeoxycholic acid monotherapy indefinitely in a patient who has already demonstrated an inadequate response at the one-year assessment denies that patient the disease-modifying benefit second-line therapy can provide during a window when treatment escalation carries the greatest potential to alter the disease trajectory.

**Decision Anchor:** Formally apply validated biochemical response criteria at the one-year assessment for every primary biliary cholangitis patient, and escalate to second-line therapy promptly upon identifying an inadequate response rather than continuing monotherapy by default.

## Primary Sclerosing Cholangitis

### Diagnosis, Inflammatory Bowel Disease Association, and Cholangiocarcinoma Risk

Primary sclerosing cholangitis, producing progressive inflammation and fibrosis of the intrahepatic and extrahepatic bile ducts, is diagnosed primarily by the characteristic multifocal stricturing and dilation pattern on magnetic resonance cholangiopancreatography, generally without requiring liver biopsy except in cases of suspected small-duct disease, a variant confined to the intrahepatic small ducts not visible on standard cholangiographic imaging, or when an overlap with autoimmune hepatitis is suspected. The strong, well-established association between primary sclerosing cholangitis and inflammatory bowel disease, predominantly ulcerative colitis though also occurring with Crohn colitis, discussed in the ninth chapter, means that every newly diagnosed primary sclerosing cholangitis patient should undergo colonoscopic evaluation for inflammatory bowel disease even in the absence of gastrointestinal symptoms, since a substantial proportion of patients have subclinical or minimally symptomatic colitis at the time of their primary sclerosing cholangitis diagnosis that would otherwise go unrecognized. Cholangiocarcinoma risk, discussed in the previous chapter, is substantially elevated in primary sclerosing cholangitis relative to the general population and relative to most other chronic liver diseases, and this risk, combined with the frequently difficult diagnostic distinction between a dominant benign stricture and an early malignant one in this specific disease, makes cholangiocarcinoma surveillance and dominant stricture evaluation a central, ongoing component of primary sclerosing cholangitis management discussed further below. The small-duct variant, in which biopsy confirms histologic features compatible with primary sclerosing cholangitis despite normal cholangiography, carries a somewhat more favorable natural history overall, including a lower cholangiocarcinoma risk, than classic large-duct disease, though it still requires the ongoing surveillance framework developed throughout this chapter given the persistent, if lower, risk this variant carries. This colonoscopic evaluation, once completed at the time of primary sclerosing cholangitis diagnosis, should also be repeated periodically even if initially negative, since inflammatory bowel disease can develop after the primary sclerosing cholangitis diagnosis in a patient whose index colonoscopy was unremarkable. Repeat imaging over time in small-duct disease is reasonable to monitor for potential progression to large-duct involvement, which occurs in a subset of these patients, converting the surveillance approach toward the standard large-duct protocol once this progression is confirmed. Vigilant, ongoing follow-up remains essential regardless of variant.

**Management and Surveillance**

No pharmacologic therapy has demonstrated clear disease-modifying benefit for primary sclerosing cholangitis itself, distinguishing it from the other cholestatic conditions developed earlier in this chapter, and management centers instead on surveillance for the disease's major complications, colorectal cancer surveillance at the intensified interval already established in the ninth chapter given the coexisting inflammatory bowel disease, hepatocellular carcinoma surveillance once cirrhosis develops, and cholangiocarcinoma surveillance using a combination of periodic cross-sectional or cholangiographic imaging and serum tumor markers, with any new dominant stricture warranting endoscopic evaluation, including brush cytology and, where available, fluorescence in situ hybridization testing, to distinguish a benign fibrotic stricture from an early malignant transformation. Endoscopic dilation of a symptomatic dominant stricture producing cholestatic symptoms or recurrent cholangitis can provide meaningful palliation, though this intervention does not alter the underlying disease's progressive natural history, and liver transplantation remains the only treatment capable of altering long-term survival once the disease has progressed to decompensated cirrhosis, discussed further in the following chapter. Ursodeoxycholic acid, despite its established benefit in primary biliary cholangitis, has not demonstrated a survival or disease-modifying benefit in primary sclerosing cholangitis specifically and, at higher doses, has been associated with worse outcomes in some studies, meaning its use in primary sclerosing cholangitis, unlike primary biliary cholangitis, is not routinely recommended as standard disease-directed therapy. Recurrent bacterial cholangitis, a complication that can develop even without an identifiable dominant stricture, particularly in patients with more advanced disease, requires prompt antibiotic treatment following the same principles established in an earlier chapter, and recurrent episodes may warrant longer-term or prophylactic antibiotic strategies in appropriately selected patients.

Figure 17.2: MRCP Findings in Primary Sclerosing Cholangitis

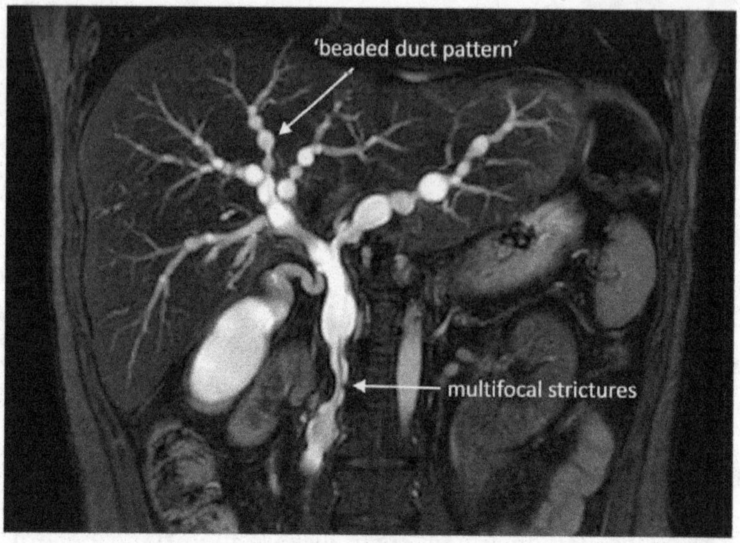


## Overlap Syndromes and Diagnostic Uncertainty

Overlap syndromes, in which a patient demonstrates features of both autoimmune hepatitis and either primary biliary cholangitis or primary sclerosing cholangitis simultaneously, present genuine diagnostic and management complexity, since no single validated diagnostic framework has achieved universal acceptance for these overlap presentations, and management is generally individualized, often combining the immunosuppressive approach used for autoimmune hepatitis with the disease-specific approach appropriate for the coexisting cholestatic condition, guided by which features predominate in a given patient's specific clinical, biochemical, and histologic presentation. Recognizing an overlap syndrome rather than forcing a patient's presentation into a single, cleaner diagnostic category matters practically, since a patient with unrecognized autoimmune hepatitis features superimposed on primary biliary cholangitis, for example, may not respond adequately to ursodeoxycholic acid alone and would benefit from the addition of immunosuppressive therapy directed at the autoimmune hepatitis component specifically. The Paris criteria, one of the more widely referenced frameworks for defining primary biliary cholangitis-autoimmune hepatitis overlap specifically, illustrate the type of structured approach clinicians can apply, though no such framework has achieved the same universal validation and adoption as the diagnostic scoring systems developed for autoimmune hepatitis or primary biliary cholangitis individually. Similarly, a primary sclerosing cholangitis-autoimmune hepatitis overlap, encountered more commonly in pediatric and younger adult patients than in the broader primary sclerosing cholangitis population, may respond partially to immunosuppressive therapy directed at the autoimmune hepatitis component even though the underlying primary sclerosing cholangitis itself, as established earlier in this chapter, lacks disease-modifying pharmacotherapy of its own. Multidisciplinary case review, involving hepatology and, where a rheumatologic or pathology consultation would add value, those specialties as well, is a reasonable step for genuinely difficult overlap cases where the optimal treatment combination remains unclear despite thorough individual evaluation. Care taken here pays dividends.

### When to Reconsider the Working Diagnosis

An inadequate response to appropriately dosed, disease-specific first-line therapy in any of the conditions developed throughout this chapter should prompt reconsideration of the working diagnosis, including the possibility of an overlap syndrome, rather than simply escalating the same treatment approach or extending the observation period indefinitely, applying the same diagnostic-reconsideration principle emphasized throughout this book whenever an expected treatment response does not materialize within a reasonable timeframe. Documenting this reconsideration explicitly, including which alternative diagnoses were considered and excluded, supports transparent clinical reasoning that any subsequent clinician reviewing the case can follow and build upon. Always.

## Pruritus Management in Cholestatic Liver Disease

Cholestatic pruritus, a frequently distressing and functionally impairing symptom in both primary biliary cholangitis and primary sclerosing cholangitis, is managed with a stepwise pharmacologic approach beginning with bile acid sequestrants such as cholestyramine, which bind pruritogenic substances within the intestinal lumen, though these agents require careful timing relative to other medications, particularly ursodeoxycholic acid, given their potential to bind and reduce absorption of concurrently administered oral medications if not appropriately separated in timing. Rifampin, though used off-label for this specific indication in many practice settings, is a reasonable second-line option for pruritus refractory to bile acid sequestrants, with regular liver chemistry monitoring given its own recognized hepatotoxicity potential, and third-line options, including naltrexone and sertraline, target the central and peripheral neurologic pathways thought to contribute to cholestatic pruritus through mechanisms distinct from the luminal bile acid binding mechanism of first-line therapy. Cholestyramine should generally be taken separately from other oral medications by at least a few hours, and patients should be counseled explicitly about this timing requirement, since inadvertent co-administration can meaningfully reduce the absorption and effectiveness of other important medications, including ursodeoxycholic acid itself. Baseline and periodic liver chemistry monitoring after starting rifampin for this indication allows early detection of drug-induced liver injury, applying the same monitoring principle already established in an earlier chapter for other medications carrying recognized hepatotoxicity potential.

### Refractory Pruritus and Emerging Therapies

Ileal bile acid transporter inhibitors, a newer drug class interrupting bile acid recirculation through the enterohepatic circulation, have shown efficacy for refractory cholestatic pruritus and represent an evolving addition to the treatment armamentarium for patients who have not achieved adequate relief with the more established stepwise approach described above, and referral to a hepatologist with specific experience managing refractory pruritus is reasonable for patients whose symptom burden remains severe despite this sequential treatment approach, since quality-of-life impact from unremitting pruritus can be substantial and merits the same dedicated attention as the underlying liver disease itself. Insurance coverage for this newer therapeutic class may vary, and awareness of local access and prior-authorization requirements helps set realistic expectations with patients about how quickly this treatment option could actually be initiated once the decision to pursue it has been made.

## Pregnancy Considerations in Autoimmune and Cholestatic Liver Disease

Autoimmune hepatitis in pregnancy requires careful medication management, since azathioprine, generally considered compatible with pregnancy based on accumulated safety experience, should typically be continued rather than discontinued given the substantial relapse risk that treatment discontinuation carries, both during pregnancy and in the postpartum period specifically, when autoimmune hepatitis relapse risk is recognized to be particularly elevated, making proactive counseling about this postpartum risk an important component of prenatal planning for women with this condition. Primary biliary cholangitis and primary sclerosing cholangitis similarly require individualized pregnancy management, with ursodeoxycholic acid generally continued given its established safety profile in pregnancy, and intrahepatic cholestasis of pregnancy, discussed in an earlier chapter, should be distinguished from a flare or new presentation of one of these underlying chronic cholestatic conditions in a pregnant patient with new pruritus and cholestatic biochemistry, since the diagnostic and management implications differ meaningfully between a pregnancy-specific condition and a chronic disease flare. Corticosteroids, when needed for a flare during pregnancy, are generally considered acceptable given accumulated safety experience, and the decision to escalate treatment during pregnancy should weigh the risk of undertreated maternal disease against medication exposure, applying the same balanced risk-benefit framework already established in earlier chapters for other conditions requiring treatment during pregnancy. Obeticholic acid, in contrast, given its more limited pregnancy safety data, is generally avoided during pregnancy, reinforcing the value of proactive family planning discussions with women of reproductive age before this specific second-line agent is initiated. Postpartum monitoring, given the specific elevated relapse risk during this window, should be scheduled proactively rather than left to occur only at a routine, non-accelerated follow-up interval. Truly.

### Coordinated Prenatal Care for Chronic Liver Disease

Coordinated care between hepatology and maternal-fetal medicine throughout pregnancy, applying the same multidisciplinary coordination model already established in earlier chapters for other complex conditions during pregnancy, supports medication decisions and monitoring that account for both the underlying chronic liver disease and pregnancy-specific considerations simultaneously, and this coordination should ideally begin at preconception counseling whenever a pregnancy is being planned rather than only once pregnancy has already been confirmed. Documenting this coordinated plan explicitly, including which specialty is responsible for which specific monitoring component throughout pregnancy, prevents the ambiguity that can otherwise arise when multiple specialties are simultaneously involved in a single patient's care during this physiologically dynamic period. Revisiting this plan explicitly at each trimester's visit ensures it remains current as pregnancy progresses and circumstances evolve. Yes.

## Pediatric-Onset Autoimmune and Genetic Liver Disease

Autoimmune hepatitis in children and adolescents follows a broadly similar diagnostic and treatment framework to adult disease, though pediatric-specific considerations, including growth monitoring during corticosteroid therapy and the specific psychosocial challenges of managing a chronic disease and its treatment during childhood and adolescence, require dedicated pediatric hepatology expertise, and the transition from pediatric to adult care for these patients benefits from the same structured, gradually shifting-responsibility transition process already developed in earlier chapters for other pediatric-onset chronic conditions. Wilson disease and alpha-1 antitrypsin deficiency are both frequently first identified in childhood, sometimes presenting with isolated, otherwise unexplained aminotransferase elevation on routine pediatric laboratory testing, and maintaining these genetic conditions on the differential for unexplained pediatric liver disease, rather than assuming pediatric liver disease more commonly reflects an acquired rather than genetic cause, supports timely diagnosis in this population. Educational and social support needs specific to a child managing a chronic illness, including coordination with school staff regarding medication administration and any activity accommodations that might be needed, should be part of a comprehensive pediatric management plan beyond the medical treatment alone. A family history of unexplained liver disease, even when not previously formally diagnosed, should specifically prompt consideration of these genetic conditions in a child presenting with new, otherwise unexplained liver test abnormalities, since a positive family history, even an informal one, can be an important diagnostic clue easily overlooked if not specifically elicited. Involving the adolescent patient directly in these discussions as they mature, rather than communicating solely through parents, prepares them for the independent self-management the eventual transition to adult care will require. Always.

### Genetic Counseling for Hereditary Liver Disease in Families With Children

When a genetic liver disease, whether Wilson disease, hereditary hemochromatosis, or alpha-1 antitrypsin deficiency, is confirmed in a parent, genetic counseling should address testing considerations for children specifically, balancing the potential benefit of early identification and, where applicable, early treatment against the psychological and practical considerations of testing a child for an adult-onset or variably penetrant condition, and this conversation is best had collaboratively with the family and, where age-appropriate, the child themselves, rather than a unilateral recommendation imposed without this shared discussion. In hereditary hemochromatosis specifically, given its adult-onset presentation and generally treatable nature once identified, many genetic counselors favor delaying testing until the child reaches an age where they can meaningfully participate in the decision themselves, distinct from Wilson disease, where earlier identification and treatment initiation carries more immediate clinical benefit. Documenting the family's decision, whatever it is, respects their autonomy and avoids repeated, unwelcome revisiting of a settled choice. Reassessing this preference periodically as the child ages ensures the decision reflects current, not outdated, family circumstances. Yes.

## Psychosocial Impact and Long-Term Coordination in Chronic Autoimmune and Genetic Liver Disease

Living with a chronic, lifelong liver disease requiring ongoing monitoring and, frequently, indefinite pharmacotherapy, whether autoimmune hepatitis, a cholestatic condition, or a genetic liver disease, imposes a substantial psychosocial burden that deserves the same routine screening and supportive attention already established throughout this book for other chronic gastrointestinal and hepatic conditions, and this screening should specifically account for disease-related anxiety about eventual progression to cirrhosis or the need for transplantation, a concern that patients may not always raise proactively even when it significantly affects their day-to-day wellbeing. Patient support organizations specific to these individual conditions, where available, provide valuable peer connection and disease-specific educational resources that a busy clinical practice may not have the time to fully provide, and referral to these resources, alongside the medical management developed throughout this chapter, represents a low-cost, high-value addition to comprehensive care for patients navigating these often rare and unfamiliar diagnoses. Normalizing this screening as a routine part of ongoing follow-up, applied consistently regardless of how well-controlled the underlying liver disease appears biochemically, communicates that psychological wellbeing is considered an integral part of comprehensive care rather than a secondary concern addressed only when a patient happens to raise it unprompted. Providing a brief, curated list of reputable resources, rather than leaving patients to search independently and potentially encounter less reliable sources of information online, ensures they are directed toward accurate, medically vetted content specific to their diagnosis. Small, consistent gestures of care compound over years of ongoing follow-up. Truly.

### Long-Term Monitoring Coordination

Long-term monitoring for these chronic conditions, spanning periodic biochemical assessment, imaging surveillance where indicated, and screening for the specific complications and comorbidities developed throughout this chapter, benefits from a clearly documented, shared monitoring plan accessible to any clinician involved in the patient's care, applying the same plan-anchored coordination principle emphasized throughout this book, since the number of distinct monitoring components required for conditions like primary sclerosing cholangitis, spanning colorectal, hepatocellular, and cholangiocarcinoma surveillance simultaneously, creates genuine risk of a component being inadvertently overlooked without this explicit, shared documentation. Reviewing this shared monitoring plan at each visit, rather than assuming it remains accurate without periodic confirmation, catches any component that may have been inadvertently missed or that requires updating as the patient's clinical status evolves over time. Consistency across visits protects patients from preventable gaps. Yes.

## Cascade Screening for Family Members in Genetic Liver Disease

First-degree relatives of a patient confirmed with hereditary hemochromatosis should be offered genetic testing for the specific HFE variant identified in the index patient, applying the same cascade testing principle already developed in earlier chapters for other hereditary conditions, and this testing, given the condition's incomplete penetrance discussed later in this chapter, should be accompanied by counseling that a positive genetic result predicts elevated risk rather than certain future disease, helping relatives understand the actionable but probabilistic nature of this information. Family screening in Wilson disease similarly extends to siblings specifically, given the autosomal recessive inheritance pattern this condition follows, meaning parents of an affected child are obligate carriers rather than typically affected themselves, while siblings each carry a meaningful probability of also being affected and should be offered biochemical or genetic screening even in the complete absence of symptoms, since early identification before symptomatic disease develops meaningfully improves long-term outcomes in this specific condition. This penetrance-related counseling nuance is important to communicate accurately, since a relative who tests positive for the HFE variant but never develops clinical iron overload should not be labeled or treated as though they carry active disease requiring the same phlebotomy schedule as an affected index patient; periodic biochemical monitoring alone is generally sufficient for this asymptomatic, genetically positive population. Because untreated, symptomatic Wilson disease can progress rapidly and cause irreversible neurologic or hepatic damage, the urgency of sibling screening in this specific condition should be communicated clearly, distinguishing it from the more measured, non-urgent timeline appropriate for hemochromatosis screening, so families understand why one genetic condition warrants prompt testing while another can reasonably be deferred. Providing written summary materials for family members to share among themselves further supports this cascade process beyond a single verbal conversation with the index patient alone. Indeed.

### Coordinating Cascade Testing Across a Genetics Clinic

Formal referral to a genetics clinic or genetic counselor, rather than the primary hepatology or gastroenterology team attempting to coordinate family-wide cascade testing independently, is a reasonable approach in complex family situations, particularly when multiple relatives across different households and, potentially, different healthcare systems require coordinated outreach and testing, since genetic counselors bring specific expertise in this family-communication and testing-coordination process that extends beyond the scope of most general hepatology practice. Establishing a standing referral relationship with a genetics clinic before this need arises, rather than searching for an appropriate referral only once a complex family situation is already underway, allows the hepatology or gastroenterology team to make this connection efficiently when the need does arise.

## Liver Transplantation Considerations Across This Chapter's Conditions

Liver transplantation remains the definitive treatment once any of the conditions developed throughout this chapter progresses to decompensated cirrhosis, and recognizing the specific transplant-relevant considerations for each condition supports appropriately timed referral: autoimmune hepatitis carries a recognized risk of disease recurrence in the transplanted liver, requiring ongoing immunosuppression management post-transplant tailored to this specific recurrence risk; primary sclerosing cholangitis similarly carries a meaningful post-transplant recurrence risk and, given its association with inflammatory bowel disease, requires coordinated post-transplant colorectal cancer surveillance continuing at the intensified interval this combination of conditions warrants; and the genetic and metabolic conditions, hereditary hemochromatosis, Wilson disease, and alpha-1 antitrypsin deficiency, are each effectively cured of their hepatic manifestation by transplantation, since the underlying metabolic defect resides in the native liver being replaced, though hemochromatosis-associated extrahepatic organ damage, once established, does not reverse with transplantation alone. Discussing these condition-specific transplant considerations proactively with a patient approaching this stage of disease, rather than only once transplant evaluation is formally underway, helps set realistic expectations about what transplantation can and cannot resolve for their specific underlying condition. Clear expectations reduce disappointment after an otherwise successful surgery. Truly.

### Timing of Transplant Referral

Referral for transplant evaluation should occur once a patient meets standard decompensation or model for end-stage liver disease score criteria, discussed in detail in the following chapter, rather than delayed until the patient has become critically ill, and this timing principle applies equally across all the conditions developed in this chapter despite their differing underlying mechanisms, since the shared endpoint of decompensated cirrhosis, once reached, requires the same proactive, rather than reactive, referral approach regardless of the specific disease that produced it. Building this referral threshold into standard clinical practice patterns, rather than relying on individual clinician judgment to recognize the moment a patient has crossed it, supports more consistent, timely referral across a broader patient population managed by clinicians with varying levels of transplant-specific experience. Timely, well-coordinated referral remains the single most impactful action a treating clinician can take. Yes.

## Genetic and Metabolic Liver Diseases

### Hereditary Hemochromatosis

Hereditary hemochromatosis, introduced in an earlier chapter as a screening consideration in the abnormal liver chemistry workup, most commonly results from a homozygous HFE gene pathogenic variant producing progressive, pathologic iron accumulation across multiple organs, and clinical penetrance is notably incomplete, meaning that many individuals with the homozygous genotype never develop clinically significant iron overload or organ damage, a nuance important for accurate patient counseling once genetic confirmation is obtained, since a positive genetic test does not guarantee eventual clinical disease. Established iron overload, confirmed through elevated ferritin and transferrin saturation alongside the genetic confirmation, is treated with therapeutic phlebotomy, generally performed at a defined frequency until ferritin reaches a target range, followed by less frequent maintenance phlebotomy to sustain this target long-term, and this treatment, when initiated before advanced organ damage, particularly cirrhosis, has developed, substantially reduces or eliminates the excess mortality this condition would otherwise carry. Non-HFE forms of hereditary hemochromatosis, resulting from pathogenic variants in genes other than HFE, are less common but should be considered in a patient with a compatible iron overload phenotype and a negative HFE genotype, since these rarer genetic causes require different confirmatory testing and, in some subtypes, carry a distinct clinical course from classic HFE-related disease. Dietary iron restriction plays a comparatively minor role relative to phlebotomy in managing established iron overload, and patients should understand that phlebotomy, not dietary modification alone, is the primary and most effective treatment, though avoiding iron supplementation and excessive vitamin C intake, which enhances iron absorption, remain reasonable adjunctive recommendations. Referral to a center with genetics expertise in these rarer variants is reasonable when a compatible phenotype and negative standard HFE testing together suggest this less common diagnostic possibility, since the specific confirmatory testing required extends beyond the standard HFE genotype panel used in routine practice. Precision here changes real outcomes.

**Wilson Disease**

Wilson disease, introduced in an earlier chapter in its acute liver failure presentation, more commonly presents with a chronic, insidious hepatic or, in some patients, predominantly neuropsychiatric course, and Kayser-Fleischer rings, copper deposition visible at the periphery of the cornea, while a classic and specific finding when present, are absent in a meaningful proportion of confirmed cases, particularly those presenting primarily with hepatic rather than neurologic manifestations, meaning their absence does not exclude the diagnosis in a patient with otherwise compatible clinical and laboratory findings. Chronic medical therapy uses copper chelation, most commonly with penicillamine or trientine, or zinc, which reduces intestinal copper absorption, and treatment is generally lifelong given the underlying genetic defect in copper metabolism, with regular monitoring of copper studies and clinical status to confirm adequate ongoing disease control and to detect the specific complications, including a described risk of neurologic worsening with certain chelating agents, particularly during the initial treatment period, that this population's treating clinicians should specifically monitor for. Neuropsychiatric manifestations, including dystonia, tremor, dysarthria, and, in some patients, prominent psychiatric symptoms such as personality change or depression, can predominate over hepatic findings and may lead to an initial misdiagnosis as a primary psychiatric or neurologic condition if Wilson disease is not specifically considered, particularly in a younger patient presenting with these atypical neuropsychiatric features. Zinc therapy, generally preferred for maintenance treatment or in presymptomatic, genetically confirmed patients given its more favorable side effect profile compared to the chelating agents, works through a distinct mechanism, inducing intestinal metallothionein production that binds dietary copper and prevents its absorption, rather than mobilizing copper already deposited in tissue as the chelating agents do. Formal neurologic and psychiatric assessment at diagnosis, regardless of which presentation predominates, establishes a baseline against which treatment response and any subsequent progression can be tracked more objectively than relying on informal clinical impression alone. Vigilance changes outcomes here.

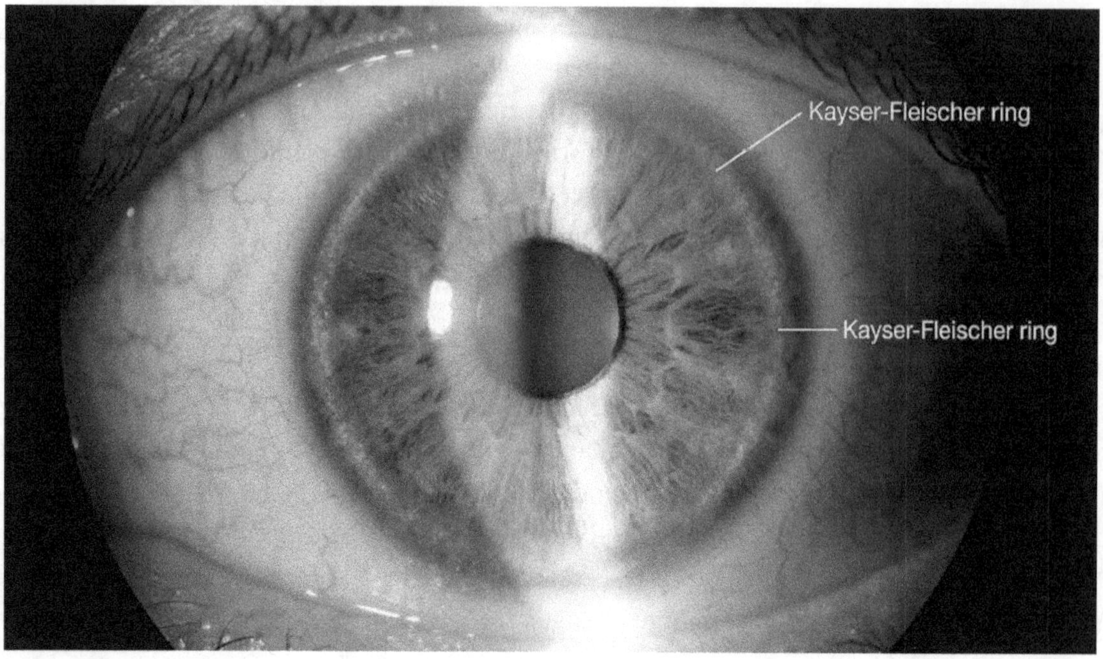


**Alpha-1 Antitrypsin Deficiency**

Alpha-1 antitrypsin deficiency, introduced in an earlier chapter as a screening consideration, produces liver disease through the accumulation of misfolded protein within hepatocytes rather than through the loss of the protein's normal protective pulmonary function, meaning that liver disease severity in this condition does not correlate directly with the degree of any coexisting pulmonary involvement, and patients should understand that these two organ manifestations, while arising from the same underlying genetic defect, follow largely independent disease courses requiring separate monitoring and management. No specific pharmacologic therapy is currently available to prevent or reverse the hepatic manifestations of alpha-1 antitrypsin deficiency, and management centers on monitoring for disease progression using the same fibrosis assessment tools developed in an earlier chapter, avoiding additional hepatotoxic exposures including excessive alcohol use, and liver transplantation for patients who progress to decompensated cirrhosis, which is notably curative for the hepatic manifestation specifically, since the transplanted liver does not carry the recipient's own genetic defect, though it does not address any coexisting pulmonary manifestations that require their own independent, ongoing management. Smoking cessation counseling remains especially important in this population given the substantially accelerated pulmonary decline smoking produces in patients with this underlying genetic vulnerability, and this specific counseling point deserves emphasis distinct from generic smoking cessation advice given the disproportionate harm smoking causes in this specific genetic context. Investigational RNA-targeted therapies aiming to reduce hepatic production of the misfolded protein at its source, rather than addressing downstream consequences alone, are under active clinical investigation and represent a potential future treatment avenue that patients may inquire about given growing awareness of this emerging research direction. Pulmonary function testing at baseline and periodically thereafter, in coordination with pulmonology, supports monitoring of the coexisting pulmonary manifestation independently from the hepatic disease course tracked by hepatology. Coordination protects both organs.

Case Presentation: A 54-year-old woman with confirmed primary biliary cholangitis has been on ursodeoxycholic acid therapy for fourteen months. Applying the reasoning developed in this chapter, formal biochemical response criteria are calculated using her alkaline phosphatase and bilirubin values, revealing an inadequate response despite confirmed medication adherence. Rather than continuing ursodeoxycholic acid monotherapy, she is started on obeticholic acid as second-line therapy added to her existing regimen. At follow-up eight months later, her biochemical parameters have improved substantially, now meeting response criteria. This case illustrates the chapter's central treatment-escalation principle: formal, criteria-based response assessment at the defined one-year interval, rather than continuing monotherapy indefinitely or relying on subjective clinical impression, identified her need for escalation at the point in her disease course when this intervention could most meaningfully alter her long-term trajectory.

Case Presentation: A 38-year-old man with primary sclerosing cholangitis and known ulcerative colitis undergoes routine surveillance MRCP, which demonstrates a new dominant stricture in the common hepatic duct not present on prior imaging. Applying the reasoning developed in this chapter, this new dominant stricture prompts endoscopic evaluation with brush cytology and fluorescence in situ hybridization testing to distinguish a benign fibrotic stricture from early cholangiocarcinoma, given the substantially elevated cancer risk this disease carries and the genuine diagnostic difficulty distinguishing these two possibilities on imaging alone. Cytology and fluorescence in situ hybridization testing are both negative, and the stricture is managed with endoscopic dilation, achieving symptomatic improvement in his mild associated cholestatic symptoms. He continues scheduled surveillance imaging at a shortened interval given this new finding. This case illustrates the chapter's core primary sclerosing cholangitis surveillance principle: any new dominant stricture warrants active investigation for malignancy rather than assumption of benignity, given how consequential a missed early cholangiocarcinoma would be in this specific high-risk population.

## Bone Health and Extrahepatic Manifestations in Cholestatic Liver Disease

Metabolic bone disease, including osteoporosis, is common in both primary biliary cholangitis and primary sclerosing cholangitis given the impaired fat-soluble vitamin absorption that chronic cholestasis produces, discussed in principle in earlier chapters, and periodic bone density monitoring with appropriate calcium, vitamin D, and, where indicated, bisphosphonate therapy should be a routine component of comprehensive management in both conditions, applying the same proactive screening philosophy already established throughout this book rather than addressing bone health only after a fracture has already occurred. Fat-soluble vitamin deficiency more broadly, encompassing vitamins A, D, E, and K, should be screened for periodically in patients with significant, sustained cholestasis, and repletion, using the same principles developed in the seventh chapter for malabsorptive fat-soluble vitamin deficiency, addresses a component of these patients' symptom burden and long-term complication risk that liver-directed therapy alone does not resolve. Weight-bearing exercise and adequate protein intake, alongside the specific supplementation and pharmacologic measures already discussed, provide additional, low-cost, low-risk support for bone health that should be discussed as part of a comprehensive approach rather than relying on pharmacotherapy alone to address this multifactorial complication. Vitamin K deficiency specifically warrants attention given its role in coagulation, and correcting this deficiency before any planned invasive procedure, including liver biopsy where indicated, reduces avoidable bleeding risk that might otherwise be misattributed solely to underlying liver dysfunction rather than a correctable nutritional deficiency.

### Sicca Syndrome and Autoimmune Comorbidities

Sicca syndrome, dry eyes and dry mouth from coexisting autoimmune involvement of the lacrimal and salivary glands, occurs commonly alongside primary biliary cholangitis, reflecting shared autoimmune susceptibility, and other autoimmune conditions, including autoimmune thyroid disease and Raynaud phenomenon, are similarly overrepresented in this population, meaning a comprehensive review of systems for these commonly co-occurring conditions, rather than a narrow focus on liver-related symptoms alone, provides more complete, patient-centered care for this population. Referral to ophthalmology and rheumatology, as appropriate, for these coexisting conditions ensures each receives the dedicated, specialty-specific management it requires rather than being addressed only superficially within a hepatology-focused visit primarily concerned with the underlying liver disease.

| Disease | Key Diagnostic Marker | First-Line Treatment |
|---|---|---|
| Autoimmune hepatitis | ANA/ASMA or anti-LKM, elevated IgG, interface hepatitis | Corticosteroids + azathioprine |
| Primary biliary cholangitis | Antimitochondrial antibody | Ursodeoxycholic acid |
| Primary sclerosing cholangitis | Beaded pattern on MRCP | No disease-modifying therapy; surveillance-focused |
| Hereditary hemochromatosis | HFE genotype + elevated ferritin/transferrin saturation | Therapeutic phlebotomy |
| Wilson disease | Low ceruloplasmin, elevated urinary copper | Chelation (penicillamine/trientine) or zinc |

### THE GI THRESHOLD DECISION SYSTEM — Autoimmune and Cholestatic Liver Disease Thresholds

**Presentation Signature:** This chapter's threshold instances addressed treatment withdrawal timing in autoimmune hepatitis and treatment escalation criteria in primary biliary cholangitis.

**Threshold Point:** Sustained biochemical and histologic remission gates treatment withdrawal in autoimmune hepatitis; formal one-year biochemical response criteria gate second-line therapy addition in primary biliary cholangitis.

**The Call:** Both thresholds replace an open-ended, indefinite treatment default with a criteria-based reassessment point that determines whether treatment can be safely withdrawn or must be escalated.

**Trap Logic:** Withdrawing autoimmune hepatitis treatment based on biochemical remission alone without histologic confirmation, and continuing primary biliary cholangitis monotherapy indefinitely despite a documented inadequate response, are this chapter's most consequential threshold misapplications.

**Decision Anchor:** Require both biochemical and histologic remission before attempting autoimmune hepatitis treatment withdrawal, and apply formal response criteria at the one-year assessment in primary biliary cholangitis to trigger prompt escalation upon inadequate response.

## Summary and Key Concepts

Autoimmune hepatitis diagnosis integrates aminotransferase elevation, autoantibodies, elevated IgG, and characteristic histology, and treatment withdrawal requires both sustained biochemical remission and histologic confirmation rather than biochemical improvement alone.

Primary biliary cholangitis is diagnosed by a cholestatic pattern with positive antimitochondrial antibody, and formal one-year biochemical response assessment to ursodeoxycholic acid determines whether second-line therapy is added.

Primary sclerosing cholangitis is diagnosed primarily by characteristic multifocal stricturing on MRCP, strongly associates with inflammatory bowel disease requiring colonoscopic evaluation at diagnosis, and carries substantially elevated cholangiocarcinoma risk.

No disease-modifying pharmacotherapy exists for primary sclerosing cholangitis, and management centers on surveillance for colorectal cancer, hepatocellular carcinoma, and cholangiocarcinoma, with any new dominant stricture warranting active malignancy evaluation.

Hereditary hemochromatosis shows incomplete clinical penetrance despite homozygous genotype, and confirmed iron overload is treated with therapeutic phlebotomy before advanced organ damage develops.

Wilson disease can present chronically without Kayser-Fleischer rings, requiring lifelong copper chelation or zinc therapy, while alpha-1 antitrypsin deficiency's hepatic and pulmonary manifestations follow independent courses, with transplantation curative for the hepatic manifestation specifically.

# CHAPTER 18: CIRRHOSIS, PORTAL HYPERTENSION, AND DECOMPENSATED LIVER DISEASE

**Learning Objectives**

1. Distinguish compensated from decompensated cirrhosis and apply Child-Pugh and MELD scoring to prognosis and management decisions.
2. Apply variceal screening and primary prophylaxis criteria in patients with cirrhosis and portal hypertension.
3. Evaluate and manage ascites and diagnose and treat spontaneous bacterial peritonitis, including prophylaxis indications.
4. Diagnose and manage hepatic encephalopathy using a structured, precipitant-focused approach.
5. Diagnose hepatorenal syndrome and describe its management and the criteria for liver transplantation evaluation in decompensated cirrhosis.

**Chapter Outline**

This chapter develops cirrhosis and its major decompensating complications as a threshold-driven, interconnected system: the distinction between compensated and decompensated disease and its prognostic scoring, portal hypertension and variceal screening and prophylaxis, ascites and spontaneous bacterial peritonitis, hepatic encephalopathy, hepatorenal syndrome, and the criteria guiding liver transplantation evaluation. Each section connects a specific severity or diagnostic threshold to a defined management pathway.

## Cirrhosis and Compensated Versus Decompensated Disease

### Diagnosis and Staging

Cirrhosis, the histologic endpoint of sustained hepatic fibrosis from any of the etiologies developed in earlier chapters, viral hepatitis, alcohol-associated liver disease, metabolic dysfunction-associated steatotic liver disease, and the autoimmune, cholestatic, and genetic conditions discussed in the previous chapter, is increasingly diagnosed noninvasively using the fibrosis assessment tools introduced in earlier chapters, reserving liver biopsy for cases where the diagnosis remains genuinely uncertain despite this noninvasive evaluation. The compensated-versus-decompensated distinction, defined by the presence or absence of the specific complications developed throughout this chapter, ascites, variceal hemorrhage, hepatic encephalopathy, and jaundice from hepatic synthetic failure, is the single most important prognostic determination in cirrhosis, since decompensation marks a fundamental shift in disease trajectory and mortality risk that should trigger the more intensive monitoring and transplant evaluation pathway discussed later in this chapter. Determining the specific underlying etiology remains important even after cirrhosis itself has been confirmed, since etiology-specific treatment, discussed throughout earlier chapters, can still meaningfully alter disease trajectory in many cases, and a diagnosis of cirrhosis without a clearly identified cause should prompt continued diagnostic effort rather than acceptance of an unexplained cirrhosis label. Recompensation, a more recently recognized concept in which a patient who has experienced decompensation subsequently achieves sustained improvement following successful treatment of the underlying etiology, particularly after alcohol cessation or viral cure, represents an important, evolving area of understanding, though a history of prior decompensation still generally warrants the intensified monitoring and transplant-evaluation threshold discussed later in this chapter, even in a patient who has since recompensated clinically.

**Figure 18.1: Compensated Versus Decompensated Cirrhosis**

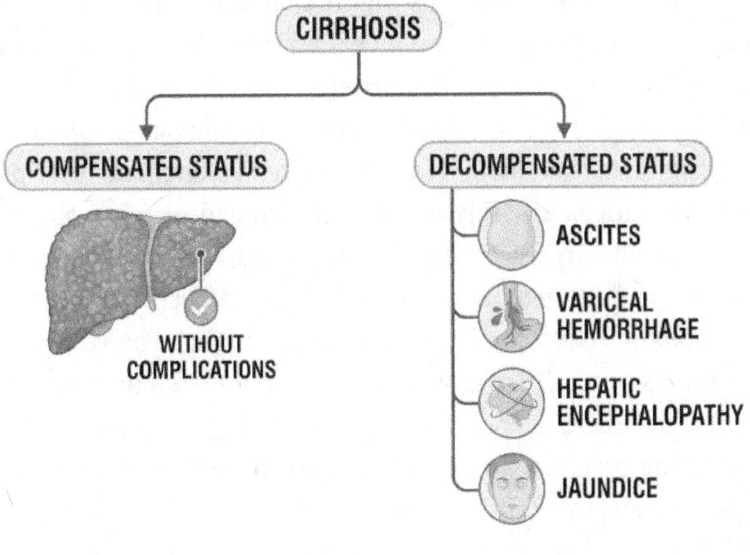


## Compensated Cirrhosis Management

The Child-Pugh score, incorporating bilirubin, albumin, prothrombin time, and the clinical presence and severity of ascites and encephalopathy, and the model for end-stage liver disease score, calculated from bilirubin, creatinine, and the international normalized ratio, both provide standardized prognostic staging, with the model for end-stage liver disease score additionally serving as the primary allocation tool for liver transplantation in most systems, making familiarity with both scoring systems essential for any clinician managing this patient population. Compensated cirrhosis management centers on etiology-specific treatment, discussed in earlier chapters for each underlying cause, alongside the screening measures developed throughout this chapter, variceal screening, hepatocellular carcinoma surveillance introduced in earlier chapters, and vaccination against hepatitis A and B, pneumococcus, and influenza given this population's increased infection vulnerability, reflecting a proactive, rather than purely reactive, management philosophy applied before decompensation has occurred. The model for end-stage liver disease score has itself evolved over time, with newer versions incorporating sodium given its independent prognostic significance in this population, and clinicians should confirm they are applying the current, validated version of this score rather than an older iteration that may no longer reflect current allocation practice. Alcohol and other hepatotoxic exposures should be explicitly reviewed and addressed at every visit regardless of the specific underlying etiology, since even a cirrhosis diagnosis unrelated to alcohol can be meaningfully worsened by superimposed alcohol use, reinforcing why this counseling deserves universal application rather than being reserved only for patients whose cirrhosis etiology is specifically alcohol-related.

## Portal Hypertension and Variceal Bleeding

### Pathophysiology and Screening for Varices

Portal hypertension, resulting from increased resistance to portal blood flow through the fibrotic, distorted hepatic architecture combined with increased splanchnic blood flow, produces the formation of portosystemic collateral vessels, most clinically significant among them esophageal and gastric varices, and screening endoscopy is recommended for patients with newly diagnosed cirrhosis to identify varices before they bleed, since the first variceal hemorrhage carries substantial mortality risk that primary prophylaxis, discussed below, can meaningfully reduce. Noninvasive tools, including platelet count, spleen size, and liver stiffness measurement by elastography, can help identify patients at sufficiently low risk of clinically significant varices to safely defer screening endoscopy, applying the same noninvasive-first, risk-stratified approach already established in earlier chapters for other diagnostic decisions, though endoscopy remains the definitive method for identifying and characterizing varices once screening is undertaken. Hepatic venous pressure gradient measurement, an invasive but highly informative direct measure of portal pressure, is generally reserved for specific research or complex clinical scenarios rather than routine clinical practice, where the noninvasive tools and endoscopic findings developed throughout this section provide adequate practical guidance for most management decisions. Periodic reassessment of these noninvasive parameters, rather than a single evaluation at the time of cirrhosis diagnosis alone, is important since portal hypertension and the associated variceal risk can progress over time even in a patient who initially met criteria for deferring screening endoscopy.

### Primary Prophylaxis

Primary prophylaxis against a first variceal hemorrhage is indicated for patients with medium-to-large varices or small varices with high-risk stigmata identified on screening endoscopy, and the choice between nonselective beta-blocker therapy, reducing portal pressure through decreased cardiac output and splanchnic vasoconstriction, and endoscopic variceal band ligation is generally guided by patient preference, comorbidities affecting beta-blocker tolerability, and local expertise, since both approaches have demonstrated comparable efficacy in reducing first bleeding risk in appropriately selected patients. Heart rate reduction to a specific target, generally to around 55 to 60 beats per minute or the maximally tolerated dose, confirms adequate beta-blocker dosing, and titrating to this objective physiologic endpoint, rather than a fixed dose applied uniformly regardless of individual response, ensures the medication is providing its intended pharmacologic effect.

**THE GI THRESHOLD DECISION SYSTEM — Hepatic Thresholds — Variceal Screening and Primary Prophylaxis Initiation**

**Presentation Signature:** A patient with newly diagnosed cirrhosis requires an initial assessment to determine whether variceal screening is indicated and, if varices are identified, whether primary prophylaxis should be initiated.

**Threshold Point:** Noninvasive risk stratification using platelet count, spleen size, or liver stiffness defines the threshold below which screening endoscopy can be safely deferred; once endoscopy is performed, variceal size and the presence of high-risk stigmata define the threshold for primary prophylaxis initiation.

**The Call:** Patients meeting low-risk noninvasive criteria defer screening endoscopy with periodic noninvasive reassessment; patients undergoing endoscopy with medium-to-large varices or high-risk small varices are started on primary prophylaxis, either nonselective beta-blocker therapy or endoscopic band ligation based on individual patient factors.

**Trap Logic:** Applying screening endoscopy uniformly to every cirrhosis patient regardless of noninvasive risk stratification, or conversely failing to initiate primary prophylaxis once high-risk varices are identified, both fail to match intervention intensity to the actual, individualized bleeding risk a given patient presents.

**Decision Anchor:** Apply noninvasive risk stratification to guide the need for screening endoscopy, and initiate primary prophylaxis promptly once high-risk varices are identified rather than deferring treatment or applying screening indiscriminately regardless of risk stratification.

## Ascites and Spontaneous Bacterial Peritonitis

### Diagnosis and Management of Ascites

New-onset ascites warrants diagnostic paracentesis to confirm the cause and exclude infection, with the serum-ascites albumin gradient, calculated by subtracting the ascitic fluid albumin from the serum albumin, distinguishing portal hypertension-related ascites, a gradient of 1.1 grams per deciliter or greater, from other causes including malignancy or infection-related ascites without portal hypertension, and this gradient, rather than the older total-protein-based classification it has largely replaced, provides superior diagnostic accuracy for this specific distinction. Management of cirrhosis-related ascites follows a stepwise approach beginning with sodium restriction and diuretic therapy, typically combining spironolactone and furosemide in a fixed ratio to maintain potassium balance while achieving adequate natriuresis, and escalating to large-volume paracentesis with albumin replacement for refractory ascites not adequately controlled by maximal diuretic therapy, reflecting the same stepwise, response-based escalation principle already established throughout this book for other chronic conditions. Ascitic fluid cell count and culture, ideally with the culture bottles inoculated at the bedside rather than sent to the laboratory for later inoculation, given the substantially higher culture yield this bedside technique achieves, should be obtained on essentially every diagnostic paracentesis regardless of the clinical suspicion for infection, since spontaneous bacterial peritonitis, discussed further below, can present with minimal or atypical symptoms. Regular monitoring of renal function and electrolytes during diuretic titration is essential given the risk of overdiuresis producing acute kidney injury or clinically significant electrolyte derangement, and this monitoring should intensify during any period of dose escalation or when the patient reports symptoms suggestive of intravascular volume depletion.

Figure 18.3: Paracentesis Technique and Serum-Ascites Albumin Gradient Interpretation

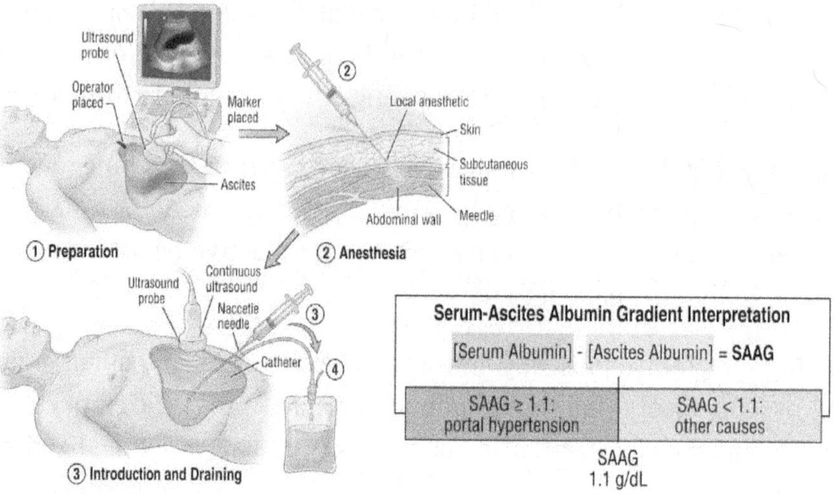


## Spontaneous Bacterial Peritonitis: Diagnosis and Treatment

Spontaneous bacterial peritonitis, an infection of ascitic fluid without an identifiable intra-abdominal surgical source, is diagnosed by an ascitic fluid absolute neutrophil count of 250 cells per cubic millimeter or greater, and diagnostic paracentesis should be performed promptly in any hospitalized cirrhotic patient with ascites, given the substantial mortality risk of untreated spontaneous bacterial peritonitis and the nonspecific, sometimes minimal symptoms this infection can produce, meaning a low threshold for paracentesis, rather than reserving the procedure only for patients with classic peritonitis symptoms, is essential to avoid missing this diagnosis. Empiric antibiotic therapy, typically a third-generation cephalosporin, should be initiated promptly once the diagnosis is confirmed or strongly suspected, and albumin administration alongside antibiotics in patients with more severe presentations, meeting specific bilirubin or creatinine criteria, reduces the risk of hepatorenal syndrome developing as a complication of the infection itself, a specific adjunctive measure that should not be overlooked in appropriately selected patients.

## THE GI THRESHOLD DECISION SYSTEM — Hepatic Thresholds — Spontaneous Bacterial Peritonitis Prophylaxis Indications

**Presentation Signature:** A patient with cirrhosis and ascites is being evaluated for long-term management, and the clinician must determine whether antibiotic prophylaxis against spontaneous bacterial peritonitis is indicated.

**Threshold Point:** A prior episode of spontaneous bacterial peritonitis defines the threshold for secondary prophylaxis, generally indefinite; low ascitic fluid protein combined with advanced liver disease severity or renal impairment defines a threshold for primary prophylaxis in patients without a prior episode; and acute gastrointestinal hemorrhage in a cirrhotic patient defines a threshold for short-term prophylaxis regardless of ascitic fluid protein level.

**The Call:** Patients meeting any of these specific criteria receive prophylactic antibiotics, typically a fluoroquinolone or trimethoprim-sulfamethoxazole for the primary and secondary indications, or a short course of a different agent specifically during acute variceal hemorrhage; patients without any of these specific risk criteria do not require prophylaxis despite having ascites.

**Trap Logic:** Applying prophylactic antibiotics to every patient with any ascites regardless of these specific criteria risks unnecessary antibiotic exposure and resistance development, while failing to apply prophylaxis in a patient who has already had one spontaneous bacterial peritonitis episode exposes them to a substantial risk of a life-threatening recurrence.

**Decision Anchor:** Apply antibiotic prophylaxis specifically to patients meeting the defined primary, secondary, or hemorrhage-related indications rather than a uniform prophylaxis policy applied to every ascites patient or withheld from every patient regardless of these specific risk criteria.

## Hepatic Encephalopathy and Hepatorenal Syndrome

### Hepatic Encephalopathy: Diagnosis and Management

Hepatic encephalopathy, a spectrum of neurocognitive dysfunction resulting from the accumulation of gut-derived toxins, most notably ammonia, that an insufficient or bypassed liver fails to adequately clear, is graded using a standardized clinical scale from minimal, subclinical impairment detectable only by specific psychometric testing through overt confusion to coma, and every episode of overt hepatic encephalopathy should prompt an active, systematic search for a specific precipitating factor, including infection, gastrointestinal bleeding, constipation, medication noncompliance, or a new sedating medication, rather than attributing the episode to the underlying liver disease alone without this precipitant-focused evaluation. Lactulose, a non-absorbable disaccharide that acidifies the colonic lumen and promotes ammonia excretion, is first-line therapy, titrated to achieve a specific target stool frequency, and rifaximin, a minimally absorbed antibiotic reducing ammonia-producing gut bacteria, is added for patients with recurrent episodes despite adequately dosed lactulose, reflecting the same stepwise, response-based escalation principle applied throughout this chapter's other conditions. Minimal hepatic encephalopathy, the subclinical form detectable only through specific psychometric or neurophysiologic testing, is easily missed on routine clinical assessment yet carries meaningful implications for driving safety and daily functioning, and screening for this subclinical form should be considered in patients whose family reports subtle cognitive changes not obviously explained by overt confusion on standard bedside evaluation. Inadequate lactulose dosing, whether from underdosing that fails to achieve the target stool frequency or overdosing that produces excessive diarrhea and dehydration, both undermine effective treatment, and titrating the dose based on the patient's actual stool output, typically targeting two to three soft bowel movements daily, is essential to achieving genuine therapeutic benefit.

**Hepatorenal Syndrome: Diagnosis and Management**

Hepatorenal syndrome, a functional renal failure resulting from the severe splanchnic and systemic vasodilation characteristic of advanced cirrhosis rather than from intrinsic structural kidney disease, is a diagnosis of exclusion requiring the systematic exclusion of other causes of acute kidney injury, including volume depletion, addressed with an albumin challenge before this diagnosis is confirmed, and nephrotoxic medications or structural renal disease, discussed further in the differential, and this exclusionary diagnostic process, rather than a reflexive attribution of any new renal impairment in a cirrhotic patient to hepatorenal syndrome, prevents both a missed alternative, potentially more readily treatable cause and inappropriate treatment of a patient who does not actually have this specific syndrome. Treatment combines a vasoconstrictor, most commonly terlipressin where available or, in regions where terlipressin is not approved, a combination of midodrine and octreotide, with albumin, and this vasoconstrictor-albumin combination addresses the underlying splanchnic vasodilation directly, while liver transplantation remains the only treatment capable of definitively resolving hepatorenal syndrome, since the syndrome's underlying driver, the cirrhotic circulatory state itself, persists as long as the native liver disease remains untreated. Recent diagnostic criteria have shifted toward incorporating a more dynamic assessment of creatinine trajectory rather than a single static threshold value, reflecting evolving understanding that the rate of renal function decline, not simply the absolute creatinine value at a single time point, carries important diagnostic and prognostic significance in distinguishing hepatorenal syndrome from other causes of acute kidney injury in this population. Terlipressin carries a recognized risk of ischemic complications given its potent vasoconstrictive effect, and appropriate patient selection, along with careful monitoring for signs of peripheral or cardiac ischemia during treatment, is essential to using this effective but not risk-free therapy safely in an already medically complex patient population. In regions where terlipressin has only recently become available, teams accustomed to the midodrine-octreotide combination may need dedicated protocol updates and staff education to transition confidently to this newer, generally more effective agent. Champion clinicians who lead this transition can help colleagues adapt more smoothly. Change management matters as much as the medicine itself. Always.

## Refractory Ascites and Advanced Interventions

Refractory ascites, defined as fluid accumulation not adequately controlled by maximal diuretic therapy or that recurs rapidly after therapeutic paracentesis, warrants consideration of a transjugular intrahepatic portosystemic shunt in appropriately selected patients, a procedure creating a direct connection between the portal and hepatic venous systems to reduce portal pressure, and this intervention, while effective at controlling ascites, carries a recognized risk of precipitating or worsening hepatic encephalopathy given the diversion of portal blood flow away from the liver's detoxifying function, meaning careful patient selection, excluding those with poorly controlled baseline encephalopathy or advanced synthetic dysfunction, is essential before proceeding. Repeated large-volume paracentesis remains a reasonable alternative to transjugular intrahepatic portosystemic shunt placement in patients who are not appropriate candidates for the procedure given comorbidities or baseline encephalopathy risk, and this decision, weighing procedural risk against the burden of recurrent large-volume paracentesis, should be individualized collaboratively with the patient rather than defaulting uniformly to either approach. Post-procedure monitoring for encephalopathy over the following weeks is essential given that this complication, when it occurs, typically manifests within this early post-procedure window, and educating both the patient and their family about this specific risk before the procedure supports early recognition should it develop. Albumin replacement following large-volume paracentesis, generally recommended once the removed fluid volume exceeds a specific threshold, reduces the risk of post-paracentesis circulatory dysfunction, a complication that can itself precipitate hepatorenal syndrome or worsen hyponatremia if this replacement is omitted. Shunt patency should also be periodically reassessed after TIPS placement, since shunt stenosis or occlusion, when it occurs, can lead to recurrence of the ascites the procedure was intended to control, prompting revision if this complication develops. Alternatives to albumin, including synthetic plasma expanders, have generally shown inferior outcomes in this specific setting and are not recommended as substitutes, reinforcing why albumin specifically, despite its higher cost relative to these alternatives, remains the standard of care for this indication. Awareness of local supply considerations for albumin, given periodic shortages some institutions have experienced, is a practical operational consideration worth building into departmental planning. Doppler ultrasound provides a convenient, noninvasive means of following shunt function over time. This routine follow-up should not be overlooked. Always. Truly.

### Hepatic Hydrothorax

Hepatic hydrothorax, pleural fluid accumulation, most commonly right-sided, resulting from the same portal hypertensive physiology producing ascites, transmitted through microscopic diaphragmatic defects, is managed with the same sodium restriction and diuretic approach used for ascites, and thoracentesis, rather than chest tube placement, is preferred when drainage is needed, since chest tubes in this specific setting carry a substantially elevated complication risk given the ongoing, rapid fluid reaccumulation this condition produces, an important distinction from how pleural effusions from other causes are typically managed. Transjugular intrahepatic portosystemic shunt placement is also an option for refractory hepatic hydrothorax not adequately controlled by sodium restriction and diuretics, applying the same portal-pressure-reduction rationale used for refractory ascites discussed above, given the shared underlying pathophysiology these two fluid accumulation patterns share. Video-assisted thoracoscopic pleurodesis is an option for patients not responding to less invasive measures and not candidates for or not responding to a shunt, though this more invasive procedure is generally reserved for cases where the less invasive options have already been reasonably tried. This graduated escalation pathway mirrors the same stepwise philosophy applied consistently throughout this chapter's other complications. Always.

## Cirrhotic Cardiomyopathy and Hepatopulmonary Syndrome

Cirrhotic cardiomyopathy, a subclinical or overt cardiac dysfunction distinct from other structural heart disease, characterized by blunted contractile response to stress despite normal or even elevated resting cardiac output, reflects the same systemic circulatory disturbance underlying the vasodilation driving ascites and hepatorenal syndrome discussed elsewhere in this chapter, and this condition can become clinically apparent particularly during the hemodynamic stress of liver transplantation surgery itself, making pre-transplant cardiac assessment an important component of the comprehensive transplant evaluation discussed later in this chapter. Hepatopulmonary syndrome, resulting from intrapulmonary vascular dilation that impairs oxygen exchange, produces a distinctive symptom pattern including platypnea, worsened dyspnea specifically when upright, and orthodeoxia, worsened oxygen saturation when upright, and recognizing this specific positional pattern, rather than attributing dyspnea in a cirrhotic patient to a more generic cause, is important given that hepatopulmonary syndrome carries specific implications for transplant prioritization in many allocation systems given its otherwise progressive, transplant-responsive natural history. Echocardiography as part of routine pre-transplant evaluation should specifically assess for the diastolic dysfunction and prolonged QT interval characteristic of this condition, findings that might otherwise be overlooked on a standard echocardiographic report not specifically tailored to this population's distinct cardiac phenotype. Contrast echocardiography, using agitated saline to detect intrapulmonary shunting, is the standard screening test for hepatopulmonary syndrome, and this test should be considered in any cirrhotic patient reporting the characteristic positional dyspnea pattern rather than pursued only after more common cardiopulmonary causes have already been exhaustively excluded. Cardiology consultation before transplant listing is reasonable for any patient with abnormal findings on this specialized cardiac assessment, ensuring perioperative cardiac risk is fully characterized before the patient proceeds through the remainder of the transplant evaluation process. Yes.

### Portopulmonary Hypertension

Portopulmonary hypertension, pulmonary arterial hypertension occurring in the setting of portal hypertension, is a distinct entity from hepatopulmonary syndrome despite the similar-sounding names, and distinguishing between them, generally through echocardiography followed by right heart catheterization when pulmonary hypertension is suspected, matters significantly since portopulmonary hypertension, unlike hepatopulmonary syndrome, can represent a contraindication to transplantation if sufficiently severe and inadequately controlled with pulmonary vasodilator therapy prior to the planned surgery, given the substantial perioperative mortality risk uncontrolled severe pulmonary hypertension carries during major surgery. Coordinating this evaluation with pulmonology or cardiology given the specialized nature of pulmonary vasodilator therapy and right heart catheterization interpretation, rather than managing it in isolation within hepatology alone, reflects the same multidisciplinary collaboration model already established throughout this book for other conditions requiring specialized expertise beyond a single specialty's scope. Longitudinal monitoring during pulmonary vasodilator therapy, including repeat right heart catheterization at defined intervals, tracks treatment response and informs the ongoing reassessment of transplant candidacy as therapy progresses. Truly.

## Coagulopathy and Bleeding Risk Management in Cirrhosis

Cirrhosis-related coagulopathy, reflected in an elevated international normalized ratio, does not straightforwardly indicate bleeding risk in the way this same laboratory abnormality would in other clinical contexts, since cirrhosis produces a complex, rebalanced hemostatic state involving concurrent deficiencies in both procoagulant and anticoagulant factors, and reflexive correction of an elevated international normalized ratio with fresh frozen plasma before routine procedures, a once-common practice, is now recognized as generally unnecessary and potentially harmful given the volume load this correction imposes without reliably reducing actual bleeding risk. Platelet count and fibrinogen level provide additional information relevant to periprocedural bleeding risk assessment beyond the international normalized ratio alone, and thromboelastography, where available, offers a more comprehensive, global assessment of the actual hemostatic balance in an individual patient than any single laboratory value considered in isolation, supporting more accurate, individualized periprocedural risk assessment than reliance on the international normalized ratio alone would provide. Communicating this updated understanding to proceduralists from other specialties who may still default to the older, more reflexive fresh frozen plasma correction practice supports safer, more evidence-based periprocedural management across the full care team rather than only within hepatology itself. Access to thromboelastography remains limited to certain specialized centers, meaning most practices will continue to rely on the standard laboratory panel and clinical judgment for most periprocedural decisions, reserving this more sophisticated testing for genuinely uncertain, higher-stakes cases where the additional information would meaningfully change management.

### Portal Vein Thrombosis

Portal vein thrombosis, an increasingly recognized complication of cirrhosis given growing evidence that the underlying hemostatic rebalancing described above can favor thrombosis as readily as bleeding in certain circumstances, is generally identified on routine surveillance imaging performed for hepatocellular carcinoma screening, discussed in an earlier chapter, and anticoagulation is considered in appropriately selected patients, particularly those who are transplant candidates, since untreated, progressive portal vein thrombosis can complicate the technical aspects of the transplant surgery itself, though this decision requires careful, individualized weighing of thrombosis progression risk against bleeding risk given the underlying coagulopathy this population also carries. Direct oral anticoagulants have shown promise as an alternative to traditional agents like warfarin or low molecular weight heparin in this population, offering the convenience of oral, fixed dosing without the monitoring burden traditional agents require, though experience with these newer agents specifically in cirrhotic patients remains more limited than with the traditional options. Individualized case discussion at a multidisciplinary hepatology-hematology conference, where available, can support this nuanced anticoagulation decision in genuinely complex cases where the risk-benefit balance is not straightforward. Yes.

## Psychosocial Impact and Palliative Care in Decompensated Cirrhosis

Decompensated cirrhosis carries a substantial symptom burden and prognostic uncertainty comparable to many advanced malignancies, yet palliative care involvement has historically lagged behind oncology in this population, and integrating palliative care alongside disease-directed management and transplant evaluation, rather than only once transplantation is no longer a viable option, applies the same early-integration principle already established in earlier chapters for other serious, life-limiting conditions, addressing symptom burden, psychosocial distress, and goals-of-care conversations throughout the disease course rather than only at its terminal stage. Encephalopathy, discussed earlier in this chapter, presents unique challenges for goals-of-care discussions given its potential to impair a patient's decision-making capacity during exactly the periods when important treatment decisions may need to be made, making advance care planning conversations, held proactively during periods of clear cognitive function rather than deferred until a crisis arises, particularly valuable in this specific population. Establishing a referral pathway to palliative care that operates in parallel with, rather than as a replacement for, active transplant evaluation communicates to patients that pursuing comfort and quality-of-life support does not mean abandoning hope for transplantation or other disease-directed treatment. Documenting a patient's expressed wishes clearly and making this documentation readily accessible to any clinician who may need to reference it during a subsequent encephalopathy episode ensures these carefully considered preferences are honored even when the patient cannot personally restate them at the moment of clinical need. Framing this integration explicitly as complementary rather than competing supports genuine patient trust in both the transplant team and the palliative care team simultaneously. Truly.

### Caregiver Support in Decompensated Cirrhosis

Family members and caregivers of patients with decompensated cirrhosis, particularly those managing recurrent hepatic encephalopathy episodes at home, carry a substantial caregiving burden that deserves the same dedicated attention already emphasized throughout this book for caregivers of patients with other serious chronic illnesses, and providing caregivers with clear, written guidance on recognizing early encephalopathy signs and when to seek urgent evaluation empowers them to respond appropriately to a condition that can fluctuate unpredictably between clinic visits. Connecting caregivers with support resources, including caregiver support groups where available, acknowledges that they too are navigating a difficult, ongoing situation alongside the patient and deserve dedicated attention to their own wellbeing rather than being viewed solely as an extension of the patient's care team. Even a brief acknowledgment of the caregiving burden at each visit, without requiring a formal referral every time, communicates ongoing attentiveness to their wellbeing alongside the patient's. Yes.

## Acute-on-Chronic Liver Failure

Acute-on-chronic liver failure, a distinct clinical entity characterized by acute decompensation of cirrhosis accompanied by multi-organ failure and a high short-term mortality risk, is increasingly recognized as a specific syndrome warranting its own dedicated assessment framework rather than being managed identically to a routine decompensation episode, and identifying the specific precipitating event, most commonly infection, alcohol relapse, or superimposed viral or drug-induced injury, is essential since addressing this precipitant, alongside aggressive organ support, meaningfully influences the trajectory of this otherwise often rapidly progressive condition. Prognostic scoring systems specific to acute-on-chronic liver failure, incorporating the number and severity of organ failures present, provide more accurate short-term mortality prediction in this specific population than the standard Child-Pugh or MELD scores developed earlier in this chapter, which were derived from and validated in a more stable, chronically decompensated population rather than this acutely, rapidly deteriorating one.

### Intensive Care Coordination in Acute-on-Chronic Liver Failure

Management of acute-on-chronic liver failure requires close coordination between hepatology and critical care given the multi-organ support this condition frequently demands, and early, proactive discussion with a transplant center is warranted even before the full extent of organ failure has stabilized, since some patients with acute-on-chronic liver failure can be successfully bridged to transplantation if referral and evaluation are not delayed until the patient has become too unstable for safe transfer or surgery.

## Medication Considerations and Dosing Adjustments in Cirrhosis

Medication selection and dosing in cirrhosis requires specific consideration beyond standard prescribing practice, since impaired hepatic metabolism can alter drug clearance unpredictably, and several medication classes deserve particular caution, including nonsteroidal anti-inflammatory drugs, which can precipitate both gastrointestinal bleeding, given the coagulopathy and portal hypertensive gastropathy risk already present in this population, and renal impairment, given the already precarious renal hemodynamics characteristic of advanced cirrhosis, meaning these agents are generally avoided in patients with cirrhosis, particularly once any degree of decompensation has occurred. Sedating medications, including benzodiazepines and opioids, warrant similarly careful consideration given both their potential to precipitate or worsen hepatic encephalopathy, discussed earlier in this chapter, and their altered, often prolonged pharmacokinetics in the setting of impaired hepatic clearance, meaning that when these medications are genuinely necessary, starting at reduced doses with close monitoring for oversedation or emerging encephalopathy is the appropriate default approach rather than standard, non-adjusted dosing.

### Antibiotic Selection Considerations

Antibiotic selection in cirrhotic patients, particularly for infections beyond spontaneous bacterial peritonitis discussed earlier in this chapter, should account for the specific nephrotoxicity risk certain agents carry in a population already predisposed to renal impairment, and consultation with infectious disease or clinical pharmacy specialists for complex or prolonged antibiotic courses can help navigate this additional layer of dosing complexity that general antibiotic selection principles applied to patients without underlying liver disease do not fully capture.

## Gastric Varices and Non-Variceal Portal Hypertensive Bleeding Sources

Gastric varices, classified by their location relative to the esophagogastric junction and whether they represent an extension of esophageal varices or an isolated gastric finding, carry a distinct management approach from esophageal varices, with endoscopic injection of a tissue adhesive, most commonly cyanoacrylate, generally preferred over band ligation for the isolated gastric fundal variant given band ligation's higher rebleeding risk in this specific anatomic location, and recognizing this distinction prevents applying the esophageal-variceal treatment paradigm uniformly to a gastric variceal finding where it is less effective. Portal hypertensive gastropathy, a diffuse mucosal change distinct from discrete varices, producing a characteristic mosaic or snakeskin appearance on endoscopy, can itself be a source of chronic, low-grade blood loss or, less commonly, acute hemorrhage, and this entity is managed with nonselective beta-blocker therapy, the same portal-pressure-reducing approach used for variceal prophylaxis, rather than the endoscopic techniques appropriate for discrete variceal bleeding sources. Combination therapy, using both endoscopic and pharmacologic approaches together for gastric variceal management, may be considered in select higher-risk patients, reflecting the same combined-modality principle already applied elsewhere in this chapter's approach to esophageal variceal prophylaxis. Iron supplementation may be needed in patients with chronic blood loss from portal hypertensive gastropathy, and monitoring for iron deficiency anemia over time in a patient with this known finding supports proactive identification before it produces more pronounced symptomatic anemia. Ongoing clinical trials continue to refine best practice in this area, and clinicians managing gastric variceal disease should remain attentive to evolving evidence given the relative paucity of large, definitive studies compared to the more extensively studied esophageal variceal literature. Consistent, periodic laboratory monitoring makes this slow, low-grade process visible before it becomes symptomatic. This is a low-cost, high-value habit worth building into every visit. Indeed.

### Distinguishing Gastric Varices From Portal Hypertensive Gastropathy

Correctly distinguishing gastric varices from portal hypertensive gastropathy on endoscopy matters significantly for treatment selection, since applying endoscopic variceal-directed therapy to gastropathy, or conversely relying on beta-blocker therapy alone for an actively bleeding gastric varix, both represent a mismatch between the specific portal hypertensive complication present and the treatment approach it requires, reinforcing the value of careful endoscopic characterization rather than a generic label of portal hypertensive bleeding applied without this specific distinction. Clear documentation of the specific finding, using precise terminology rather than a generic description of portal hypertensive changes, supports accurate communication to any subsequent endoscopist or clinician reviewing prior reports when planning future management. This is a simple but consequential documentation discipline that costs nothing and pays real dividends in continuity of care. Small habits, repeated consistently, compound into real quality of care. It sets the tone for everything after.

## Muscle Cramps, Umbilical Hernia, and Other Common Cirrhosis Complications

Muscle cramps are a common, often underrecognized complaint in cirrhosis that meaningfully affects quality of life, and while several pharmacologic options have been studied, none carries strong, consistent evidence of benefit, meaning management often centers on addressing contributing factors, including electrolyte derangements from diuretic therapy discussed earlier in this chapter, and validating the symptom's genuine impact on the patient rather than dismissing it as a minor complaint unworthy of dedicated attention. Umbilical hernia, common in patients with significant ascites given the sustained increase in intra-abdominal pressure this fluid accumulation produces, requires careful surgical timing consideration, since elective repair is generally deferred until ascites is well controlled given the substantially elevated wound complication and recurrence risk when surgery is performed in the setting of poorly controlled, ongoing fluid accumulation, while incarcerated or ruptured umbilical hernia constitutes a surgical emergency regardless of ascites control status. Referral to physical therapy for a structured stretching and conditioning program may provide symptomatic benefit for some patients, representing a low-risk, nonpharmacologic option worth considering alongside the more limited pharmacologic choices available for this bothersome symptom. Patient education about warning signs of incarceration, including increasing pain, redness, or an inability to reduce the hernia manually, empowers patients to seek urgent evaluation promptly rather than delaying care for a complication that can rapidly become surgically emergent. Setting realistic expectations that this specific symptom may only partially improve, rather than fully resolve, helps patients approach management with appropriate, sustainable expectations rather than frustration when a complete resolution is not achieved. Written instructions covering these specific warning signs, provided at the time the hernia is first identified, give patients a reliable reference they can consult later if concerning symptoms develop.

### Coordinating Elective Surgical Care in Cirrhosis

Any elective surgical procedure in a patient with cirrhosis, not only umbilical hernia repair specifically, warrants careful preoperative risk assessment using the same Child-Pugh and model for end-stage liver disease scoring already established earlier in this chapter, since surgical risk correlates strongly with the severity of underlying liver disease, and this assessment should inform a shared decision about whether, and when, an elective procedure is safely pursued, ideally in coordination with hepatology input before the surgical team proceeds. Optimizing ascites control, correcting significant coagulopathy where feasible, and ensuring nutritional status is as favorable as possible before an elective procedure, rather than proceeding with surgery in a suboptimally prepared patient, meaningfully improves perioperative outcomes across the range of elective procedures this population may require. Coordinating this preoperative optimization timeline with the surgical team well in advance of the planned procedure avoids the disruption of a last-minute delay discovered only once surgery has already been scheduled. Small logistical steps like this often make the biggest practical difference. Truly.

## Liver Transplantation Evaluation

Referral for liver transplantation evaluation is generally appropriate once a patient develops their first major decompensating event or reaches a model for end-stage liver disease score threshold indicating meaningfully elevated one-year mortality risk, and this referral, applying the same proactive-rather-than-reactive timing principle already established in the previous chapter, should occur promptly once these criteria are met rather than delayed until the patient has deteriorated further, since the transplant evaluation process itself, including the comprehensive medical, surgical, and psychosocial assessment this process requires, takes meaningful time to complete. Transplant candidacy assessment extends beyond liver disease severity alone to encompass overall medical fitness for major surgery, psychosocial support and, where relevant, substance use history applying the same structured assessment framework already discussed in an earlier chapter for alcohol-associated liver disease specifically, and this comprehensive, multidisciplinary evaluation reflects the reality that transplantation success depends on far more than the recipient's liver disease severity alone. Regional variation in organ availability and waitlist times should also inform the timing of this referral discussion, and clinicians practicing in areas with longer expected waitlist times may reasonably consider earlier referral relative to the same MELD threshold applied in a region with shorter typical wait times. A dedicated transplant social worker, engaged early in the evaluation process, can help identify and address practical barriers, including housing stability, transportation to follow-up appointments, and caregiver availability, that might otherwise only surface later in the process when they could delay an already time-sensitive evaluation. Financial counseling regarding the substantial costs of transplantation and post-transplant care, though ultimately handled by dedicated financial coordinators, benefits from early, transparent conversation so patients are not blindsided by these considerations partway through an already demanding evaluation process. Even a brief mention of these resources at the outset reduces anxiety later in the process. Early identification of these barriers prevents wasted time later. Proactive planning respects the patient's time. Truly.

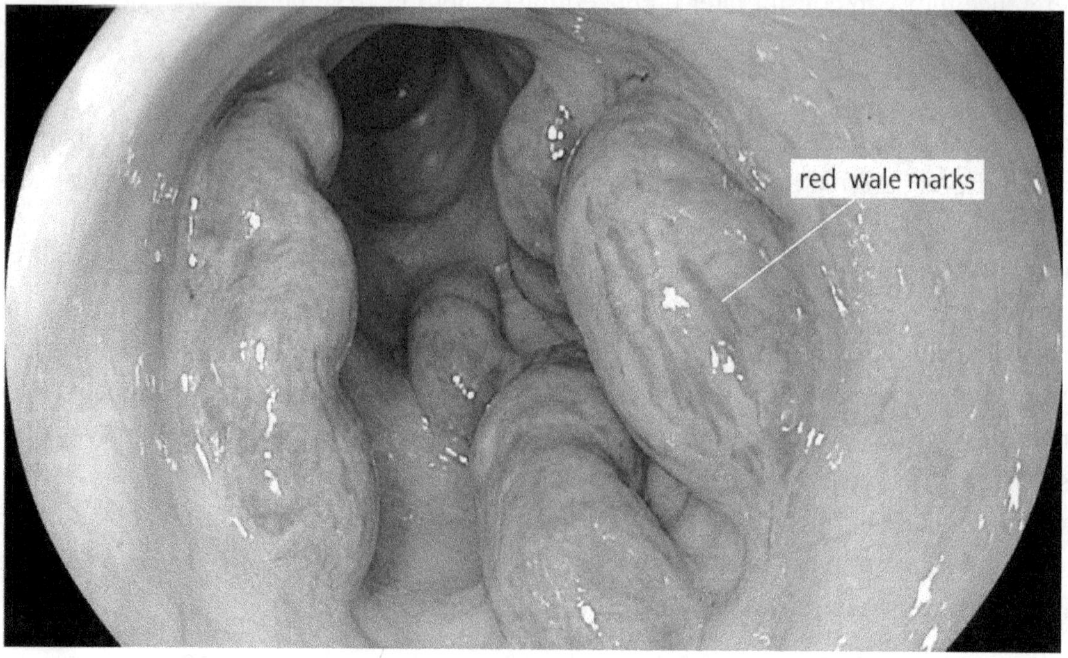


Case Presentation: A 61-year-old man with known cirrhosis from chronic hepatitis C, previously treated and cured, presents with new abdominal distension. Diagnostic paracentesis confirms ascites with a serum-ascites albumin gradient of 1.4 grams per deciliter, consistent with portal hypertension, and ascitic fluid absolute neutrophil count returns at 340 cells per cubic millimeter, meeting criteria for spontaneous bacterial peritonitis despite his relatively mild presenting symptoms. Applying the reasoning developed in this chapter, empiric third-generation cephalosporin therapy is initiated promptly given this diagnosis, and albumin is administered given his bilirubin and creatinine values meeting criteria for this specific adjunctive therapy. He improves clinically over the following days, and given this confirmed episode, he is discharged on indefinite secondary prophylaxis with a fluoroquinolone. This case illustrates the chapter's central low-threshold diagnostic paracentesis principle: his minimal presenting symptoms did not preclude a confirmed, clinically significant infection, reinforcing why paracentesis should be pursued liberally in any cirrhotic patient with ascites presenting for any reason, rather than reserved for patients with more dramatic peritonitis symptoms.

Case Presentation: A 55-year-old woman is newly diagnosed with compensated cirrhosis from metabolic dysfunction-associated steatohepatitis. Noninvasive risk stratification using platelet count and liver stiffness measurement suggests a meaningful probability of clinically significant varices, and she proceeds to screening endoscopy, which identifies medium-sized esophageal varices without high-risk stigmata. Applying the reasoning developed in this chapter, these findings meet criteria for primary prophylaxis, and after discussing both nonselective beta-blocker therapy and endoscopic band ligation, she elects beta-blocker therapy given her preference to avoid a repeat endoscopic procedure. She tolerates the medication well with an appropriate heart rate response confirming adequate dosing. This case illustrates the chapter's core variceal prophylaxis principle: identifying medium-sized varices on screening endoscopy defined a clear threshold for primary prophylaxis initiation, and the specific modality chosen reflected informed patient preference between two comparably effective options rather than a single default approach applied uniformly.

## Nutritional Assessment and Sarcopenia in Cirrhosis

Malnutrition and sarcopenia, muscle mass loss, are common in cirrhosis and carry independent prognostic significance beyond the standard severity scoring systems developed earlier in this chapter, and formal nutritional assessment, incorporating both dietary intake history and objective measures of muscle mass where available, should be a routine component of comprehensive cirrhosis management rather than addressed only once overt malnutrition becomes clinically apparent through unintentional weight loss or visible muscle wasting. Protein restriction, a historically common but now recognized as counterproductive practice once believed to reduce ammonia production and encephalopathy risk, is no longer recommended, since adequate protein intake is essential to prevent and treat sarcopenia, and current guidance instead favors frequent, small meals with a late-evening snack to minimize the prolonged overnight fasting period that accelerates muscle catabolism in this population. Bioelectrical impedance analysis and, where available, cross-sectional imaging-based muscle measurement offer more objective assessment tools than clinical impression alone, though these specialized techniques are not universally available, meaning a careful clinical history focused on functional decline and unintentional weight change remains a valuable, widely accessible screening approach even where these more objective tools are not accessible. Communicating this updated guidance clearly to patients and families who may have received older, now outdated protein-restriction advice helps prevent unnecessary, potentially harmful ongoing protein limitation that could otherwise persist based on outdated information. Involving the patient's family in dietary planning, particularly when a spouse or other household member typically prepares meals, extends the practical impact of nutritional counseling beyond the clinic visit itself into the patient's actual daily eating environment. Indeed.

### Coordinating Nutritional Support

Referral to a dietitian with specific experience managing cirrhosis-related nutritional needs, rather than generic nutritional counseling not tailored to this population's distinct requirements, supports more effective, individualized dietary planning, and this referral should be considered proactively for any patient with decompensated cirrhosis or evidence of sarcopenia rather than reserved only for patients who have already developed severe, clinically obvious malnutrition. Setting concrete, achievable dietary goals collaboratively with the patient, rather than delivering generic nutritional guidance detached from their specific circumstances, supports better adherence and more meaningful improvement in nutritional status over time.

| Complication | Key Diagnostic Threshold | First-Line Management |
|---|---|---|
| Esophageal varices | Medium-large size or high-risk stigmata | Nonselective beta-blocker or band ligation |
| Spontaneous bacterial peritonitis | Ascitic fluid ANC ≥250 cells/mm³ | Third-generation cephalosporin ± albumin |
| Hepatic encephalopathy | Clinical grading + precipitant identification | Lactulose, add rifaximin if recurrent |
| Hepatorenal syndrome | Exclusion of other AKI causes + no response to albumin challenge | Vasoconstrictor (terlipressin) + albumin |

**THE GI THRESHOLD DECISION SYSTEM — Decompensated Cirrhosis Thresholds**

**Presentation Signature:** This chapter's threshold instances addressed variceal screening and primary prophylaxis initiation, and spontaneous bacterial peritonitis prophylaxis indications.

**Threshold Point:** Noninvasive risk stratification and endoscopic variceal characteristics gate screening and prophylaxis decisions; specific prior-episode, ascitic-fluid-protein, and hemorrhage-related criteria gate SBP prophylaxis.

**The Call:** Both thresholds replace uniform, one-size-fits-all screening or prophylaxis policies with criteria-based, individualized risk assessment that matches intervention intensity to the patient's actual risk profile.

**Trap Logic:** Applying screening or prophylaxis uniformly regardless of these specific criteria, in either direction, either exposes low-risk patients to unnecessary intervention or leaves high-risk patients inadequately protected against a preventable, life-threatening complication.

**Decision Anchor:** Apply noninvasive risk stratification before committing to screening endoscopy, initiate primary prophylaxis promptly once high-risk varices are identified, and apply SBP prophylaxis specifically to patients meeting the defined primary, secondary, or hemorrhage-related criteria.

## Summary and Key Concepts

The compensated-to-decompensated transition, defined by ascites, variceal hemorrhage, hepatic encephalopathy, or jaundice, marks the single most important prognostic shift in cirrhosis, and Child-Pugh and MELD scores provide standardized staging and transplant allocation.

Variceal screening can be deferred in patients meeting low-risk noninvasive criteria, and primary prophylaxis with beta-blockers or band ligation is indicated once medium-large varices or high-risk stigmata are identified on screening endoscopy.

The serum-ascites albumin gradient, not total ascitic protein, most accurately distinguishes portal hypertension-related ascites from other causes, and refractory ascites is managed with large-volume paracentesis and albumin replacement.

Spontaneous bacterial peritonitis, diagnosed by an ascitic fluid neutrophil count of 250 cells/mm³ or greater, requires a low threshold for diagnostic paracentesis given its often minimal symptoms, and specific criteria define primary, secondary, and hemorrhage-related antibiotic prophylaxis indications.

Hepatic encephalopathy management requires active identification of a specific precipitating factor for every episode, with lactulose as first-line therapy and rifaximin added for recurrent episodes.

Hepatorenal syndrome is a diagnosis of exclusion requiring an albumin challenge and exclusion of other causes, treated with a vasoconstrictor plus albumin, with liver transplantation the only definitive treatment; transplant referral should occur promptly at the first major decompensating event.

# CHAPTER 19: ACUTE GASTROINTESTINAL HEMORRHAGE AND VASCULAR DISORDERS

**Learning Objectives**

1. Apply pre-endoscopic risk stratification and initial resuscitation principles for acute upper gastrointestinal hemorrhage.
2. Manage variceal and non-variceal upper gastrointestinal hemorrhage using evidence-based, threshold-driven pathways.
3. Evaluate and manage acute lower gastrointestinal hemorrhage, including timing of colonoscopy.
4. Recognize acute mesenteric ischemia promptly and apply an appropriate diagnostic and management pathway.
5. Diagnose and manage ischemic colitis and distinguish it from other causes of lower gastrointestinal bleeding and abdominal pain.

**Chapter Outline**

This chapter develops the acute, time-sensitive gastrointestinal emergencies that integrate concepts from throughout this book: upper gastrointestinal hemorrhage, variceal and non-variceal, with its pre-endoscopic risk stratification threshold; lower gastrointestinal hemorrhage and its timing-of-colonoscopy threshold; and the vascular emergencies, acute mesenteric ischemia and ischemic colitis. Each section connects a specific severity or diagnostic threshold to a defined, time-sensitive management pathway.

## Upper Gastrointestinal Hemorrhage

### Initial Resuscitation and Risk Stratification

Acute upper gastrointestinal hemorrhage presents with hematemesis, melena, or, in severe, rapid bleeding, hematochezia, and initial management prioritizes hemodynamic resuscitation, intravenous access, and restrictive red blood cell transfusion, generally targeting a hemoglobin threshold rather than a specific hemoglobin normalization, since a restrictive transfusion strategy has demonstrated improved outcomes compared to a more liberal approach in this population, reflecting a meaningful departure from older, more permissive transfusion practices historically applied in acute hemorrhage of any cause. Pre-endoscopic risk stratification, most commonly using the Glasgow-Blatchford score, incorporating blood urea nitrogen, hemoglobin, systolic blood pressure, heart rate, and clinical findings including melena or syncope, identifies patients at sufficiently low risk to be considered for outpatient management or early discharge without inpatient endoscopy, while higher-scoring patients require inpatient admission and more urgent endoscopic evaluation, and this score, calculated before any endoscopic information is available, provides an evidence-based alternative to relying on clinical gestalt alone for this critical early triage decision. Coagulopathy correction, when genuinely indicated, should be individualized rather than reflexive, applying the same nuanced approach to correcting an elevated international normalized ratio already established in the previous chapter for cirrhotic patients specifically, since overcorrection carries its own risks without necessarily improving actual bleeding control. The Rockall score, incorporating both pre-endoscopic clinical variables and post-endoscopic findings, complements the Glasgow-Blatchford score by adding prognostic information once the endoscopic source has been identified, and using both scores at their respective, appropriate time points provides the most complete risk assessment across the full course of a patient's hospitalization.

### Variceal Hemorrhage Management

Variceal hemorrhage, discussed in the previous chapter's portal hypertension section, requires specific additional management beyond the general upper gastrointestinal hemorrhage approach, including prompt initiation of a vasoactive agent, most commonly octreotide, reducing splanchnic blood flow and portal pressure, and antibiotic prophylaxis, typically a third-generation cephalosporin, given the substantially elevated infection risk this specific bleeding source carries in cirrhotic patients and the demonstrated mortality benefit antibiotic prophylaxis provides in this population, both of which should be initiated promptly, ideally before endoscopy, rather than delayed until the variceal source is endoscopically confirmed. Endoscopic variceal band ligation is the primary endoscopic treatment for esophageal variceal hemorrhage, generally performed within twelve hours of presentation once the patient is hemodynamically stabilized, and balloon tamponade or a self-expanding esophageal stent serves as a temporizing bridge measure for hemorrhage refractory to endoscopic and pharmacologic therapy, reserved for this specific rescue scenario given the significant complication risk these bridging measures carry. Octreotide is generally continued for three to five days following the acute bleeding episode, reflecting the observation that rebleeding risk remains elevated during this early window, and premature discontinuation before this recommended duration has elapsed risks exposing the patient to a preventable rebleeding episode during a period when continued pharmacologic portal pressure reduction still provides meaningful protective benefit. Repeat band ligation sessions at defined intervals following the acute hemorrhage episode, continued until variceal eradication is achieved, are essential to reducing recurrent bleeding risk, and this ongoing endoscopic surveillance and treatment program should be scheduled proactively before the patient is discharged rather than left to informal, unstructured follow-up.

### THE GI THRESHOLD DECISION SYSTEM — Hemorrhage Thresholds — Pre-Endoscopic Risk Stratification in Upper GI Bleeding

---

**Presentation Signature:** A patient presents with suspected acute upper gastrointestinal hemorrhage, and the clinician must determine the appropriate triage pathway before endoscopy is performed.

**Threshold Point:** The Glasgow-Blatchford score, calculated from readily available clinical and laboratory data without requiring endoscopic information, defines the threshold separating patients at sufficiently low risk for consideration of outpatient management from those requiring inpatient admission and more urgent endoscopic evaluation.

**The Call:** Patients meeting the low-risk threshold may be considered for outpatient management with close follow-up in appropriately selected circumstances; patients above this threshold are admitted, resuscitated, and undergo endoscopy within the timeframe their clinical severity and suspected bleeding source, variceal versus non-variceal, dictates.

**Trap Logic:** Relying on clinical impression alone, without calculating this validated score, risks both unnecessarily admitting genuinely low-risk patients and, more consequentially, underestimating risk in a patient whose presentation seems reassuring but whose objective score indicates a meaningfully elevated risk profile.

**Decision Anchor:** Calculate the Glasgow-Blatchford score for every patient with suspected acute upper gastrointestinal hemorrhage before triage disposition is finalized, rather than relying on clinical gestalt alone for this consequential early decision.

Figure 19.1: Forrest Classification of Peptic Ulcer Hemorrhage

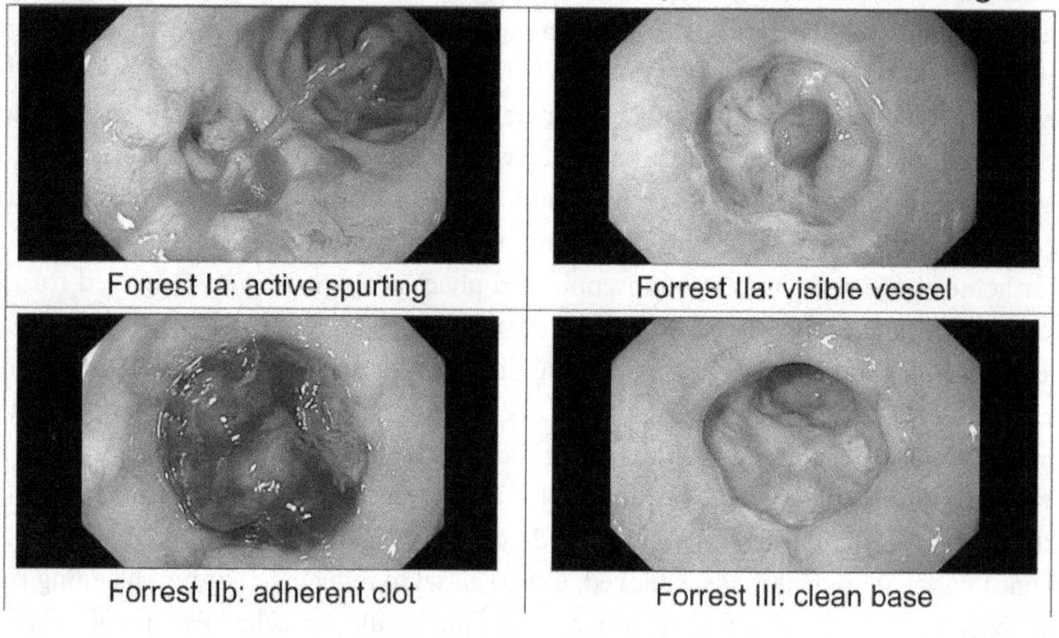


**Non-Variceal Upper Gastrointestinal Hemorrhage Management**

Peptic ulcer disease, discussed in an earlier chapter, remains the most common cause of non-variceal upper gastrointestinal hemorrhage, and the Forrest classification, describing the specific endoscopic appearance of the ulcer base, active spurting or oozing hemorrhage, a visible vessel, an adherent clot, or a clean base, stratifies rebleeding risk and directly determines whether endoscopic therapy is indicated, with high-risk stigmata warranting endoscopic hemostasis, typically combining injection therapy with a mechanical or thermal modality, while a clean-based ulcer carries sufficiently low rebleeding risk that endoscopic therapy is not required. High-dose proton pump inhibitor therapy, initiated promptly and continued for a defined course following endoscopic hemostasis in high-risk lesions, reduces rebleeding risk, and this pharmacologic therapy, alongside the endoscopic intervention itself, should be understood as a complementary rather than either-or component of comprehensive non-variceal hemorrhage management.

An adherent clot, a specific Forrest category carrying intermediate rebleeding risk, is generally managed with vigorous irrigation to attempt clot dislodgement, followed by endoscopic treatment of any underlying high-risk stigmata revealed beneath the clot, rather than either leaving the clot entirely undisturbed or reflexively treating it without this attempted dislodgement step. Once oral intake resumes and the initial high-risk period has passed, transitioning from intravenous to oral proton pump inhibitor therapy at a standard dose, continued for the duration recommended based on the specific ulcer etiology and any identified Helicobacter pylori infection, completes this treatment course appropriately.

## Lower Gastrointestinal Hemorrhage

### Etiology and Initial Evaluation

Acute lower gastrointestinal hemorrhage, presenting with hematochezia in the substantial majority of cases, arises most commonly from diverticular bleeding, discussed in the eleventh chapter, followed by hemorrhoidal bleeding, ischemic colitis, discussed later in this chapter, and, less commonly, neoplastic or inflammatory bowel disease-related bleeding, and initial evaluation should specifically exclude an upper gastrointestinal source, since brisk upper gastrointestinal hemorrhage can present with hematochezia rather than the more typical melena, and this distinction meaningfully changes the diagnostic and management pathway pursued. A nasogastric lavage, while historically used for this purpose, has largely fallen out of favor given its imperfect sensitivity and the discomfort it causes, with clinical assessment of hemodynamic stability, the specific stool description, and risk factors for an upper source now generally favored over this now less commonly performed test to guide the decision about whether upper endoscopy should precede colonoscopy in a given presentation. A careful history focused on recent colonoscopy, known diverticulosis, prior similar bleeding episodes, and specific medication use, particularly anticoagulants and nonsteroidal anti-inflammatory drugs, meaningfully narrows this differential before any diagnostic testing has even been performed, and this history-taking step should not be abbreviated simply because the presentation seems straightforward on initial impression. When genuine diagnostic uncertainty remains about whether an upper source might be contributing, particularly in a patient with risk factors for peptic ulcer disease or known varices, proceeding with upper endoscopy first, even in a patient presenting with hematochezia, is a reasonable, cautious approach rather than assuming a lower source based on the presenting symptom alone.

### Diagnostic and Therapeutic Approach

Colonoscopy, generally performed within twenty-four hours of presentation in hemodynamically stable patients following adequate bowel preparation, is both diagnostic and, when a bleeding source is identified, potentially therapeutic, and this specific timing window balances the improved diagnostic yield adequate preparation provides against the value of not delaying intervention excessively in a patient with active or recent bleeding, reflecting an evidence-based compromise between these competing considerations. For patients with ongoing, hemodynamically significant hemorrhage in whom colonoscopy cannot be performed promptly or does not identify a treatable source, computed tomography angiography or catheter-directed angiography with embolization, and, when these approaches are unsuccessful or unavailable, surgical intervention, provide escalating diagnostic and therapeutic options, reflecting the same stepwise, severity-matched escalation principle already established throughout this book for other acute conditions. Endoscopic treatment options once a definitive bleeding source is identified at colonoscopy, including clip placement, thermal coagulation, and injection therapy, are selected based on the specific lesion and its accessibility, mirroring the same technique selection considerations already developed for upper gastrointestinal hemostasis earlier in this chapter. Tagged red blood cell scintigraphy, historically used to help localize an intermittent, lower-volume bleeding source before proceeding to angiography, has become less commonly utilized as computed tomography angiography technology has improved, though it remains available in some centers as an additional localization tool for genuinely difficult cases.

Figure 19.2: CT Angiography Findings in Acute Mesenteric Ischemia

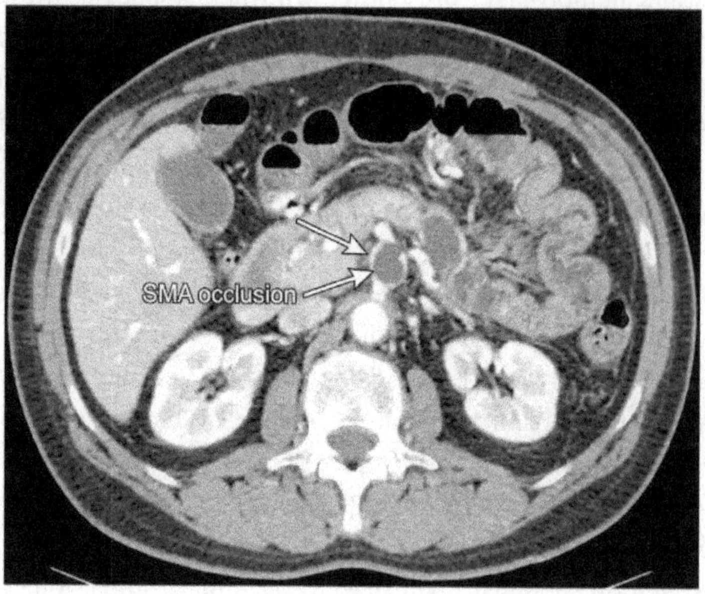


**THE GI THRESHOLD DECISION SYSTEM — Hemorrhage Thresholds — Colonoscopy Timing in Lower GI Bleeding**

**Presentation Signature:** A patient presents with acute lower gastrointestinal hemorrhage, and the clinician must determine the timing and sequence of diagnostic evaluation.

**Threshold Point:** Hemodynamic stability and the ability to complete adequate bowel preparation define the threshold for proceeding with colonoscopy within the standard twenty-four-hour window; ongoing hemodynamically significant hemorrhage precluding this preparation defines a threshold for escalation to angiographic or surgical intervention instead.

**The Call:** Hemodynamically stable patients able to complete adequate preparation undergo colonoscopy within twenty-four hours; unstable patients or those in whom bleeding precludes adequate preparation proceed directly to computed tomography angiography or catheter angiography, reserving surgery for cases where these less invasive options fail or are unavailable.

**Trap Logic:** Pursuing colonoscopy without adequate preparation in an attempt to avoid delay produces poor visualization that can miss the actual bleeding source, while delaying escalation to angiography in a hemodynamically unstable patient in hope that colonoscopy will eventually become feasible risks continued, potentially fatal hemorrhage during this delay.

**Decision Anchor:** Assess hemodynamic stability and bowel preparation feasibility explicitly at presentation, and escalate promptly to angiographic or surgical intervention in patients who do not meet the threshold for standard, prepared colonoscopy rather than pursuing an unprepared or excessively delayed colonoscopic examination.

## Obscure and Occult Gastrointestinal Bleeding

Obscure gastrointestinal bleeding, defined as bleeding of unclear source persisting or recurring after negative upper endoscopy and colonoscopy, warrants small bowel evaluation, most commonly with video capsule endoscopy, given the small bowel's relative inaccessibility to standard bidirectional endoscopy, and this stepwise evaluation, upper and lower endoscopy first, followed by small bowel investigation only when these initial studies are unrevealing, avoids unnecessarily jumping to more specialized, resource-intensive small bowel evaluation before the more common, more accessible bleeding sources have been adequately excluded. Occult gastrointestinal bleeding, presenting as iron deficiency anemia or a positive fecal occult blood test without overt bleeding, similarly warrants bidirectional endoscopy as the standard initial evaluation, and identifying a source, whether a colorectal neoplasm, discussed in an earlier chapter, or another cause, carries importance extending beyond correcting the anemia itself, since occult bleeding can be the first presenting sign of a colorectal malignancy that would otherwise go undetected until a more advanced, symptomatic stage. Repeat upper and lower endoscopy, performed by an experienced endoscopist with specific attention to commonly missed areas, is sometimes warranted before proceeding to small bowel evaluation, since a meaningful proportion of lesions ultimately attributed to obscure bleeding are later found to have been within reach of standard endoscopy but were missed on the initial examination. Age-appropriate colorectal cancer screening intervals, discussed in the eleventh chapter, should be confirmed as up to date whenever a patient presents with newly identified iron deficiency anemia, since this presentation itself functions as an indication for colonoscopy regardless of the patient's age-based screening interval.

### Small Bowel Bleeding Sources

Small bowel angioectasias represent the most common identifiable cause of obscure gastrointestinal bleeding in older adults, and these vascular lesions, when identified on capsule endoscopy or, when therapeutic intervention is needed, device-assisted enteroscopy, can be treated endoscopically with thermal ablation, though recurrent bleeding from multiple or diffusely distributed angioectasias sometimes requires additional pharmacologic approaches, including somatostatin analogues or, in refractory cases, other systemic therapies aimed at reducing the underlying angiogenic process driving lesion formation. Iron replacement, whether oral or, when oral therapy is poorly tolerated or ineffective, intravenous, should accompany any specific bleeding-source treatment, since correcting the resulting anemia is itself an important therapeutic goal independent of achieving definitive hemostasis at the identified vascular lesion.

## Second-Look Endoscopy and Rebleeding Management

Second-look endoscopy, a planned repeat examination performed within roughly twenty-four hours of the initial hemostatic procedure, is not routinely recommended for every high-risk lesion given adequate initial endoscopic therapy and appropriate proton pump inhibitor therapy, though it may be considered in specific circumstances where initial hemostasis was technically incomplete or uncertain, reflecting a selective rather than universal application of this additional procedure. Rebleeding after initial successful endoscopic hemostasis, occurring in a meaningful minority of high-risk lesions despite appropriate initial treatment, is generally managed with a repeat endoscopic attempt in the first instance, reserving angiographic embolization or surgery for cases where this repeat endoscopic attempt fails to achieve durable hemostasis, applying the same stepwise escalation principle already established throughout this book for other conditions with a graduated intervention hierarchy. Clear documentation of the specific initial hemostatic technique used and the endoscopist's assessment of its adequacy supports a subsequent, more informed decision about whether second-look endoscopy is genuinely warranted in a given case rather than defaulting reflexively to either universal repeat examination or complete omission of this consideration. Recognizing rebleeding promptly requires vigilant, structured monitoring, and any recurrence of the presenting symptoms, hematemesis, melena, or hemodynamic instability, following apparent initial hemostatic success should prompt immediate reassessment rather than assumption that these findings reflect a benign, self-limited process.

### Helicobacter Pylori Testing and Eradication After Bleeding Ulcer

Every patient with a bleeding peptic ulcer should be tested for Helicobacter pylori, discussed in the fifth chapter, and eradication therapy should be provided when this infection is confirmed, since eradication substantially reduces the risk of ulcer recurrence and rebleeding, and testing performed during the acute bleeding episode itself can produce false-negative results given reduced test sensitivity in this specific acute setting, meaning a negative test obtained during active bleeding should be confirmed with repeat testing once the acute episode has resolved rather than accepted as definitively excluding this infection. Documenting both the timing of initial testing relative to the acute bleeding episode and the plan for confirmatory retesting, where indicated, ensures this important step is not inadvertently lost between the acute hospitalization and subsequent outpatient follow-up, a transition point where important but non-urgent follow-up items can sometimes fall through the cracks. Both invasive testing at the time of endoscopy, biopsy-based rapid urease testing or histology, and noninvasive testing, stool antigen or urea breath testing, are acceptable approaches, with the choice generally guided by whether endoscopic biopsy is already being performed for another indication during the same procedure. Documenting the eradication confirmation test result, generally performed at least four weeks after completing treatment, ensures the treatment's success is formally verified rather than assumed based on symptom improvement alone. A missed confirmation test represents a genuine, preventable gap in secondary prevention that this simple documentation step closes. Simple but essential.

## NSAID-Related Bleeding and Prevention Strategies

Nonsteroidal anti-inflammatory drug use is a major, modifiable risk factor for both peptic ulcer disease and its bleeding complications, and patients with a history of an ulcer-related bleeding event who require ongoing nonsteroidal anti-inflammatory drug therapy for another condition should receive concurrent proton pump inhibitor prophylaxis and, where feasible, transition to a cyclooxygenase-2 selective agent, which carries a somewhat lower gastrointestinal bleeding risk than nonselective agents, though this reduced gastrointestinal risk must be weighed against this drug class's own cardiovascular risk profile in appropriately selected patients. Assessing the ongoing necessity of nonsteroidal anti-inflammatory drug therapy itself, in collaboration with the prescribing clinician, and pursuing alternative analgesic strategies where clinically reasonable, represents the most direct risk-reduction strategy available, since no amount of gastroprotective co-therapy fully eliminates the risk this drug class carries, particularly in a patient who has already demonstrated vulnerability to this specific complication. Patients often underestimate the gastrointestinal risk of over-the-counter nonsteroidal anti-inflammatory drug products, mistakenly assuming that a medication available without a prescription necessarily carries a lower risk profile, and directly correcting this common misconception is an important, straightforward part of effective patient counseling around this specific class of medication. Nonpharmacologic approaches to pain management, including physical therapy and topical agents where clinically appropriate, deserve consideration alongside pharmacologic alternatives, since reducing overall reliance on any single analgesic class provides the most durable risk reduction over the long term. Reassessing this need periodically, rather than assuming the initial decision remains appropriate indefinitely, ensures ongoing alignment between actual clinical necessity and continued exposure to this modifiable risk. Always worth revisiting.

### Aspirin for Cardiovascular Prophylaxis After GI Bleeding

Low-dose aspirin used for cardiovascular prophylaxis presents a similarly nuanced risk-benefit calculation after a gastrointestinal bleeding event, and current evidence generally supports resuming aspirin promptly after bleeding has been controlled in patients with a genuine, ongoing cardiovascular indication, given data suggesting that prolonged aspirin discontinuation carries meaningful cardiovascular risk that outweighs the modest rebleeding risk increase resumption produces, particularly when resumed alongside appropriate proton pump inhibitor co-therapy. This resumption decision should be made collaboratively with the prescribing cardiologist or primary care clinician, ensuring the specific cardiovascular indication and its associated risk are fully weighed alongside the gastrointestinal considerations developed throughout this chapter. Communicating this evidence-based resumption timeline clearly to patients who may feel understandably anxious about restarting a medication so soon after a bleeding episode reassures them that this decision reflects careful weighing of their overall risk profile rather than a casual or inconsistent recommendation.

## Dieulafoy Lesion and Other Uncommon Bleeding Sources

Dieulafoy lesion, a large, aberrant submucosal artery that erodes through an otherwise normal-appearing overlying mucosa, produces sudden, often dramatic hemorrhage from a lesion that can be genuinely difficult to identify endoscopically given its typically small mucosal defect and intermittent bleeding pattern, and this diagnosis should be considered when a source is not immediately apparent on initial endoscopy in a patient with significant, otherwise unexplained upper gastrointestinal hemorrhage, sometimes requiring a repeat examination or specialized techniques, including endoscopic ultrasound, to identify the underlying vessel definitively. Gastric antral vascular ectasia, producing a characteristic endoscopic appearance sometimes described as watermelon stomach given its longitudinal red stripes, causes chronic, often occult blood loss rather than the acute, dramatic hemorrhage more typical of Dieulafoy lesion, and endoscopic thermal therapy, applied over multiple sessions given the diffuse nature of this vascular abnormality, is the primary treatment approach for this specific, distinct entity. Endoscopic clipping or thermal coagulation, once the lesion is identified, generally achieves durable hemostasis, and marking the lesion location with an endoscopic tattoo at the time of treatment supports easier relocation should repeat evaluation become necessary given this lesion's characteristically subtle mucosal appearance. Gastric antral vascular ectasia occurs with increased frequency in patients with cirrhosis and certain autoimmune conditions, and considering these associations when the diagnosis is established can prompt appropriate additional evaluation for a coexisting condition that might otherwise go unrecognized. Given how uncommon this specific lesion is, referral to an endoscopist with particular experience in its recognition and treatment is reasonable when initial identification proves genuinely difficult despite a strong clinical suspicion for this diagnosis. Correctly distinguishing gastric antral vascular ectasia from portal hypertensive gastropathy, discussed in the previous chapter, matters given their differing endoscopic appearance and treatment approach, and this distinction should be made explicit in the endoscopy report. Truly.

### Aortoenteric Fistula

Aortoenteric fistula, an uncommon but catastrophic cause of gastrointestinal hemorrhage occurring in a patient with a history of aortic aneurysm repair, particularly with a prior aortic graft, should be considered specifically in this population given the extremely high mortality this diagnosis carries if unrecognized, and a herald bleed, a smaller, self-limited bleeding episode preceding the eventual, often fatal massive hemorrhage this condition produces, should prompt urgent evaluation and surgical or vascular consultation in any patient with this specific surgical history presenting with even modest gastrointestinal bleeding, rather than the more routine evaluation appropriate for a patient without this specific risk factor. Computed tomography with contrast is generally the initial imaging study of choice when this diagnosis is suspected, though a negative or equivocal study does not fully exclude the diagnosis given this condition's recognized difficulty to definitively confirm on imaging alone, meaning surgical consultation should proceed based on clinical suspicion even when imaging is not immediately confirmatory. A high index of suspicion combined with a low threshold for surgical exploration, even without definitive imaging confirmation, is warranted given the catastrophic consequences of a delayed diagnosis in this specific, high-mortality condition. Vigilance saves lives here. Indeed. Yes, always.

## Hemodynamic Monitoring and Critical Care Coordination in Severe GI Hemorrhage

Patients with severe, hemodynamically significant gastrointestinal hemorrhage warrant intensive care unit-level monitoring and, where appropriate, early critical care or surgical consultation rather than management confined solely within a general medical or gastroenterology-only framework, since the resuscitation and airway protection needs of a severely bleeding patient, particularly one with a compromised mental status from hypovolemia or hepatic encephalopathy in cirrhotic patients, frequently exceed what a general ward setting can safely provide. Massive transfusion protocols, activated in the most severe hemorrhage presentations, provide a coordinated, pre-established framework for delivering blood products in a balanced ratio, and familiarity with the local massive transfusion protocol, including how to activate it and what products it provides, is essential for any clinician who may encounter a patient with this level of hemorrhage severity, since delay in recognizing the need for this coordinated response can meaningfully worsen outcomes in the most critical presentations. Establishing clear, predefined communication and escalation pathways between gastroenterology, critical care, and surgery before a critical presentation actually arises supports a faster, more coordinated response than improvising this collaboration for the first time during an acute, high-stakes hemorrhage episode. Periodic mock activation drills, conducted as part of routine institutional preparedness, can help ensure that when a genuine massive transfusion scenario arises, the involved teams execute the protocol efficiently rather than encountering unfamiliar logistics for the first time during an actual life-threatening emergency. Investing in this preparation before it is needed pays real dividends when a genuine emergency arises.

### Airway Protection Before Endoscopy in Severe Hemorrhage

Airway protection, including consideration of endotracheal intubation before endoscopy in a patient with significant hematemesis, altered mental status, or both, protects against aspiration during the endoscopic procedure itself, and this decision should be made proactively based on the patient's presenting risk factors rather than reactively only after an aspiration event has already occurred during an unprotected endoscopic examination. This proactive assessment should be revisited if the patient's clinical status changes during the resuscitation period, since a patient who initially seemed stable enough for unprotected endoscopy may deteriorate before the procedure actually begins, requiring reassessment of this decision rather than proceeding based solely on the initial evaluation. Vigilance here protects patients from a preventable, serious complication.

## Post-Discharge Follow-Up and Secondary Prevention After GI Hemorrhage

Every patient discharged after an acute gastrointestinal hemorrhage benefits from a clearly documented follow-up plan addressing the specific etiology identified, whether that means scheduled variceal band ligation sessions for a cirrhotic patient, Helicobacter pylori eradication confirmation for a peptic ulcer patient, or colonoscopic surveillance for a patient with a bleeding colonic polyp, and this plan should be communicated explicitly to both the patient and their primary care clinician, since gaps in this handoff communication are a recognized, preventable source of missed secondary prevention opportunities across many acute care transitions, not only gastrointestinal hemorrhage specifically. Medication reconciliation at discharge deserves particular attention in this population, given how frequently anticoagulants, antiplatelet agents, and nonsteroidal anti-inflammatory drugs are implicated in the presenting hemorrhage, and a deliberate, documented review of which medications are being resumed, discontinued, or modified, with clear rationale for each decision, protects against the confusion that can otherwise arise when multiple specialists have each independently weighed in on a single medication list during the hospitalization. Building this discharge communication into a standardized template or checklist, rather than relying on individual clinician memory to include every relevant detail, supports consistency across a busy inpatient service where many patients with varying etiologies and follow-up needs are discharged simultaneously. Providing the patient with a written, updated medication list at discharge, rather than relying on verbal instruction alone, gives them and any subsequent clinician a reliable reference that reduces the risk of an inadvertent medication error during this vulnerable care transition. Consistency here protects patients during a genuinely vulnerable transition. Truly.

### Patient Education on Warning Signs of Rebleeding

Clear, plain-language education about the specific warning signs of rebleeding, recurrent dark or bloody stool, lightheadedness, or recurrent vomiting of blood, delivered before discharge and reinforced in writing, empowers patients to seek care promptly rather than delaying evaluation out of uncertainty about whether their symptoms warrant urgent attention, and this education deserves the same dedicated time and attention as the medical management itself, since a well-informed patient who returns promptly for a genuine rebleeding episode achieves a meaningfully better outcome than one who delays care out of uncertainty or reluctance to seek help again so soon after a difficult hospitalization. This same education should specifically address when to call for guidance versus when to seek emergency care directly, since patients uncertain about this distinction may either delay appropriately urgent care or, conversely, seek emergency evaluation unnecessarily for symptoms that could be addressed through a phone call to their care team instead. These small details compound to genuinely safer care over time. Yes.

## Pediatric and Elderly Considerations in GI Hemorrhage

Gastrointestinal hemorrhage in children follows a different etiologic distribution than the adult presentations developed throughout this chapter, with causes including Meckel diverticulum, intussusception, and juvenile polyps figuring more prominently, and this distinct differential, alongside the specific technical and sedation considerations pediatric endoscopy requires, generally warrants involvement of a pediatric gastroenterologist rather than management under an adult-oriented framework applied without modification to a pediatric patient. Elderly patients, conversely, often present with less dramatic hemodynamic compensation for a given volume of blood loss given age-related changes in cardiovascular reserve, meaning a seemingly modest degree of tachycardia or blood pressure change in an older patient may actually represent more significant hemorrhage than the same vital sign findings would suggest in a younger patient, and this age-related blunting of the typical compensatory response should be factored into risk stratification and resuscitation decisions in this population. Meckel scan, a nuclear medicine study using technetium-99m pertechnetate to identify ectopic gastric mucosa within a Meckel diverticulum, remains a valuable diagnostic tool specifically in pediatric patients with suspected occult or overt bleeding from this congenital anomaly, illustrating a specialized diagnostic approach not typically required in the adult bleeding evaluations developed throughout the rest of this chapter. Cognitive impairment, common in elderly patients, can further complicate history-taking and symptom reporting, meaning collateral history from family members or caregivers becomes especially valuable when evaluating an elderly patient with suspected gastrointestinal hemorrhage who cannot reliably provide a complete account of their symptoms independently. Pretreatment with an H2-receptor antagonist can improve the sensitivity of the Meckel scan by enhancing tracer retention within the ectopic gastric mucosa, an important technical detail that should not be overlooked when ordering this specific study. This same principle applies broadly whenever an elderly patient's history is incomplete for any reason, not only in the specific context of gastrointestinal hemorrhage. Precision matters most for the youngest patients.

### Polypharmacy Considerations in Elderly GI Bleeding Patients

Polypharmacy, common in elderly patients and frequently including multiple medications that individually or in combination elevate gastrointestinal bleeding risk, anticoagulants, antiplatelet agents, nonsteroidal anti-inflammatory drugs, and selective serotonin reuptake inhibitors among them, warrants a comprehensive medication review at the time of an acute bleeding episode, since identifying and addressing this cumulative risk burden, rather than focusing narrowly on a single presumed causative agent, supports more effective secondary prevention going forward. Involving a clinical pharmacist in this comprehensive review, where available, can provide additional expertise identifying interactions and cumulative risk that might not be immediately apparent from a standard medication list review alone. Deprescribing conversations, revisiting whether each medication remains necessary given the patient's current clinical situation, are a valuable, underutilized tool in this population that deserves as much attention as the acute bleeding management itself. A brief, structured medication review at every follow-up visit, not only immediately after the acute hemorrhage episode, sustains this attention over the longer term. Always worth the extra minute.

## Psychosocial Impact of Acute GI Hemorrhage

An acute, severe gastrointestinal hemorrhage episode, particularly one requiring intensive care admission or a life-threatening presentation, can produce significant psychological distress extending well beyond the hospitalization itself, including anxiety about recurrence, and screening for this distress at follow-up visits, applying the same routine screening standard already established throughout this book for other serious acute illnesses, supports patients through a recovery process that is not purely physical. Patients with cirrhosis who experience variceal hemorrhage face a particularly compounded psychological burden, since this event often serves as a stark, frightening confirmation of their disease's severity and a reminder of the underlying condition's potential for further, life-threatening complications, and acknowledging this specific emotional weight directly, rather than focusing exclusively on the biomedical management already developed throughout this chapter, supports a more complete, patient-centered recovery process. Post-traumatic stress symptoms specifically, including intrusive memories of the bleeding episode or heightened anxiety around subsequent medical procedures, deserve dedicated screening attention, given how a genuinely frightening acute medical event can produce lasting psychological effects distinct from ordinary situational anxiety. Connecting these patients with the same integrated hepatology-palliative care model discussed in the previous chapter can provide continuity of psychosocial support extending beyond the acute hemorrhage episode into their broader, ongoing cirrhosis management. Attentiveness to this dimension of recovery is not optional. Truly.

### Supporting Family Members During Acute Hemorrhage Episodes

Family members witnessing a loved one's acute, sometimes visually alarming gastrointestinal hemorrhage, particularly hematemesis, often experience significant acute distress themselves, and providing clear, timely updates throughout the acute management process, using the same crisis-communication principles already established in earlier chapters for other rapidly evolving medical emergencies, supports the family through this acutely frightening experience alongside the patient. Debriefing conversations after the acute crisis has resolved, offering both the patient and their family an opportunity to ask questions and process the experience once the immediate danger has passed, can support a more complete emotional recovery than focusing exclusively on the acute medical needs alone. This care extends the healing well beyond the hospital stay. Yes.

## Radiation-Induced and Post-Procedural Bleeding

Radiation proctitis and radiation-induced gastrointestinal bleeding, occurring in patients with a history of pelvic or abdominal radiation therapy, most commonly for prostate, cervical, or rectal malignancy, present a distinct etiology from the more common causes developed throughout this chapter, and endoscopic argon plasma coagulation has emerged as the preferred first-line treatment for the characteristic telangiectasias radiation injury produces, applied over multiple sessions given the diffuse, chronic nature of this radiation-related vascular change. Post-polypectomy bleeding, whether occurring immediately during the procedure or delayed by days to weeks afterward, requires prompt recognition and, in the delayed presentation specifically, active consideration in any patient with a recent colonoscopic polypectomy who presents with new hematochezia, since this temporal association can be easily overlooked if the recent procedure is not specifically elicited during the patient's history. Coordination with the treating radiation oncologist can provide valuable context about the specific radiation field and dose, information that may help predict the likely severity and expected clinical course of the resulting proctitis in a given patient. Managing post-polypectomy bleeding generally begins with repeat colonoscopy for endoscopic hemostasis when a discrete bleeding site can be identified, mirroring the same endoscopy-first approach already established for other lower gastrointestinal bleeding sources throughout this chapter. This collaborative approach reflects the same cross-specialty coordination emphasized consistently throughout this book. Every detail here matters for the patient in front of us. Truly. Indeed.

### Post-Sphincterotomy and Post-Biopsy Bleeding

Bleeding following endoscopic sphincterotomy, discussed in the context of biliary interventions in earlier chapters, and bleeding following mucosal or submucosal biopsy elsewhere in the gastrointestinal tract, while both generally uncommon and often self-limited, should be anticipated specifically in patients with underlying coagulopathy or those on antithrombotic therapy, reinforcing why the periprocedural risk assessment developed throughout this book for other invasive procedures applies equally to these specific endoscopic interventions, not only to more obviously high-risk procedures. Proactive counseling before the procedure about this recognized possibility, however uncommon, supports informed consent and reduces the alarm a patient might otherwise feel if this complication does occur without having been forewarned of the possibility beforehand. This same principle of informed, transparent risk communication applies broadly across every invasive procedure discussed throughout this book, not only the specific interventions named here. It is a closing reminder worth carrying forward into every future clinical encounter. Care taken here reflects care taken everywhere. Yes.

## Acute Mesenteric Ischemia and Vascular Disorders

### Acute Mesenteric Ischemia: Recognition and Management

Acute mesenteric ischemia, resulting from arterial embolism, arterial thrombosis, mesenteric venous thrombosis, or nonocclusive mesenteric ischemia from severe hypoperfusion, classically presents with pain out of proportion to physical examination findings, a specific, high-yield clinical clue that should prompt urgent evaluation even when the abdominal examination itself is deceptively unremarkable, since this specific disconnect between severe pain and a benign-appearing examination reflects the early, pre-infarction phase of this condition before peritoneal signs from bowel necrosis have developed. Computed tomography angiography is the diagnostic study of choice, and time-sensitive surgical or endovascular intervention, restoring mesenteric blood flow before irreversible bowel infarction occurs, is essential given the extremely high mortality this condition carries once diagnosis or intervention is delayed, making acute mesenteric ischemia one of the genuine gastrointestinal emergencies where diagnostic delay directly and dramatically worsens survival. Atrial fibrillation is a major risk factor for the embolic subtype specifically, and this history should be specifically elicited in any patient presenting with a clinical picture concerning for acute mesenteric ischemia, since it meaningfully raises pretest probability and can help justify pursuing urgent imaging even when the presentation is not yet fully classic. Serum lactate elevation, while a nonspecific marker that rises only once significant bowel ischemia has already occurred, can support the diagnosis when positive but should never be relied upon to exclude acute mesenteric ischemia when clinical suspicion remains high, since a normal lactate early in the disease course does not rule out this diagnosis.

### Ischemic Colitis

Ischemic colitis, distinct from acute mesenteric ischemia in both its generally less severe presentation and its typically more favorable prognosis, results from transient, nonocclusive hypoperfusion to the colon, most commonly affecting watershed areas between major arterial territories, and presents with crampy abdominal pain and hematochezia, generally milder in severity than the presentation of acute mesenteric ischemia, and most cases resolve with supportive management alone, including bowel rest and intravenous fluids, without requiring the urgent surgical or endovascular intervention that acute mesenteric ischemia demands. Distinguishing ischemic colitis from acute mesenteric ischemia matters significantly given their markedly different management urgency and prognosis, and the combination of clinical presentation, the milder pain-to-examination relationship characteristic of ischemic colitis rather than the dramatic pain-out-of-proportion finding of mesenteric ischemia, and imaging findings, generally supports this distinction, though a small subset of ischemic colitis cases progress to a more severe, gangrenous form requiring surgical intervention, meaning close monitoring rather than uniform reassurance is still warranted even in this generally more favorable condition. Colonoscopy, performed cautiously and with limited insufflation once the patient is hemodynamically stable, can help confirm the diagnosis and assess severity, typically showing segmental mucosal edema, hemorrhage, and, in more severe cases, ulceration, with the watershed distribution pattern, most notably at the splenic flexure, providing an additional supportive clue to this diagnosis. Clinical warning signs suggesting progression toward the more severe, gangrenous form, including worsening pain, fever, rising white blood cell count, or the development of peritoneal signs on repeat examination, should prompt urgent surgical consultation rather than continued observation alone.

Case Presentation: A 58-year-old man with known cirrhosis and prior esophageal varices presents with hematemesis. His Glasgow-Blatchford score, calculated on arrival, is markedly elevated. Applying the reasoning developed in this chapter, octreotide and a third-generation cephalosporin are initiated promptly, before endoscopy is performed, given the strong suspicion for variceal hemorrhage in this specific clinical context. He is resuscitated using a restrictive transfusion strategy, and upper endoscopy performed within twelve hours confirms actively bleeding esophageal varices, treated successfully with band ligation. He completes his antibiotic course and continues nonselective beta-blocker therapy for secondary prophylaxis at discharge. This case illustrates the chapter's central variceal hemorrhage principle: octreotide and antibiotic prophylaxis, initiated before endoscopic confirmation based on strong clinical suspicion alone, and a restrictive transfusion approach, together reflect the evidence-based, threshold-driven management this specific bleeding source requires.

Case Presentation: A 74-year-old woman presents with painless hematochezia and known diverticulosis on prior colonoscopy. She is hemodynamically stable, and upper gastrointestinal sources are considered unlikely given her stable vital signs and the absence of any melena or upper gastrointestinal symptoms. Applying the reasoning developed in this chapter, she completes an expedited bowel preparation and undergoes colonoscopy within eighteen hours of presentation, identifying a diverticulum with active bleeding successfully treated with endoscopic clip placement. This case illustrates the chapter's core lower gastrointestinal hemorrhage principle: her hemodynamic stability and ability to complete adequate bowel preparation met the threshold for standard, prepared colonoscopy within the standard timing window, rather than requiring escalation to angiographic intervention, and this timely, well-prepared examination successfully identified and treated the actual bleeding source.

Figure 19.3: Endoscopic Variceal Band Ligation Technique

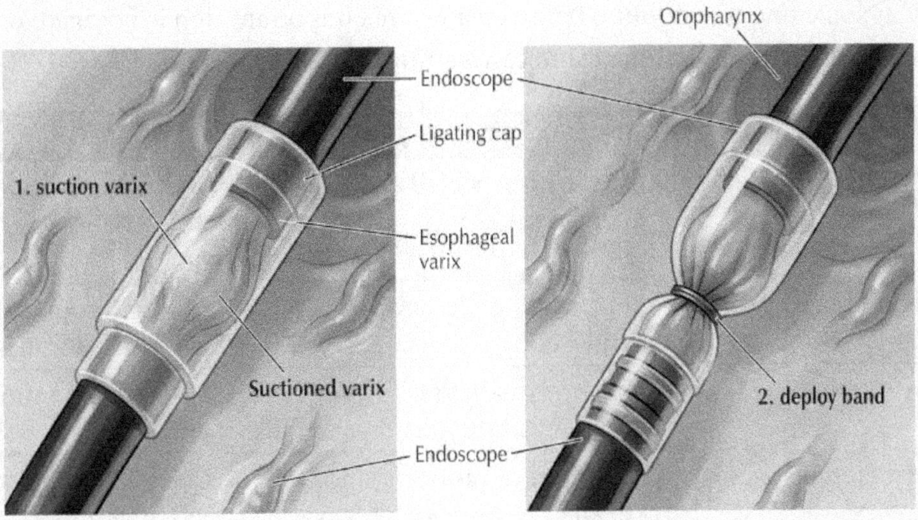


## Anticoagulation and Antiplatelet Management in Acute GI Bleeding

Patients on anticoagulation or antiplatelet therapy who present with acute gastrointestinal hemorrhage require individualized decisions about reversal and resumption timing, balancing the immediate bleeding risk against the thrombotic risk that the underlying indication for this therapy carries, and this decision should generally involve the prescribing specialty, cardiology for a recent coronary stent or atrial fibrillation management, or neurology for a recent stroke, given the significant, sometimes life-threatening consequences of inappropriately prolonged anticoagulation interruption in a patient with a high-risk thrombotic indication. Reversal agents, specific to the anticoagulant class involved, vitamin K and prothrombin complex concentrate for warfarin, and the specific reversal agents now available for certain direct oral anticoagulants, should be used judiciously, reserved for genuinely life-threatening hemorrhage rather than applied reflexively to any gastrointestinal bleeding episode regardless of severity, given both the cost and the thrombotic risk reversal itself can carry in some cases. Documenting the specific rationale for a reversal or continuation decision in the medical record supports clear communication among the multiple specialties typically involved in managing this competing-risk scenario, and this documentation becomes particularly valuable if the patient's clinical course subsequently changes and the original decision needs to be revisited. Consulting a pharmacist familiar with the specific reversal agent options and their appropriate dosing and administration can support safer, more accurate use of these specialized agents, particularly for clinicians who encounter this scenario infrequently.

### Resumption Timing After Bleeding Control

Resumption of anticoagulation or antiplatelet therapy after bleeding has been controlled should occur as soon as the bleeding risk has reasonably diminished, generally within days rather than weeks in most circumstances, since excessively prolonged discontinuation exposes the patient to their underlying thrombotic risk without ongoing benefit, and this resumption timing decision, like the initial reversal decision, benefits from the same collaborative, cross-specialty input given the competing risks involved. A specific, documented resumption date agreed upon at the time of discharge, rather than a vague plan to resume therapy at some undefined future point, ensures this important step is not inadvertently delayed or overlooked once the patient has left the acute care setting.

| Condition | Key Diagnostic Threshold | First-Line Management |
|---|---|---|
| Variceal UGIB | Known/suspected cirrhosis + hematemesis | Octreotide + antibiotics before endoscopy, then band ligation |
| Non-variceal UGIB | Forrest classification on endoscopy | PPI + endoscopic hemostasis if high-risk stigmata |
| Lower GI bleeding | Hemodynamic stability + prep feasibility | Colonoscopy within 24 hours if stable |
| Acute mesenteric ischemia | Pain out of proportion to exam | Urgent CT angiography + revascularization |

## THE GI THRESHOLD DECISION SYSTEM — Acute Hemorrhage and Vascular Emergency Thresholds

**Presentation Signature:** This chapter's threshold instances addressed pre-endoscopic risk stratification in upper GI bleeding and colonoscopy timing in lower GI bleeding.

**Threshold Point:** The Glasgow-Blatchford score gates triage disposition before endoscopy in upper GI bleeding; hemodynamic stability and preparation feasibility gate colonoscopy timing versus angiographic escalation in lower GI bleeding.

**The Call:** Both thresholds replace clinical gestalt alone with validated, criteria-based triage decisions that determine the urgency and modality of intervention before the bleeding source itself has even been identified.

**Trap Logic:** Relying on clinical impression rather than the Glasgow-Blatchford score for upper GI bleeding triage, and pursuing unprepared or excessively delayed colonoscopy in an unstable lower GI bleeding patient, are this chapter's most consequential threshold misapplications.

**Decision Anchor:** Calculate the Glasgow-Blatchford score for every suspected upper GI bleed before triage disposition, and assess hemodynamic stability and preparation feasibility explicitly in lower GI bleeding to determine whether standard colonoscopy or angiographic escalation is warranted.

## Summary and Key Concepts

Restrictive transfusion strategy and Glasgow-Blatchford score-based pre-endoscopic risk stratification, calculated before any endoscopic information is available, guide initial triage in acute upper gastrointestinal hemorrhage.

Variceal hemorrhage requires prompt octreotide and antibiotic prophylaxis initiated before endoscopic confirmation, followed by endoscopic band ligation, while non-variceal hemorrhage management is guided by the Forrest classification determining endoscopic hemostasis need.

Lower gastrointestinal hemorrhage evaluation should exclude an upper source, and colonoscopy within twenty-four hours is appropriate for hemodynamically stable patients able to complete adequate bowel preparation, with angiographic or surgical escalation for unstable patients.

Acute mesenteric ischemia presents with pain out of proportion to examination findings and requires urgent CT angiography and time-sensitive revascularization given its extremely high mortality when diagnosis or intervention is delayed.

Ischemic colitis, distinct from acute mesenteric ischemia in both presentation severity and prognosis, generally resolves with supportive management alone, though a small subset progresses to a more severe form requiring surgical intervention.

# THE GI THRESHOLD MASTER INDEX

This index consolidates every named score, classification system, and clinical threshold introduced throughout this textbook's Rhythm Layer into a single, cross-referenced navigator, organized by the same eight clinical domains the book itself follows. Each entry states the governing threshold in the same compact form used at the point of care: the specific cutoff or classification, the decision it triggers, and the chapter in which the full clinical reasoning is developed. This section is a scanning tool, not a substitute for the chapter discussion; a clinician who needs the mechanism, the exceptions, or the supporting evidence behind a given threshold should return to the cross-referenced chapter, while a clinician who needs only to confirm a cutoff or recall which decision it triggers can do so here without paging through the full text. Entries are grouped by domain in the same order the chapters themselves proceed, from foundational diagnostic reasoning through the acute hemorrhage and vascular emergencies that close the book, so that a reader already oriented to a chapter's content can locate its corresponding threshold entries quickly.

## Foundational and Endoscopic Diagnostic Thresholds

These thresholds govern the earliest decision points in gastroenterology practice, before a specific organ-system diagnosis has been established, and the endoscopic classification that converts a bleeding lesion's appearance into a reproducible management decision.

| Threshold System | Threshold Point | Decision Anchor | Chapter |
|---|---|---|---|
| Shock Index | Heart rate divided by systolic blood pressure greater than 1.0 | Identifies compensated hemorrhagic shock before resting vital signs become abnormal; triggers immediate resuscitation over further history-taking | Ch. 1 |
| Tokyo Guidelines (Cholangitis Severity) | Systemic inflammation + cholestasis + imaging evidence of obstruction; hypotension, altered mentation, or organ dysfunction defines severe grade | Antibiotics started on clinical suspicion before cultures return; severity grade, not the complete Charcot triad, determines urgency of drainage | Ch. 1 |
| Forrest Classification | Ia/Ib active hemorrhage or IIa visible vessel = high | Forrest grade at index endoscopy, not initial hemoglobin, | Ch. 2 |

| | | | |
|---|---|---|---|
| | rebleeding risk; IIc/III = low risk; IIb adherent clot = intermediate | determines need for endoscopic hemostasis and length of inpatient monitoring | |

## Esophageal Thresholds

These thresholds govern reflux disease severity, motility disorder classification, Barrett esophagus surveillance, and the structural interventions used across esophageal disease.

| Threshold System | Threshold Point | Decision Anchor | Chapter |
|---|---|---|---|
| Age/Alarm-Feature Threshold (GERD) | Age 60+ at onset, or any alarm feature (dysphagia, weight loss, bleeding, anemia) | Defines the line between an empiric PPI trial and upfront endoscopy; symptom severity alone does not cross this threshold | Ch. 3 |
| Prague Classification | Circumferential (C) and maximal (M) extent of columnar-appearing mucosa above the GE junction | Segment length, not qualitative description, sets the surveillance biopsy protocol and interval | Ch. 3 |
| Barrett Dysplasia Grade | Indefinite/low-grade dysplasia = intermediate zone requiring expert pathology confirmation; high-grade/intramucosal carcinoma = eradication threshold | Confirmed dysplasia grade, not segment length or symptoms, determines surveillance vs. endoscopic eradication therapy | Ch. 3 |
| Chicago Classification (Achalasia Subtyping) | Integrated relaxation pressure and peristaltic pattern define Type I, II, or III achalasia | Subtype, not symptom severity, determines whether pneumatic dilation, myotomy, or a tailored approach is preferred | Ch. 4 |
| Safe Esophageal Dilation Increments | Incremental, graded dilation with a defined maximum | Exceeding the safe per-session increment materially | Ch. 4 |

| | | | |
|---|---|---|---|
| | single-session increase | raises perforation risk regardless of stricture appearance | |

## Gastric and Duodenal Thresholds

These thresholds govern the dyspepsia diagnostic pathway, NSAID-related gastrointestinal risk stratification, and the sequencing of therapy in functional dyspepsia and gastroparesis.

| Threshold System | Threshold Point | Decision Anchor | Chapter |
|---|---|---|---|
| Age/Alarm-Feature Threshold (Dyspepsia) | Age cutoff (regionally variable) plus any alarm feature | Below threshold: test-and-treat for H. pylori; above threshold: endoscopy-first regardless of symptom response to empiric therapy | Ch. 5 |
| NSAID GI Risk Stratification | Combination of prior ulcer history, age, concurrent anticoagulant/antiplatelet/corticosteroid use, and dose | Risk category, not NSAID class alone, determines whether gastroprotection, agent substitution, or NSAID avoidance is warranted | Ch. 5 |
| Functional Dyspepsia Treatment Sequencing | Predominant subtype (postprandial distress vs. epigastric pain) after H. pylori testing and PPI trial | Subtype, confirmed after first-line testing, determines whether a prokinetic or a neuromodulator is the appropriate next step | Ch. 6 |
| Gastroparesis Severity Staging | Symptom severity and degree of gastric emptying delay on scintigraphy | Severity stage, not symptom description alone, determines whether dietary modification, prokinetic therapy, or a more invasive intervention is escalated to | Ch. 6 |

## Small Bowel Thresholds

These thresholds govern celiac disease diagnosis in equivocal presentations, the sequencing of a malabsorption workup, breath testing interpretation, and the threshold for intestinal rehabilitation or transplant referral in intestinal failure.

| Threshold System | Threshold Point | Decision Anchor | Chapter |
|---|---|---|---|
| Seronegative Celiac Diagnostic Threshold | Negative serology with high clinical suspicion or equivocal biopsy findings | HLA typing and gluten challenge protocol, not serology alone, resolve the seronegative or equivocal case | Ch. 7 |
| Malabsorption Workup Sequencing | Stepwise exclusion of pancreatic, mucosal, and bacterial causes before a rarer diagnosis is pursued | Sequence, not parallel testing of every possible cause, is the efficient and evidence-based approach | Ch. 7 |
| Breath Testing Interpretation (SIBO) | Rise in breath hydrogen or methane above a defined threshold within a specified time window | Threshold crossing, and its timing, determines antibiotic selection and whether SIBO or another motility disorder is the more likely explanation | Ch. 8 |
| Intestinal Rehabilitation/Transplant Referral Threshold | Failure of nutritional autonomy despite optimized intestinal rehabilitation, or recurrent central line complications | These specific failure criteria, not remaining bowel length alone, define the threshold for transplant referral | Ch. 8 |

## Colorectal and Functional Bowel Disease Thresholds

These thresholds govern acute severe ulcerative colitis management, Crohn disease risk stratification, the distinction between IBS-D and its organic mimics, dyssynergic defecation testing, and colorectal cancer screening initiation by risk category.

| Threshold System | Threshold Point | Decision Anchor | Chapter |
|---|---|---|---|
| Acute Severe Ulcerative Colitis Day-Three Decision | Truelove and Witts-type severity criteria reassessed on day three of intravenous corticosteroids | Day-three response, not clinical impression alone, determines continuation of steroids versus rescue therapy (infliximab or cyclosporine) or colectomy | Ch. 9 |
| Crohn Disease Risk Stratification | Presence of specific poor-prognosis features (perianal disease, deep ulcers, extensive involvement, early surgery) | Risk category at diagnosis, not symptom severity alone, determines whether early biologic therapy is initiated rather than a conventional step-up approach | Ch. 9 |
| Harvey-Bradshaw Index / Mayo Score | Composite clinical and endoscopic activity scores for Crohn disease and ulcerative colitis, respectively | Objective mucosal healing, not symptom resolution alone, confirms remission and guides treatment de-escalation decisions | Ch. 9 |
| IBS-D vs. Organic Mimic Threshold | Presence of alarm features, atypical age of onset, or specific serologic/inflammatory markers | These specific discriminating features, not symptom pattern alone, separate IBS-D from celiac disease, microscopic colitis, or IBD | Ch. 10 |
| Rome IV Criteria | Symptom-based diagnostic criteria for disorders of gut-brain interaction, applied only after organic | Rome IV criteria are a diagnostic framework, not a substitute for excluding alarm- | Ch. 10 |

| | | | |
|---|---|---|---|
| | disease has been reasonably excluded | feature-driven organic disease first | |
| Dyssynergic Defecation Testing Threshold | Chronic constipation refractory to first-line fiber and osmotic laxative therapy | This refractoriness threshold, not constipation duration alone, triggers anorectal manometry to distinguish dyssynergia from slow-transit constipation | Ch. 10 |
| Colorectal Cancer Screening Initiation by Risk Category | Average risk (age-based), family history-based, or hereditary syndrome-based risk tier | Risk category, not age alone, determines both the initiation age and the appropriate screening modality and interval | Ch. 11 |
| Hereditary Cancer Syndrome Red Flags | Multiple affected relatives, early age of onset, or a specific tumor spectrum suggestive of a hereditary syndrome | These red flags, not a single affected relative alone, define the threshold for genetic counseling and germline testing referral | Ch. 11 |

## Pancreaticobiliary Thresholds

These thresholds govern acute pancreatitis severity stratification, chronic pancreatitis pain management escalation, surgical timing in acute cholecystitis, biliary decompression urgency, and pancreatic and biliary neoplasia management.

| Threshold System | Threshold Point | Decision Anchor | Chapter |
|---|---|---|---|
| BISAP / Ranson Criteria | Composite clinical and laboratory criteria assessed within the first 48 hours of acute pancreatitis | Severity-stratified score, not a single laboratory value, determines resuscitation intensity and level-of-care monitoring | Ch. 12 |
| Chronic Pancreatitis Pain Escalation Threshold | Inadequate response to a defined trial of first-line analgesic and enzyme-replacement therapy | This defined nonresponse, not pain severity alone, triggers escalation to neuromodulator | Ch. 12 |

| | | | |
|---|---|---|---|
| | | therapy, celiac plexus block, or endoscopic/surgical intervention | |
| Tokyo Guidelines (Cholecystitis Grading) | Local inflammatory signs plus systemic inflammatory response and organ dysfunction grading | Grade, not symptom duration alone, determines candidacy and timing for early cholecystectomy versus percutaneous drainage | Ch. 13 |
| Biliary Decompression Urgency (Cholangitis) | Severity grade and response to antibiotics within 24 hours | Severity, not diagnostic certainty alone, determines whether ERCP drainage is emergent or can be sequenced after an antibiotic trial | Ch. 13 |
| Pancreatic Adenocarcinoma Resectability Classification | Specific vascular contact criteria on dedicated pancreatic protocol imaging (SMA, celiac axis, SMV/portal vein) | Vascular relationship, not tumor size or general impression, classifies resectable, borderline resectable, or unresectable disease | Ch. 14 |
| IPMN Surgical Referral Threshold | Presence of high-risk stigmata (obstructive jaundice, enhancing mural nodule, main duct dilation above threshold) | High-risk stigmata, not cyst size alone, define the threshold for surgical referral versus continued surveillance | Ch. 14 |

## Hepatology Thresholds

These thresholds govern the interpretation of abnormal liver chemistries, acute liver failure transplant referral, chronic hepatitis B treatment initiation, severe alcohol-associated hepatitis corticosteroid response, autoimmune hepatitis treatment withdrawal, primary biliary cholangitis treatment escalation, variceal prophylaxis, and spontaneous bacterial peritonitis prophylaxis.

| Threshold System | Threshold Point | Decision Anchor | Chapter |
|---|---|---|---|
| R-Value (Liver Injury Pattern) | ALT elevation relative to ULN divided by ALP elevation relative to ULN; >5 hepatocellular, <2 cholestatic | Calculated R-value, not noting that enzymes are simply elevated, determines the entire subsequent diagnostic pathway | Ch. 15 |
| Acute Liver Failure Transplant Criteria | Established prognostic criteria incorporating etiology, coagulopathy degree, and encephalopathy grade | Meeting these criteria, not further clinical deterioration, triggers immediate transplant center referral | Ch. 15 |
| Chronic Hepatitis B Phase Classification | HBV DNA level, HBeAg status, and ALT elevation define immune-tolerant, immune-active, or inactive carrier phase | Phase, reassessed at each visit, not a single HBV DNA value, determines antiviral treatment initiation | Ch. 16 |
| Maddrey Discriminant Function / MELD (Alcohol-Associated Hepatitis) | Severity score at presentation defining severe alcohol-associated hepatitis | Severity score, not clinical impression, determines corticosteroid candidacy | Ch. 16 |
| Lille Score (Day-Seven Reassessment) | Bilirubin trajectory from baseline calculated at day seven of corticosteroid therapy | Day-seven Lille score, not day-one severity, determines corticosteroid continuation versus futility and discontinuation | Ch. 16 |
| Autoimmune Hepatitis Treatment Withdrawal Threshold | Sustained biochemical remission (2-3+ years) plus histologic | Both biochemical AND histologic remission, not biochemical | Ch. 17 |

| | | | |
|---|---|---|---|
| | remission on repeat biopsy | normalization alone, must be met before withdrawal is attempted | |
| Primary Biliary Cholangitis Treatment Escalation | Formal biochemical response criteria (ALP, bilirubin) assessed at approximately one year of UDCA therapy | One-year response assessment, not continued monotherapy by default, determines second-line therapy addition | Ch. 17 |
| Child-Pugh Score / MELD(-Na) | Bilirubin, albumin, INR, ascites, encephalopathy (Child-Pugh); bilirubin, creatinine, INR, sodium (MELD-Na) | Standardized staging and primary transplant allocation tool; decompensation, not a single lab value, marks the prognostic shift | Ch. 18 |
| Variceal Screening/Prophylaxis Threshold | Noninvasive risk stratification (platelets, spleen size, elastography) for screening; variceal size/stigmata for prophylaxis | Noninvasive criteria guide screening necessity; medium-large varices or high-risk stigmata trigger primary prophylaxis | Ch. 18 |
| SBP Prophylaxis Indications | Prior SBP episode (secondary); low ascitic protein + advanced disease/renal impairment (primary); acute GI hemorrhage (peri-hemorrhage) | These specific criteria, not ascites presence alone, define antibiotic prophylaxis indications | Ch. 18 |
| Ascitic Fluid Absolute Neutrophil Count | $\geq$250 cells/mm³ | Low threshold for diagnostic paracentesis given often-minimal SBP symptoms; this count, not symptom severity, confirms diagnosis | Ch. 18 |

## Acute Hemorrhage and Vascular Emergency Thresholds

These thresholds govern pre-endoscopic risk stratification in upper gastrointestinal hemorrhage and the timing decision between standard colonoscopy and angiographic escalation in lower gastrointestinal hemorrhage.

| Threshold System | Threshold Point | Decision Anchor | Chapter |
|---|---|---|---|
| Glasgow-Blatchford Score | Composite of BUN, hemoglobin, systolic BP, heart rate, and clinical findings (melena, syncope), calculated pre-endoscopically | Calculated before endoscopic information is available; determines inpatient admission versus consideration of outpatient management | Ch. 19 |
| Rockall Score | Pre- and post-endoscopic clinical and endoscopic variables | Adds post-endoscopic prognostic information complementing the pre-endoscopic Glasgow-Blatchford triage decision | Ch. 19 |
| Lower GI Bleeding Colonoscopy Timing Threshold | Hemodynamic stability and ability to complete adequate bowel preparation | Stability and preparation feasibility, not time elapsed alone, determine standard 24-hour colonoscopy versus angiographic/surgical escalation | Ch. 19 |
| Pain-Out-of-Proportion Sign (Acute Mesenteric Ischemia) | Severe pain disproportionate to a benign-appearing abdominal examination | This specific clinical disconnect, not examination findings alone, should prompt urgent CT angiography given the extreme time sensitivity of this diagnosis | Ch. 19 |

## Using This Index

Each entry in this index summarizes a threshold in its most compact, actionable form. The full clinical reasoning behind each threshold, including the mechanism that explains why the cutoff sits where it does, the exceptions and edge cases that modify its application, and the evidence supporting the associated decision, is developed in the cross-referenced chapter and should be consulted whenever a decision carries genuine clinical stakes rather than serving only as a quick confirmatory check. This index is organized by clinical domain rather than alphabetically by score name, reflecting the observation that a clinician facing a specific clinical scenario, a patient with suspected pancreatitis or a patient with abnormal liver chemistries, is more efficiently served by a domain-organized reference than by needing to already know a score's name before locating it. A cross-reference by score name would duplicate much of this same content in a different order without adding diagnostic value beyond what the domain organization already provides, and the domain structure additionally reinforces how threshold-based reasoning recurs as a consistent pattern across every area of gastroenterology and hepatology developed throughout this book, rather than presenting each threshold as an isolated fact to be memorized independently of its clinical context.

# CONCLUSION

The preface to this book opened with a fellow moving between a variceal bleed, an abnormal liver panel, a flare of ulcerative colitis, and a vague complaint of chronic diarrhea, often within the same afternoon. The nineteen chapters that followed were written to meet that clinician at each of those bedsides, and the arc they traced was deliberate: from the foundational reasoning that converts a presenting symptom into a differential diagnosis, through each organ system in the order gastroenterology is actually taught and practiced, and closing with the acute hemorrhage and vascular emergencies that remain the single most common reason a gastroenterologist is called to see a hospitalized patient. A reader who has worked through the book in this order has moved from the general skill of clinical reasoning to its most exacting, time-pressured application, which is where that skill is tested most directly.

The GI Threshold Decision System that runs through every chapter reflects a conviction stated at the outset of this book: that gastroenterology's essential difficulty is rarely a lack of knowledge and is far more often the gap between recognizing that a threshold exists and knowing, at the bedside, which one governs the patient in front of the clinician. A shock index, a Forrest grade, a MELD score, a dysplasia grade confirmed by expert pathology, a day-seven Lille score, a Glasgow-Blatchford calculation before endoscopy has even begun; each of these converts a continuous, uncertain clinical picture into a specific, defensible decision, and each appears in this book not as an isolated fact to memorize but as one instance of a single recurring pattern. Once that pattern is internalized, an unfamiliar threshold encountered later in training or practice becomes easier to absorb, because the clinician already knows what shape the reasoning is supposed to take: name the presentation, name the threshold, name the decision it triggers, name the look-alike that gets it wrong, and anchor the whole sequence in one memorable rule.

Every specific cutoff in this book will eventually be revised. Guideline bodies update their recommendations as evidence accumulates, scoring systems are refined or replaced, and a threshold that governs practice today may carry a different number, or a different name entirely, within a few years of this book's printing. What does not change is the underlying discipline this book has tried to model throughout: that a threshold, once identified, should be applied consistently and reassessed deliberately rather than abandoned to clinical impression, and that the specific cutoff matters less than the habit of asking, at every consequential decision point, which threshold is actually in play here, and have I confirmed it rather than assumed it. A clinician who carries that habit forward will find it easier to absorb the next revised guideline than a clinician who has only memorized today's numbers without understanding why the reasoning was structured the way it was.

The GI Threshold Master Index at the end of this book exists for exactly this kind of ongoing use. It is not meant to be read once and set aside; it is meant to sit within reach during a busy consult service, a clinic day, or board preparation, functioning as the fast, cross-referenced confirmation that the full chapter discussion was written to support. When a threshold matters enough to change management, the index points back to the chapter where the mechanism, the exceptions, and the evidence behind that threshold are developed in full, and that return trip, from index to chapter and back, is the intended rhythm of how this book is used over the course of a career rather than a single reading.

Gastroenterology and hepatology touch nearly every organ system and nearly every stage of a patient's life, from a first screening colonoscopy to the final stages of decompensated liver disease, and the clinicians who practice this specialty carry a corresponding responsibility to get the threshold decisions right, because the cost of getting them wrong, a missed dominant stricture, a delayed transplant referral, an unrecognized threshold for resuscitation, is measured in outcomes that matter enormously to the patient in front of them. This book was written in the belief that making those thresholds explicit, rather than leaving them to be absorbed piecemeal over years of trial and error, gives a clinician a faster and more reliable path to the judgment that this specialty demands. The reasoning is now in the reader's hands; applying it, patient by patient, is where it becomes practice.

www.ingramcontent.com/pod-product-compliance
Lightning Source LLC
LaVergne TN
LVHW060441061126
851857LV00016B/1689
*9780557978267*